Legal
Issues
in Nursing

second edition

P9-DMX-512

Legal
Issues
in Nursing

second edition

Ginny Wacker Guido, JD, MSN, RN

Professor and Chair
Department of Nursing
Eastern New Mexico University
Portales, New Mexico

Appleton & Lange
Stamford, Connecticut

Copyright © 1997 by Appleton & Lange
A Simon & Schuster Company
Copyright © 1988 by Appleton & Lange

97 98 99 00 01 / 10 9 8 7 6 5 4 3 2 1

Prentice Hall International (UK) Limited, *London*
Prentice Hall of Australia Pty. Limited, *Sydney*
Prentice Hall Canada, Inc., *Toronto*
Prentice Hall Hispanoamericana, S.A., *Mexico*
Prentice Hall of India Private Limited, *New Delhi*
Prentice Hall of Japan, Inc., *Tokyo*
Simon & Schuster Asia Pte. Ltd., *Singapore*
Editora Prentice Hall do Brasil Ltda., *Rio de Janeiro*
Prentice Hall, *Upper Saddle River, New Jersey*

ISBN 0-8385-5647-7

90000

9 780838 556474

Acquisitions Editor: Kathleen L. Riedell
Production Editor: Jeanmarie M. Roche
Designer: Libby Schmitz

PRINTED IN THE UNITED STATES OF AMERICA

As with the first edition,
this book is dedicated to my family, without whom
it would never have been a reality:

Ed, Jenny, and Joey Guido
and
Cecelia G. Wacker.

Contents

Preface

The second edition of *Legal Issues in Nursing* reflects the continuing influence that legal issues and the law have on the professional practice of nursing. Professional accountability and responsiblity are ever increasing, particularly as nursing becomes more autonomous with the move from institutional settings to community settings and as advanced practice nurses gain more independence through state nurse practice acts. Consumers continue to become more knowledgeable about their rights within the health care delivery system. Readers familiar with the first edition will recognize that much of the content in this text is new, reflecting these changes in the practice of professional nursing.

This book is intended for nursing students as well as practicing nurses. As with the first edition, the primary function of the text is to familiarize both student and professional nurses with current legal concepts, thereby allowing for improved patient care through the knowledge and understanding of the ways in which these issues affect clinical practice. Additionally, this text is intended to: (1) educate the beginning nurse, whether in the academic or practice setting, about legal issues and the functions of laws; (2) provide a ready source of information for practicing nurses; and (3) provide a means for preventing malpractice lawsuits.

An important caveat is that this book is not meant to take the place of professional advice from practicing attorneys—nurses are cautioned to seek legal counsel before proceeding with any legal matter. The book, however, is meant to augment the role of legal counsel and assist nurses in understanding the legal process and liability issues as they relate to the practice of nursing.

While preserving the unique features of the former edition, this edition of *Legal Issues in Nursing* differs from the first in several ways. The first part of the book acquaints the reader with basic legal knowledge, such as the sources and types of laws, the role of the court system in legal matters, and the role of case law in determining standards of nursing care. Completely rewritten, this first part emphasizes the vast impact that law has on the professional practice of nursing, the important role of nurse expert witnesses in defining professional standards of care, and major legal doctrines and rules that underlie nursing practice. Included in these doctrines and rules is an expanded section on due process and equal protection of the law rights from both patient and nursing perspectives.

The second part of the book retains many of the legal concepts covered in the first edition. Some chapters in this part of the book are rewritten and incorporate many of the issues that formed the third part of the previous edition.

Included is an expanded section on patient self-determination, the role of confidentiality in documentation, abuse issues, and the rights of patients in research. Retained are sections related to negligence and malpractice, standards of care, consent issues, and professional malpractice insurance issues.

The third section of the book is completely revised and updated as well, and is easily the most exciting section for readers. New chapters in this section emphasize the vital and expanding roles of nurses in community health nursing, including home health care, occupational health, and school health nursing. Additionally, there are new chapters on federal laws, emphasizing the Americans with Disabilities Act of 1990 and the Civil Rights Act of 1991, on contract laws, and on nursing in a variety of practice settings. Nursing issues are discussed from the perspective of staff nurses in hospital and clinic settings, nurse managers in in-patient and out-patient settings, community health nurse roles, and the role of nurses in academic settings. This section incorporated the latest case law in collective bargaining and the National Labor Relations Board and in discrimination and confidentiality cases that have arisen in the area of nursing the patient with AIDS.

The final section incorporates the philosophy of ethics as it pertains to legal issues. Rather than list the types of ethical issues that could arise, this chapter has been rewritten to emphasize various ethical principles and provide a usable ethical model for decision making in clinical areas. This revision allows nurses to make realistic and individual decisions in everyday clinical settings.

Many of the features of the original edition have been enhanced. Each chapter opens with a preview of the content to be covered and a listing of the key concepts to be explored. Guidelines have been updated and placed throughout the chapters for ease of usage, with multiple guidelines in many chapters. Current case law is incorporated throughout the text, illustrating various applications of legal issues to professional nursing practice. The glossary has been expanded to include definitions of key concepts covered throughout the text.

Most exciting are the new features of the book. Exercises have been incorporated into each chapter, challenging readers to think critically as they apply newly acquired knowledge of legal principles and issues to actual clinical situations. Exercises also encourage and assist readers in exploring their own state laws. Chapters conclude with sections that reinforce the goals of the chapter: "After completing this chapter ... " reviews issues and principles identified in the chapter, and "Apply your legal knowledge" challenges readers to take their knowledge a step further.

There is so much to be learned and understood by nurses new to the field of nursing. The text and pedagogical features added to this edition of *Legal Issues in Nursing* are designed to insure that readers understand and master concepts as they complete chapter material. The text will also serve as a reference to the practicing nurse in the challenging years to come.

Ginny Wacker Guido, JD, MSN, RN

Acknowledgments

My deepest appreciation and thanks to the following persons who spent endless time both in reviewing the initial outlines and the final chapters:

Nayna Campbell Philipsen, RN, PhD, JD
Formerly an Associate Professor, School of Nursing
University of North Carolina at Greensboro
Currently with the Maryland Department of Health
and Hygiene

Eileen Kohlenberg, PhD, RN, CNAA
Associate Professor and Chair
Adult Health and Gerontological Nursing
School of Nursing
University of North Carolina at Greensboro

I would also like to thank Ms. Sandy Segovia for all of her invaluable assistance during the writing of this second edition.

Ginny Wacker Guido, JD, MSN, RN

I

INTRODUCTION TO THE LAW AND THE JUDICIAL PROCESS

• one

Legal Concepts

PREVIEW

The disciplines of law and professional nursing have been officially integrated since the first mandatory nurse practice act was passed by New York in 1938. The profession of nursing has continuously relied on statutory law for its right to exist on a licensure basis and on court decisions for interpretation of statutes. The civil rights movement of the 1960s and the malpractice crisis of the 1970s have led, seemingly quite naturally, to a heightened legal-mindedness of the 1980s and 1990s. No longer can nurses rely on a working ignorance of the law and legal doctrines. Today's professional practitioners must know, understand, and apply legal decisions and doctrines to their everyday nursing practices. This chapter presents an overview of the legal system, including the sources and types of laws.

KEY CONCEPTS

law	res judicata	misdemeanors
constitutional law	common law	felonies
statutory law	civil law	substantive law
administrative law	specific performance	procedural law
attorney general's opinions	tort law	due process of law
judicial (or decisional) law	public law	equal protection of the law
stare decisis (or precedent)	criminal law	rational basis test
landmark decision		

DEFINITION OF LAW

Law has been defined in a variety of ways. The word *law* is derived from the Anglo-Saxon term *lagu*, meaning that which is fixed or laid down. Black's *Law Dictionary* defines **law** as "that which is laid down, ordained, or established; a body of rules of action or conduct prescribed by controlling authority and having binding legal force; and that which must be obeyed and followed by citizens subject to sanctions or legal consequences" (1990, pp. 884–885). Perhaps law is better defined as the sum total of rules and regulations by which a society is governed. Law includes the rules and regulations established and enforced by custom within a given community, state, or nation. As such, law is made by society and exists to regulate society.

The actual definition of law is not as important as the impact of law on society. If law is made by society, whether by legislative bodies or by justices of the court, then it reflects the ever-changing needs and expectations of a society and is therefore dynamic and fluid. Law is not an exact science, but rather an ongoing and organized system of change in response to current conditions and public expectations.

SOURCES OF LAW

Understanding the various sources of law assists in determining their impact on the nursing profession. Each of the three branches of the government has the authority and right to create laws, and these laws form the basis of the judicial system.

ABLE 1–1. UNITED STATES CONSTITUTION, AMENDMENTS 1–10, AND 14

1. Congress shall make no law respecting an establishment of religion, or prohibiting the free exercise thereof; of abridging the freedom of speech, or of the press; or the right of the people peaceably to assemble, and to petition the Government for a redress of grievances.

2. A well-regulated Militia, being necessary to the security of a free State, the right of the people to keep and bear Arms, shall not be infringed.

3. No Soldier shall, in time of peace, be quartered in any house, without the consent of the Owner, nor in time of war, but in a manner to be prescribed by law.

4. The right of the people to be secure in their persons, houses, papers, and effects, against unreasonable searches and seizures, shall not be violated, and no Warrants shall issue, but upon probable cause, supported by Oath or affirmation, and particularly describing the place to be searched, and the persons or things to be seized.

5. No persons shall be held to answer for a capital, or otherwise infamous crime, unless a presentment or indictment of a Grand Jury, except in cases arising in the land or naval forces, or in the Militia, when in actual service in time of War or public danger; nor shall any person be subject for the same offense twice put in jeopardy of life or limb; nor shall be compelled in any criminal case to be a witness against himself, nor be deprived of life, liberty, or property, without due process of law; nor shall private property be taken for public use, without just compensation.

6. In all criminal prosecutions, the accused shall enjoy the right to a speedy and public trial by an impartial jury of the State and district wherein the crime shall have been committed, which district shall have been previously ascertained by law, and to be informed of the nature and cause of the accusation; to be confronted with the witnesses against him; to have compulsory process for obtaining witnesses in his favor, and to have the Assistance of counsel for his defense.

7. In Suits at common law, where the value in controversy shall exceed twenty dollars, the right of trial by jury shall be preserved, and no fact tried by a jury, shall be otherwise reexamined in any Court of the United States than according to the rules of the common law.

8. Excessive bail shall not be required, nor excessive fines imposed, nor cruel and unusual punishments inflicted.

9. The enumeration in the Constitution, of certain rights, shall not be construed to deny or disparage others retained by the people.

10. The powers not delegated to the United States by the Constitution, nor prohibited by it to the States, are reserved to the States respectively, or to the people.

14. Section 1. All persons born or naturalized in the United States, and subject to the jurisdiction thereof, are citizens of the United States and the State wherein they reside. No State shall make or enforce any law which shall abridge the privileges or immunities of citizens of the United States; nor shall any State deprive any person of life, liberty, or property, without due process of law; nor deny to any person within its jurisdiction the equal protection of the laws.

United States Constitution, while the states have the inherent power to act except where the Constitution reserves the power for the federal government. The states' power to legislate and govern is often referred to as *police power,* which is generally seen as allowing the states to make laws necessary to maintain public order, health, safety, and welfare.

Constitutional Law

Constitutional law is a system of fundamental laws or principles for nance of a nation, society, corporation, or other aggregate of indivi purpose of a constitution is to establish the basis of a governir The Constitution of the United States establishes the general organ the federal government, grants specific power to the federal govern places limitations on the federal government's powers.

The general organization of the U.S. Constitution is, in reality, power from the states to the federal government, and the federal gc has only the power the Constitution grants it. The federal governme lect taxes, declare war, and enact laws that are "necessary and prop ercising its powers. Constitutional law is the supreme law of the l federal law takes precedence over state and local law. Ideally, state a powers should be exercised so as not to interfere with each other, b is a conflict, federal laws prevail.

The U.S. Constitution also places limitations on the federal go These limitations have been enacted through the Bill of Rights (th amendments of the Constitution), which protects one's right to fr speech, trial by jury, the free exercise of religious preference, and free unreasonable search and seizure (United States Constitution, Am 1–10, 1787). Table 1–1 enumerates these rights and freedoms.

Constitutional law governs for the future as well as for the prese the stability of constitutional law protects a society from frequent ar fluctuations in public opinion (16 *American Jurisprudence*, 1995). tional law is also the highest form of statutory law (defined in the tion), which governs and meets existing conditions.

Each state has its own constitution, establishing the organization o government, giving the state certain powers, and placing limits on power. An important difference between federal and state constitutio that the federal government derives positive grants of power from Constitution, while states enjoy plenary powers subject only to limit their individual state constitutions, the U.S. Constitution, and any li necessary for the successful operation of the federal system.

Statutory Law

Statutory laws are those made by the legislative branch of governme tory laws are designed to declare, command, or prohibit. Generally r as *statutes*, these laws are created by the U.S. Congress, state legislativ city councils, or other elected bodies. Statutes are officially *enacted* (and passed) by legislative bodies and are compiled into codes, colle statutes, or city ordinances. Examples include the United States C Black's Statutes.

The federal and state governments have broad powers to legislat general welfare of the public. The federal government's power is grant

An example of statutory laws are licensure laws, which regulate health care providers within individual states. These laws are designed to protect the general public from incompetent health care providers. Known as *nurse practice acts*, these statutory laws give authority to qualified and licensed practitioners to practice nursing within a state, the District of Columbia, or a U.S. territory. Other statutory laws that affect the practice of professional nursing include statutes of limitations, protective and reporting laws, natural death acts, and informed consent laws. See Chapter 11 for a more complete discussion of nurse practice acts.

Administrative Law

Administrative laws are enacted by means of the decisions and rules of *administrative agencies*, which are specific governing bodies charged with implementing particular legislation. When statutes are enacted, administrative agencies are given the authority to carry out the specific intentions of the statutes, by creating rules and regulations that enforce the statutory laws. Legislative bodies pass the individual nurse practice acts (statutory laws) and create state boards of nursing (state administrative agencies). The state boards of nursing implement and enforce the state nurse practice acts by writing rules and regulations for the enforcement of the statutory law and by conducting investigations and hearings to ensure the law's continual enforcement.

This authority is given to administrative agencies by the state legislature, since the elected legislative body has neither the time nor the needed expertise to ensure that statutory laws are properly enforced. Administrative agencies are normally composed of persons with specific qualifications and experience and are given a single charge to implement and regulate the enforcement of a given statutory law. State boards of nursing are usually comprised of predominantly registered nurse members, who are actively employed in educational or practice settings within nursing, and their charge is the enforcement of the state nurse practice act.

EXERCISE 1-1

Read the table of contents of your state nurse practice act. Can you distinguish the state administrative body (board of nursing) that is created by the legislature? Which sections of your nurse practice act create the administrative body? Which sections serve to distinguish legislative intent?

Administrative rules and regulations have validity only to the extent that they are within the scope of the authority granted by the legislative body. State constitutional law places some limitations on legislative bodies. The charge given to the administrative agency must be specific, and the legislative body re-

mains ultimately responsible for the rules and regulations that the administrative body passes.

There may also be some procedural acts that govern administrative bodies.
Such procedural acts delineate how the agency promulgates rules and regulations and provides for comments from the public before the rules and regulations are enforceable. The procedural acts may also provide for publication in
a state register prior to the enforcement of the new rules and regulations.

The administrative agency has the initial authority to decide how its rules
and regulations are enforced, and the decisions of the administrative agency
may be appealed through the state court system. If appealed, the courts limit
their review of the agency's actions to one of the following five areas:

1. Was the delegation of power to the specific administrative agency constitutional and proper?
2. Did the specific administrative agency follow proper procedures in enforcing the statutory law?
3. Is there a substantial basis for the decision?
4. Did the administrative agency act in a nondiscriminatory and nonar-
   bitrary manner?
5. Was the issue under review included in the delegation to the agency?

Attorney General's Opinions

A second example of administrative law is the *attorney general's opinion.* Often
the national or state attorney general is requested to give an opinion regarding
a specific interpretation of a law. Individuals or agencies may request such an
opinion, and the opinion is binding until a subsequent statute, regulation, or
court order amends the attorney general's opinion.

The attorney general's opinions provide guidelines based on both statutory
and common law principles. Sometimes statutes are written in such vague
terms that nurses seek opinions concerning the interpretation of the statute.
Opinions can also be formal or informal. The greater the liability risks, the
more likely that a formal opinion will be issued. If legal issues then arise and
the nurse has a formal attorney general's opinion, the court will more likely
find that the nurse acted in a reasonable and responsible manner in seeking
clarification on the matter.

Judicial Law

Judicial (or *decisional*) *laws* are made by the courts and interpret legal issues
that are in dispute. Depending on the type of court involved, the judicial or decisional law may be made either by a single justice, with or without the assistance of a jury, or by a panel of justices. As a rule of thumb, the initial trial
courts have a single justice or magistrate, intermediary appeals courts have
three justices, and the highest appeals courts have a panel of nine justices.

All courts serve to rule on issues in dispute. In deciding cases, the courts interpret statutes and regulations or may decide which of two conflicting statutes

or regulations apply to a given fact situation. Courts may also decide if the statute or regulation violates a constitution (federal or state), since all statutes and regulations must be in harmony with the governing constitution. The landmark case of *Marbury v. Madison* (1803) established the power of the judiciary in interpreting constitutional law. For example, a nurse who questions the authority of the state board of nursing may file a court action if the nurse has cause to believe that there has been a legal or procedural error on the part of the board's action against him or her.

Two important legal doctrines guide courts in their decision-making role.

1. The doctrine of **precedent** or **stare decisis** literally means to "let the decision stand." This doctrine is applied by courts of law in cases with similar fact patterns that have been previously decided by the court system. The court looks at the facts of the current case before it, reviews previous decisions that applied the same rules and principles with the similar fact situation, and then arrives at a similar decision in the case currently before the court. This doctrine has great implications for nurses, because it gives them insight into how the court has previously fixed liability in given fact situations. Nurses must avoid two important pitfalls before deciding if the doctrine of precedent should apply to a given fact situation.

   a. The previous case must be within the jurisdiction of the court hearing the current case. For example, a previous New York case decided by an appellate court within New York does not set precedent for a California state court, although the California court may model its decision after the New York case. It is not compelled to do so, since two separate jurisdictions are involved. Within the same jurisdiction, the case would set precedent. A New York appellate decision would be relied on by the lower courts in New York State.

   b. The court hearing the current case may depart from precedent and set a **landmark decision,** which signifies that precedent is changed by the current court decision. Such a landmark decision is usually arrived at for one of several reasons. Societal needs may have changed, technology may have become more advanced, or following the previous decision would further harm an already injured person. A well-known example of a landmark decision was the U.S. Supreme Court holding in *Roe v. Wade* (1973). That court, for the first time in American history, recognized the right of a woman to seek and receive a legal abortion during the first two trimesters of pregnancy.

2. A second doctrine that courts employ in the duplication of litigation and seemingly apparent contradiction in decisions is **res judicata,** which means literally "a thing or matter settled by judgment." Res judicata applies only when a legal dispute has been decided by a competent court of jurisdiction and no further appeals are possible. The doctrine then prevents the same parties in the original lawsuit from retrying the same issues involved in the first lawsuit. Res judicata prevents multiple litigation by parties who have

lost in the original suit in that those parties are prevented from taking the same issues to another court in hopes of persuading a second trial court in their favor.

Res judicata does not apply to competent appeals to an appellate court, nor does it apply to parties who were not named in the original lawsuit. Res judicata likewise does not apply to issues that were not decided by the original trial court so that a second lawsuit could be filed by the same parties on different specific issues.

All laws, regardless of origin, are fluid and subject to change. Constitutional laws may be amended. Statutory laws may be amended, repealed, or expanded by future legislative action. Administrative bodies may be dissolved, expanded, or redefined. Judicial or decisional laws may be modified or completely altered by new court decisions.

CLASSIFICATIONS (TYPES) OF LAW

Laws may be further classified into several types. Many nurses may have wondered about classifications such as (1) common law, (2) civil law, (3) public law, (4) criminal law, (5) private law, (6) substantive law, and (7) procedural law.

Common Law

Law may be classified according to the court in which it was first instituted. The federal courts and 49 of the state courts in America follow the common law of England. *Common law* is law derived from principles rather than from rules and regulations, and it is based on justice, reason, and common sense. During the colonial period, the English common law was uniformly applied in the 13 original colonies. After the American Revolution, individual states adopted various parts of the common law, and differences in interpretation and enforcement began that exist to this day. Individual state statutory and judicial laws also account for the variation of common law principles from state to state.

Civil Law

Louisiana elected to adopt civil or Napoleonic laws, since the origins of that state were of a predominantly French influence. Derived from the civil laws of the French, Romans, and Spaniards, Napoleonic or *civil law* may be said to be based on rules and regulations.

Civil law may also be used to distinguish the area of the law concerned with the rights and duties of private persons and citizens. Civil law is administered between citizen and citizen (between private persons) and is enforced through the courts as damages or money compensation. No fine or imprisonment is assessed in civil law, and injured parties usually collect money damages from the private citizens who have harmed them.

The court, though, may also decide that an action, known as *specific performance,* be performed rather than allow money damages, if the court deems that specific performance best aids the injured party. For example, in a contract dispute, the court may force an employer to reinstate a previously discharged worker and to pay the worker compensation for the time he or she was without employment rather than merely paying the worker for the time spent out of work.

Civil law may be further divided into a variety of legal specialties: contract law, labor law, patent law, tort law, among others. Perhaps the most important area of law to the professional nurse, *tort law* involves compensation to those wrongfully injured by others' actions. This is the area of law that is normally involved in medical malpractice claims. Tort law is covered in more depth in Part II of this book.

Public Law

Public law is the branch of law concerned with the state in its political capacity. The relationship of a person to the state is at the crux of public law. Perhaps one of the best examples of public law is the entire field of criminal law.

Criminal Law

Criminal law refers to conduct that is offensive or harmful to society as a whole. If an act is expressly forbidden or prohibited by statute or by common law principles, it is referred to as a crime. Most often crimes are viewed as an offense against the state rather than as against an individual, and the state, city, or administrative body brings the legal action against the offender. Examples of crimes include minor traffic violations, theft, and unlawfully taking another's life. Punishment for the commission of crimes ranges from simple fines to imprisonment to execution.

Crimes can be classified in two ways: (1) *Misdemeanors* are lesser crimes and may involve fines of less than $1,000 or imprisonment of less than one year. (2) *Felonies* are more serious, involve fines of greater than $1,000, and are punishable by prison terms of greater than one year or by death.

The same action by a given individual may be the basis for both a civil lawsuit as well as a criminal wrong. For example, if a nurse removes a ventilator-dependent patient from a ventilator and the patient subsequently dies, the state board of nursing may remove the nurse's license to practice nursing, and the family may file a wrongful death suit (a civil suit) against the nurse. In the criminal case, the court would consider the intent of the defendant as well as the actual action. In the civil case filed out of the same action, the court considers only the action performed.

In certain nursing situations, the nurse may be said to have violated criminal laws, and the number of criminal cases against nurses is on the rise. Examples include falsification of narcotic records (*People v. Coe*, 1986), failure to renew nursing licenses (*Kansas State Board of Nursing v. Burkman*, 1975), withholding life support in terminally ill patients, and the administration of drugs that cause or hasten a patient's death (*Jones v. State of Texas*, 1986). In the so-called "angel of mercy" line of cases, where nurses administer fatal doses of lidocaine, insulin, or potassium chloride to elderly patients, nurses have been charged with criminal violations (*The People v. Diaz*, 1992, and *Rachals v. State of Georgia*, 1987).

Other, less common, instances of criminal charges against professional nurses include the rape of patients (*State of North Carolina v. Raines*, 1987), manslaughter (*People of the State of New York v. Simon*, 1990), and attempted murder (*Caretenders v. Commonwealth of Kentucky*, 1991).

EXERCISE 1-2

Describe instances in which the conduct of a professional nurse (with regard to treatment of a patient) might be cause for criminal charges. (For example, the administration of toxic chemotherapeutic agents may place a patient in a more life-threatening condition than the disease process does.) How would a court of law distinguish such a case?

Private Law

Private law is synonymous with civil or common law, which has been discussed earlier in this chapter.

Substantive Law

Substantive law, which defines the substance of the law, may be further classified into civil, administrative, and criminal law. Thus, substantive law concerns the specific wrong, harm, or duty that caused the lawsuit or action to be brought against an individual. Lawsuits brought to remedy violations of these laws must eventually prove the existence of the elements that comprise the actual claims.

Procedural Law

Procedural law, which governs the procedure or rules to create, implement, or enforce substantive law, may vary according to the type of substantive law involved and the jurisdiction in which the lawsuit is brought. Thus, procedural law concerns the process and rights of the individual charged with violating substantive law. Procedural issues that could be at issue include the admissibility of evidence, the time frame for initiating lawsuits, and the qualifications of expert witnesses.

DUE PROCESS OF LAW AND EQUAL PROTECTION OF THE LAW

Due process of law, a phrase often misquoted, applies only to state actions and not to the actions of private citizens. Basically, the due process clause of the U.S. Constitution is intended to prevent a person from being deprived of "life, liberty, or property" by actions of state or local governments (Amendment 14, Section 1). While difficult to define, the due process clause is founded on the fundamental principle of justice rather than on a rule of law, and its purpose is to ensure the fair and orderly administration of laws (16A *Corpus Juris Secundum,* 1984).

Due process protects the public from arbitrary actions. Laws must operate equally among all persons, and laws must be definite, not vague. Due process is violated if a particular person of a class or community is singled out by the law. A "person of ordinary intelligence who would be law abiding can tell what conduct must be to conform to [the law's] regulation, and the law is susceptible to uniform interpretation and application by those charged with enforcing it" (*State v. Schuster's Express, Inc.,* 1969, at 792).

The two primary elements of due process are that (1) the rule as applied must be reasonable and definite, and (2) fair procedures must be followed in enforcing the rule. This latter provision ensures that adequate notice be given before the rule is enforced so that persons who will be affected by it will have time to explain why the rule should or should not be enforced. Nurses become involved in the application of due process when requested to appear before state boards of nursing in that they must be given proper notice of the upcoming hearing and the charges that the board will be hearing. In the hospital setting, the concept of due process has been interpreted to include a hospital's right to licensure by the state and the right of qualified medical personnel to staff appointments in public hospitals.

Like due process, the equal protection clause of the Fourteenth Amendment also restricts state actions and has no reference to private actions. The concept of *equal protection of the law* has become the source of many civil rights (*Words and Phrases,* 1994). More than an abstract right, the equal protection clause guarantees that all similarly situated persons will be affected similarly. Laws need not affect every man, woman, and child alike, but reasonable classifications of persons must be treated similarly (*Dorsey v. Solomon,* 1984). Thus, states may not enforce rules and regulations based solely on classifications as determined by race, religion, and gender. The due process clause does not preclude states from resorting to classifications of persons for the purpose of litigation, but "the classification must be reasonable and not arbitrary and must rest upon some ground of difference having a fair and substantial relationship to the object of legislation so that all persons similarly circumstanced shall be treated alike" (*Ex Parte Tigner,* 1964, at 894–895).

In determining whether equal protection of the law has been achieved, courts use the *rational basis test,* which essentially states that persons in the same classes must be treated alike. It also states that reasonable grounds that further legitimate governmental interests exist in making distinction between those persons who fall within the class and those persons who fall outside the class (*Ohio University Faculty Association v. Ohio University,* 1984).

A recent case, decided under the equal protection clause of both the United States and Arizona Constitutions, held that it was unreasonable to allocate treatment within a service category solely on the criterion of age (*Salgado v. Kirschner,* 1994). In that case, a middle-aged Medicaid recipient was denied a life-saving liver transplant based on an Arizona statute that limits Medicaid coverage for medically necessary transplants to persons under the age of 21. The court found that age was the only criterion used and that age was medically irrelevant to liver transplant outcomes in that no evidence linking age to greater survival rate was shown. This case is significant in that age, if used to set restrictions on care, cannot be neither the sole factor considered nor medically irrelevant.

The distinction between due process and equal protection was best summarized in *Peterson v. Garvey Elevators, Inc.* (1983). In that case, the court stated "the difference between due process and equal protection of the law is that due process emphasizes fairness between state and individual regardless of how other individuals in the same situation are treated while equal protection emphasizes disparity in treatment by a state between classes on individuals whose situations arguably are indistinguishable" (at 897).

SUMMARY

A basic understanding of the legal system, though complex, protects nurses against potential litigation, while allowing them to be confident in the care they deliver. The legal system is a blend of rules and regulations, contains both federal and state laws, and may seem overwhelming at first glance. An appreciation of the legal system takes time to develop and the subsequent chapters of this book will assist individuals in understanding legal concepts in relationship to professional nursing practice.

AFTER COMPLETING THIS CHAPTER, YOU SHOULD BE ABLE TO

- Define the term *law* and describe four sources from which law is derived, including constitutional, statutory, administrative, and judicial (decisional) law.
- Compare and contrast the doctrines of precedent (stare decisis) and res judicata.
- Define and give applications of jurisdiction and landmark decision.
- List four ways in which laws can be changed.
- Define the classifications of law, including common, civil, criminal, public, and private law.

- Distinguish substantive and procedural law and state why each is important to professional nursing practice.
- Discuss due process and equal protection of the law.

APPLY YOUR LEGAL KNOWLEDGE

- Which classifications of law are commonly applied to professional nursing?
- How do attorney generals' opinions protect the practice of professional nursing?
- Do all four sources of law protect the practice of nursing? Why or why not?

REFERENCES

Black, H. C. (1990). *Law dictionary* (6th ed.). St. Paul: West Publishing.

Caretenders v. Commonwealth of Kentucky, 821 S.W. 2d 83 (Kentucky, 1991).

Dorsey v. Solomon, 435 F. Supp. 725 (DC MD 1984).

Ex Parte Tigner, 132 S.W. 2d 885, 139 Tx. Cr. Rept. 452 (Texas, 1964).

Jones v. State of Texas, 716 S.W. 2d 142 (Texas, 1986).

Kansas State Board of Nursing v. Burkman, 531 P. 2d 122 (Kansas, 1975).

Marbury v. Madison, 5 U.S. (1 Cranch) 137 (1803).

Ohio University Faculty Association v. Ohio University, 449 N.E. 2d 792, 5 Ohio App. 2d 130 (Ohio, 1984).

People of the State of New York v. Simon, 549 N.Y.S. 2d 701 (New York, 1990).

People v. Coe, 501 N.Y.S. 2d 977 (NY Super. 1986).

Peterson v. Garvey Elevators, Inc., 850 P. 2d 893, 252 Kan 976 (Kansas, 1993).

Rachals v. State of Georgia, 361 S.E. 2d 671 (Georgia, 1987).

Roe v. Wade, 410 U.S. 113 (1973).

Salgado v. Kirschner, 878 P. 2d 659 (Arizona, 1994).

16 *American Jurisprudence* (2nd ed.) (1995). Constitutional Law.

16A *Corpus Juris Secundum* (1984). Constitutional Law, Sec. 1–20, 957.

State of North Carolina v. Raines, 334 S.E. 2d 138 (1987).

State v. Schuster's Express, Inc., 5 Conn. Cir. 472, 256 A. 2d 792 (1969).

The People v. Diaz, 834 P.2d 1171 (California, 1992).

Words and Phrases (1994), Equal Protection of the Law. *14A.* St. Paul, MN: West Publishing Company.

United States Constitution, Amendments 1–10, 14 (1787).

· two

The Judicial Process

PREVIEW

To fully appreciate the doctrine of precedent and the vast impact of landmark decisions on the court, nurses must first appreciate the complexities of the American court system. The significance of majority and minority opinions becomes clearly relevant as one differentiates the court systems, tiers, and jurisdiction issues. This chapter introduces the role of courts, gives a thorough description of the American court system, and concludes with a section on analyzing a legal case.

questions of fact	state appellate court (or court of intermediate appeal)	writ of certiorari
questions of law		statutes of limitations
fact-finder	state supreme court	discovery rule
jurisdiction	U.S. district court	plaintiff
trial court	U.S. Supreme Court	defendant

QUESTIONS OF LAW OR FACT

Facts are determined by evidence presented by both sides in a legal controversy. *Questions of fact* present a factual dispute that the jury answers. Facts are not necessarily what actually happened, since persons on both sides will have perceived a given incident through their own eyes. Each party to the controversy brings unique perceptions to the trial setting. It is the responsibility of the fact-finder to weigh admissible evidence as presented and to decide where the facts of the case really lie. For example, a question of fact can concern such issues as admission to a hospital. Was the patient formally admitted to a hospital so that a patient-hospital relationship was established? Questions of fact can also include how much an operation or a hospital service cost or who was involved in an incident. To date, questions of fact have concerned practice standards in that juries have decided whether practice standards have set the standard of care for individual patients. If, as Fiesta suggests, practice standards become more widely accepted, they will meet the standard of care so that it will become a question of law as to whether the professional practitioner met or violated the standard (1994).

Sometimes facts are agreed on by both sides to the controversy prior to the trial. In these cases, the only questions left to be resolved are *questions of law,* which involve the application or interpretation of laws and are determined by the judge in the court. For example, the judge may rule that a provision in a nurse's contract was against public policy and is therefore nonenforceable. Or the judge may rule that a particular provision in the contract is reasonable and thus enforceable. Federal and state statutes, rules and regulations, prior court decisions, new technology, and societal needs may all play a part in determining the law as it applies to a specific trial.

Fact-finders, usually the jurors at the trial, determine the facts that are admissible. These selected people are charged with weighing the admitted evidence, while the judge or magistrate determines questions of law. If there is a trial without a jury, then the judge serves as both the fact-finder and the determinator of questions of law.

JURISDICTION OF THE COURTS

Jurisdiction, the authority by which courts and judicial officers accept and decide cases, is the power and authority of a court to hear and determine a judicial proceeding (Black, 1990). Jurisdiction determines the courts' ability to hear and rule on a lawsuit. Jurisdiction may be divided into two categories.

Subject matter jurisdiction refers to the court's competence to hear and to determine a case within a class of cases. For example, a court may have jurisdiction only in cases that involve probate matters (wills, estates, and the like), that involve family matters (adoptions, divorces, and child custody), or that involve criminal matters. Subject matter jurisdiction, along with the nature of the cause of action, may be determined by the amount or value of the claim as pled. For example, some courts have jurisdiction of a given case up to $1,000 or to cases that have a pled-damage figure of between $1,000 and $5,000.

Personal jurisdiction refers to the power of a given court regarding a particular person. Personal jurisdiction is the legal power of a court to render a judgment against a party or parties to the action or proceeding. For example, personal jurisdiction often involves the county of the defendant. A court situated in the county of the defendant has personal jurisdiction over the defendant. A court situated in the county of the plaintiff's residence can also have personal jurisdiction over the parties to the lawsuit.

Courts may be either state or federal in origin. Federal courts seek to ensure that laws created by the U.S. Congress are enforced, and state courts have their sole jurisdiction within the given state. Overseeing the process is the U.S. Supreme Court, which has jurisdiction over all the land.

Overlapping or *concurrent jurisdiction* may occur in that more than one court is qualified to hear a given dispute. In some areas of overlapping or concurrent jurisdiction and in some instances of specific subject matter jurisdiction, the federal constitution gives guidance. For example, the federal courts have original jurisdiction over admiralty cases, crimes involving federal laws, bankruptcy cases, and patent laws. The U.S. Constitution gives the U.S. Supreme Court original jurisdiction (that which is inherent or conferred to the court) over cases "involving ambassadors, other public ministers and consuls and those in which a state is a named party" (Article III, Section 2).

If there is no mandatory court of jurisdiction, attorneys representing the parties filing the lawsuit will advise their clients of the optimal court in which to file the lawsuit. Concurrent jurisdiction frequently occurs in cases with multiple defendants and in cases that involve parties residing in different states. One court might be more favorable to the party filing the lawsuit than another court for many reasons, including shorter length of time to trial, more favorable damage awards, and shorter distances for witnesses to travel.

STATE COURTS

Trial Courts

The court of original jurisdiction in most states is the *trial court,* and it is the first court to hear legal disputes. At this level, applicable law is determined, evidence is presented and evaluated to ascertain the facts, and either a judge or a jury (functioning under the guidance of a judge) applies the law to the admissible facts. As stated in the preceding sections, the judge determines questions of law and then guides the jury in applying this law to the questions of fact.

Even though the jury's tasks are to determine facts and, after proper instructions, to apply the law to the facts, the judge retains control over the entire trial process. The judge may find that the evidence is inadmissible or that the evidence as presented is insufficient to establish a factual issue for the jury to resolve. The judge may dismiss the case or may overrule a jury decision if he or she finds that justice has not been served.

Most state courts operate on a three-tier system. Sometimes called *inferior courts,* trial courts are the courts with original jurisdiction in most states with three-tier systems. Other names for the first court in which the lawsuit is filed include circuit courts, superior court, supreme court (New York State), courts of common pleas, chancery courts, and district courts.

State Appellate Courts

The side that loses the case at trial level may decide to pursue the case to appellate level if there are procedural or legal grounds for an appeal. In a three-tier system, these *state appellate courts,* or *courts of intermediate appeal,* do not rehear the entire trial but base their decisions on evidence as presented in a record of the trial hearing. There are no witnesses, new evidence, or jurors. The intermediate court may concur (agree) with the previous decision, reverse the prior decision, or remand (send the case back to the trial level) and reorder a new trial.

Intermediate courts of appeal have different names throughout the states. They may be called courts of appeal, intermediate appellate courts (Hawaii), appellate division of the supreme court (New York), superior court, court of special appeals (Maryland), court of civil appeals, and court of criminal appeals. States that have two-tier systems, such as North Dakota, Rhode Island, and Maine, have no intermediate appellate courts.

State Supreme Courts

The ultimate court of appeal in the state is usually named the *state supreme court.* This court hears appeals from the intermediate appellate courts and serves to adopt rules of procedure for the state and to license attorneys within the individual state. This court is the final authority for state issues, unless a federal issue or constitutional right is involved. The state supreme court may hear cases directly from the trial level. For example, if the trial court case concerned the interpretation of the state constitution or a state statute, the case can be appealed directly to the state supreme court. An example of such a direct appeal involving the interpretation of the Missouri nurse practice act occurred in *Sermchief v. Gonzales* (1983).

Other names for the highest court of appeals in the state include state court of last resort (West Virginia), supreme judicial court (Maine and Massachusetts), and court of appeals (New York and Maryland). Some states (Texas and Oklahoma) may also have separate supreme courts of criminal appeals.

EXERCISE 2-1

How is your state's court system structured? What types of trial courts exist? What are they called? What is their jurisdiction? Which court would most likely hear nursing malpractice cases?

FEDERAL COURTS

District Courts

The federal court system mimics the majority of state court systems. The original trial courts in the federal three-tier system are the **U.S. district courts** and the specialty courts such as the U.S. court of claims, the U.S. bankruptcy courts, and the U.S. patent courts. The district courts normally hear cases involving a *federal question* (a question regarding a federal statute or violations of the rights and privileges granted by the U.S. Constitution) or those involving parties with citizenships in different states (*diversity of citizenship*). In cases involving diverse citizenship, the federal court system applies rules of federal procedure in deciding applicable state law.

Courts of Appeal

The intermediary courts are the U.S. courts of appeal. These courts were known as the circuit courts of appeals prior to June 25, 1948. There are currently 12 courts of appeal, and they are frequently called U.S. circuit courts even today. These courts are located in 12 areas (or circuits) of the country. The U.S. courts of appeal are numbered 1 through 11, with the District of Columbia Court of Appeals being the 12th court. Each of the first 11 courts of appeal consists of one to five state regions. These courts function as do the intermediary courts on the state level.

Supreme Court

The highest level of the federal court system is the **U.S. Supreme Court,** whose decisions are binding in all state and federal courts. This nine-justice court hears appeals from the U.S. courts of appeals and from the various state supreme courts when state court decisions involve federal laws or constitutional questions based on a *writ of certiorari,* or written petition to hear the case.

Because most nursing practice cases concern tort law or state licensure issues, rarely are lawsuits involving nurses as primary defendants heard in the federal court system. Exceptions to this rule are nurses working in the military and veterans' hospitals or other federally funded health care centers. Cases involving these nurses are frequently settled in federal courts.

STATUTES OF LIMITATIONS

Statutes of limitations, procedural law time frames, are essentially time intervals during which a case must be filed or the injured party is *barred* (prevented legally) from bringing the lawsuit. Set by the state legislature, statutes of limitation establish a time frame within which a suit must be brought. Most states allow one to two years for the filing of a personal injury lawsuit. The majority of the states do not begin measuring time until the injured party has actually discovered the injury that will become the basis of the ensuing lawsuit. According to the so-called *discovery rule,* patients have two years from the time that they knew or should have known of the injury to file a personal injury lawsuit.

Because of the malpractice crisis of the mid-1970s, many states have moved away from open-ended discovery statutes. Some courts have distinguished between traumatic injury cases and disease cases. In *traumatic injury cases,* the injury is normally of the type that the patient knows or should have known of immediately. For example, the patient who has an operation on the opposite extremity or wrong area of the body will immediately know that an injury has occurred. In traumatic injury cases, the one- or two-year statute of limitations is strictly applied.

In *disease cases,* the statute of limitations may be less strictly applied, since it may be some time before the patient becomes aware of the possible malpractice event. The statute of limitations begins to measure time when the patient becomes aware of the injury (event) or when the reasonable patient would have become aware of the injury. For example, in *Kubrick v. United States* (1978), a war veteran became aware of the fact that his hearing loss was caused by the incorrect administration of a neomycin drug. He had two years from the time an ear specialist told him that neomycin causes hearing loss to file a malpractice suit against the prescribing physician.

The rationale behind statutes of limitations is that potential defendants should have the opportunity to defend themselves within a reasonable time period. Their purpose is to suppress fraudulent claims after the facts concerning them have become obscured from the lapse of time, defective memory, or death or removal of witnesses (*Noll v. City of Bozeman,* 1975). If too much time has elapsed between the occurrence and the lawsuit, facts become stale and witnesses cannot be identified or found.

At one time, courts uniformly allowed a major exception, in the case of minors, to the prompt filing of a lawsuit for personal injury. Because parents may not always enforce what is in the best interest of their child, the court allowed minors to reach their majority before the statute of limitations began to be measured. In most states this meant that the statute begins to be counted when the child reaches the 18th birthday. Lawsuits must be filed by the time injured minors reach their 20th birthday or the suit is barred by law. Today, a minority of states have become more restrictive, opting to disallow the right of a minor to bring suit upon reaching adulthood (majority).

ANALYZING LEGAL CASES

The entire legal system seems to be organized around the interpretation of case-law analysis. Laws are enacted by legislative and administrative bodies, and disputes are settled in courts. It seems to follow that, if you are able to analyze the decisions the courts hand down, then you truly understand the law. While nurses need not fully comprehend every procedural tactic to appreciate the doctrine of precedent and its mandate to nursing practice, they need a working knowledge of case-law interpretation.

CASE CITATIONS

A *case citation* is written as follows: *Darling v. Charleston Community Memorial Hospital*, 211 N.E.2d 53 (Illinois, 1965). All cases give the names of the plaintiff and defendant, as in *Darling v. Charleston Community Memorial Hospital*. The first listed name is the **plaintiff**, or the party bringing the lawsuit. At trial level, the plaintiff is synonymous with the injured party. The second named party is the **defendant**, or the party against whom the case is filed. Named parties may be individuals, corporations, states, or partnerships. The formal case citation lists the primary plaintiff and defendant. Multiple parties may be included in a single suit, but multiple plaintiffs and defendants are listed only on the original petition filed with the court hearing the case.

The order of listing is crucial. At any level of hearing, the party seeking restitution is named first, and the defending party is always named second. After the named parties to the suit is a string of numbers and abbreviations, for example, 211 N.E.2d 53. These abbreviations refer to a specific set of law reporters. *Law reporters* are published volumes containing the decisions and opinions of state and federal courts. Geographically the nation is divided into regions, such as the northeast (N.E.), northwest (N.W.), south (So.), southwest (S.W.), and Pacific (P.) regions. Additionally, some of the courts in a minority of states hear so many cases per year that one state may have its own reporter, as with California and New York. The "2d" or "3d" reference refers to the second and third series of the reporter. Most state reporters are now in the third series. If no series reference is given, the first series of the reporter is assumed.

The abbreviations may also refer to a set of federal reporters, as in 381 Fed.2d 811. The number listed before the reference to a specific reporter (eg, 381) is the volume of the reporter, and the number listed after the reporter (eg, 811) is the starting page of the case within that volume of the reporter. In the last example, the case would be found in volume 381 of the Federal Reporter, second series, on page 811.

Some cases refer to different sets of reporters, indicating that the case is located in more than one set of reporters. For example, in *Schloendorf v. Society of New York Hospital*, 211 N.Y. 125, 105 N.E. 92 (1914):

> 211 is the volume number.
> N.Y. stands for New York Reporter, first series.
> 125 is page 125.
> 105 is the volume number.
> N.E. means the Northeast Reporter, first series.
> 92 stands for page 92.
> 1914 is the year that the decision was published.

Many federal cases are found in more than one set of reporters, and some states have a recording system as well as the national service of reporting cases.

Case citations also list the specific court hearing the case and the year that the decision was decided. A state listed in the citation indicates that the highest court within the state heard the case. Examples include *Wyatt v. Stickney*, 344 F. Supp 387 (Alabama, 1972) and *Castillo v. United States*, 406 F. Supp 585 (DC, N.M., 1975). Understanding the state references is crucial, since the references indicate the jurisdiction of the ruling. References to the U.S. Supreme Court decisions never list the state in which the case originated because the jurisdiction of that court is nationwide.

ELEMENTS OF A CASE

The format used to report lawsuits is fairly standardized, and most cases have the following elements. (Refer to the sample case pp. 25–29 for clarification.)

1. A brief paragraph sets forth a synopsis of the case with the rulings by this specific court. The synopsis lists: (a) the judicial panel; (b) from which court the case was appealed; and (c) the final holding (finding) of the court. In the sample case, the justice is named and the final holding of the court is identified.
2. Key concepts are identified by the reporting system and numbered according to their appearance in the case. Usually these concepts concern broad fields of law, as constitutional or contract law, and key points as they are developed by the decision. These key concepts are known as *headnotes*.
3. An opinion follows the headnotes, stating why the plaintiff is appealing a lower court case and the ultimate decision of this court. In the sample

SAMPLE CASE

114 N.M. 13
Dawna Charlene Baca,
Plaintiff-Appellant,
v.
Dr. Jose VELEZ, Defendant-Apellee.
No. 11540.
Court of Appeals of New Mexico.
May 13, 1992.
Certiorari Denied June 18, 1992.

Nurse brought tort action against surgeon, alleging assault and battery. The District Court, Curry County, Peggy J. Nelson, D.J., entered judgment on jury verdict in favor of surgeon, and nurse appealed. The Court of Appeals, Chavez, J., held that: (1) there was no evidence of assault, and (2) trial court's evidentiary rulings were proper.

Affirmed.

1. Appeal and Err 863,934 (1)

In reviewing motion for summary judgment, Court of Appeals looks to whole record and views matter in light most favorable to support trial on merits.

2. Assault and Battery 2

Not all batteries include assaults; to be assault, there must have been act, threat or menacing conduct which caused another person to reasonably believe that he is in danger of receiving immediate battery. NMSA 1978, § 30-3-1, subd. B.

3. Assault and Battery 2

Physician who allegedly jabbed nurse in course of argument over surgical instruments was not liable for assault absent evidence that nurse felt scared before touching took place.

4. Appeal and Error 970(2)

Admission of character evidence is within discretion of trial court and will not be disturbed on appeal in absence of abuse of discretion.

5. Evidence 106(1)

Exclusion of evidence on defendant's character, in civil suit to recover for battery, was not abuse of discretion; defendant did not put his character into issue and such evidence was offered by plaintiff expressly on issue of propensity. SCRA 1986, Rule 11-404, subd. B.

6. Evidence 146

Exclusion of testimony of size or strength differences between plaintiff and battery defendant was not abuse of discretion; comparison would have been more prejudicial than probative and in any event, jury was able, by their own in-court observations, to view differences between parties.

7. Pretrial Procedure 45

Trial court properly allowed testimony from three lay witnesses disclosed near date of trial; defendant disclosed identity of witnesses within time frame allowed by pretrial order and there was no evidence that defendant knew he would be calling witnesses at earlier point in time and chose not to disclose their identities until it would be too late for plaintiff to depose them.

8. Pretrial Procedure 202

Unsigned deposition testimony of witness was properly excluded upon defendant's reasonably prompt objection, absent showing that defendant had waived signature requirement. SCRA 1986, Rule 1-030, subd. E.

9. Estoppel 68(2)

Party who offers deposition in support of motion for partial summary judgment effectively vouches for accuracy of that deposition and is thereafter judicially estopped from objecting to its admission when offered by opposing party.

10. Pretrial Procedure 202

Tape recording of deposition was properly excluded absent evidence that any stipulation or order regarding recording of deposition was made, or that any measures were taken to assure that recording was accurate and trustworthy. SCRA 1986, Rule 1-030, subd. B(4).

11. Evidence 150

Polygraph interview tape was properly excluded; rules of evidence concerned themselves only with admission of results of polygraph examination, which required professional skill of trained polygraph examiner. SCRA 1986, Rule 11-707.

12. Appeal and Error 1060.1(11)

Any conclusory arguments made by battery defendant's counsel in his opening statement did not warrant reversal of defense verdict absent showing that statement, in all probability, must have produced some effect on final results of trial.

OPINION

CHAVEZ, Judge.

Plaintiff appeals a jury verdict in favor of Defendant on her assault and battery claim. She raises eight issues on appeal: (1) whether the trial court erred in granting summary judgment on the assault claim; (2) whether the trial court erred in excluding evidence of the character of Defendant; (3) whether the trial court erred in excluding testimony of size and strength differences between Plaintiff and Defendant; (4) whether the trial court erred in allowing the testimony of three witnesses disclosed near the date of trial; (5) whether the trial court erred in refusing to allow the admission of the deposition or the taped testimony of a witness; (6) whether the trial court erred in refusing to allow a polygraph tape to be played to the jury; (7) whether the trial court erred in allowing Defendant to make conclusive remarks in his opening statement; and (8) whether the trial court erred in refusing to instruct the jury on assault. We affirm.

FACTS

This cause of action arose as a result of an incident alleged by Plaintiff to have occurred at Clovis High Plains Hospital in July 1986. Defendant is an orthopedic surgeon and a member of the staff of the hospital. Plaintiff, a nurse at the hospital at the time of the incident, worked with and was in charge of instruments. A disagreement occurred between Plaintiff and Defendant regarding certain instruments, including an osteotome, also known as a bone chisel. During the disagreement, Plaintiff alleges that Defendant jabbed Plaintiff in the back with the sharp end of the osteotome.

DISCUSSION

[1] Plaintiff's first issue is whether the trial court erred in granting partial summary judgement on her cause of action for assault. In reviewing a motion for summary judgment, this court looks to the whole record and views matters in the

light most favorable to support a trial on the merits. *North v. Public Serv. Co.*, 97 N.M. 406, 640 P.2d 512 (Ct. App. 1982). Defendant's motion for partial summary judgment was supported by excerpts from the depositions of Mary Jane Petty and Plaintiff. Plaintiff did not file affidavits or other material opposing the motion, but argued at the hearing, as she does on appeal, that she felt afraid "after the initial jabbing." In her deposition, when asked if she felt "any anticipation that he might injure [her] further," Plaintiff answered "I wasn't sure. I was scared then." She also stated that she left immediately after the alleged touching.

[2, 3] We determine this evidence to be sufficient to sustain the trial court's grant of partial summary judgment on the issue of assault. While assault and battery are closely related, one may exist without the other. See W. Page Keeton et al., Prosser and Keeton on the Law of Torts § 10, at 46 (5th ed. 1984). All batteries do not include an assault. For there to be an assault, there must have been an "act, threat or menacing conduct which causes another person to reasonably believe that he is in danger of receiving an immediate battery." NMSA 1978, §30-3-1(B) (Repl. Pamp. 1984). There was no evidence that Plaintiff felt scared before the touching took place. Therefore, there was no genuine issue of material fact whether, under these circumstances, an assault actually occurred.

[4, 5] Plaintiff's second issue is whether the trial court erred in excluding character evidence of Defendant. Admission of character evidence is within the discretion to the trial court and will not be disturbed on appeal in the absence of an abuse of discretion. *State v. Allen*, 19 N.M. 759, 581 P.2d 22 (Ct. App. 1978). Plaintiff cites several cases that allowed character evidence when character itself was at issue. In this case, however, Defendant did not put his character into issue. Also, Plaintiff's counsel argued to the trial court that the evidence in question was probative of Defendant's character and his propensity to be aggressive and domineering over women. SCRA 1986, 11-404(B) prohibits the use of evidence of other acts "to prove the character of a person in order to show that he acted in conformity therewith." Refusal to admit this evidence was not an abuse of discretion.

[6] Plaintiff's third issue is whether the trial court erred in refusing to admit testimony of size or strength differences between Plaintiff and Defendant. The determination of relevancy and materiality rests largely within the discretion of the trial court. *Wilson v. Hayner*, 98 N.M. 514, 650 P.2d 36 (Ct. App. 1982). In light of the nature of the charges against Defendant, we do not consider it an abuse of discretion for the trial court, under these circumstances, to have ruled that comparisons of the size and strength of the parties would be more prejudicial than probative. In addition the jury was able, by their own in-court observations, to view the differences between the parties.

[7] Plaintiff's fourth issue is whether the trial court erred in allowing testimony from three witnesses disclosed near the date of trial. In reference to the lay witnesses, SCRA 1986, 1-026(E)(1) places a duty on a party to seasonably supplement his response to a request to identify each of the persons expected to be called as a witness at trial. Plaintiff failed to provide us with facts indicating that the time frame in which Defendant informed her of the lay witnesses was not seasonable. See SCRA 1986, 12-208 (B)(3). There is nothing to indicate that Defendant knew he would be calling the two new lay witnesses at an earlier point in time and chose not to disclose their identities until it would be too late for Plaintiff to depose them. ID. Also, Defendant disclosed the identity of the witnesses

within the time frame allowed by the pre-trial order. The pre-trial order states that both counsel for Plaintiff and Defendant presented argument on Defendant's motion for a pre-trial order, which only asked that time deadlines be set by the court and did not specify what deadlines were desired. Therefore, counsel for Plaintiff could have anticipated such problems arising and argued against the deadlines that were set.

The case of *Beverly v. Conquistadores, Inc.*, 88 N.M. 119, 537 P.2d 1015 (Ct. App. 1975), is distinguishable from the case at hand. In *Beverly*, counsel for one of the parties indicated he had knowledge of an additional witness whom he might call to testify at the trial and refused to name the witness when ordered to do so by the trial court. This is not the situation here.

With regard to the expert witness, SCRA 1986, 11-707(D) requires any party who intends to use polygraph evidence at trial to serve written notice of such intention on the opposing party, not less than ten days before trial. Plaintiff admits Defendant complied with this rule. Under these circumstances, we cannot say the trial court abused its discretion in not granting Plaintiff a continuance and in allowing the expert witness to testify.

[8] Plaintiff's fifth issue is whether the trial court erred in refusing to allow the admission of the unsigned deposition or the taped testimony of witness Mary Petty. SCRA 1986, 1-030(E) states in pertinent part:

> Unless examination and reading of a deposition are waived by the witness and the parties, or unless the party requesting that a witness sign his deposition make[s] other arrangements for submitting a deposition to the witness, the court reporter shall advise the witness and the parties, in writing, when the transcript is ready for examination. Any changes in form or substance which the witness desires to make shall be entered . . . The deposition shall then be signed by the witness.

Additionally, SCRA 1986, 1-032(C)(4), which here should be read in conjunction with Rule 1-030(E), provides that "[E]rrors and irregularities in the manner in which the . . . deposition is . . . signed . . . under Rules 1-030 and 1-031 are waived unless a motion to suppress the deposition or some part thereof is made with reasonable promptness after such defect is, or with due diligence might have been, ascertained."

In this case, Defendant's objection was made with reasonable promptness upon discovery that the deposition was unsigned and Plaintiff did not claim that Defendant had waived the signature requirement. We hold that the trial court did not err in refusing to allow the unsigned deposition testimony of the witness into evidence. See *Garcia v. Co-Con, Inc.*, 96 N.M. 308, 629 P.2d 1237 (Ct. App. 1981).

[9] We note that Defendant offered the Petty deposition in support of his motion for partial summary judgment. When Defendant did so he in effect vouched for the accuracy of that deposition. We believe that having offered the deposition, Defendant should not thereafter be allowed, under the doctrine of judicial estoppel, to object to the admission of the same deposition when offered by the opposing party. See, e.g., *Citizens Bank v. S & H Constr. & Paving Co.*, 89 N.M. 360, 366, 552 P.2d 796, 802 (Ct. App. 1975) ("'Judicial estoppel' simply means that a party is not permitted to maintain inconsistent position in judicial proceedings."); *Eads Hide & Wool Co. v. Merrill*, 252 F.2d 80, 84 (10th Cir. 1958) ("Where a party assumes a certain position in a legal proceeding and succeeds in maintaining that

position, he may not thereafter, simply because his interests have changed, assume a contrary position, especially if it be to the prejudice of the party who has acquiesced in the position formerly taken by him.") Had Plaintiff argued that the first deposition should have been admitted, notwithstanding the lack of the witness's signature or express waiver of same, on the basis that defendant himself had utilized that same deposition in support of his successful motion for partial summary judgment, we would have favored reversal and remand for new trial. Plaintiff, however, has not advanced a judicial estoppel argument on appeal, nor did she invoke a ruling on this issue by the trial court. See SCRA 1986, 12-216 (party must invoke a ruling by the trial court to preserve issue for review). Because Plaintiff has not raised or preserved this issue, we cannot address it on appeal.

[10] With regard to the tape recording of the deposition, SCRA 1986, 1-030(B)($) states:

> The parties may stipulate in writing or the court may upon motion order that the testimony at a deposition be recorded by other than stenographic means. The stipulation or order shall designate the person before whom the deposition shall be taken, the manner of recording, preserving and filing the deposition, and may include other provisions to assure that the recorded testimony will be accurate and trustworthy.

There is no evidence in the record that any stipulation or order was made, or that any measures were taken to assure that the recording was accurate and trustworthy. The trial court did not err in refusing to allow the tape recording of the deposition.

[11] Plaintiff's sixth issue is whether the trial court erred in not allowing the polygraph interview tape to be played to the jury. SCRA 1986, 11-707 specifically deals with the use of polygraph examinations. Polygraph examinations are defined as "test[s] using a polygraph instrument which at a minimum simultaneously graphically records on a chart the physiological changes in human respiration, cardiovascular activity, galvanic skin resistance or reflex for the purpose of lie detection." SCRA 1986, 11-707(A)(2). A polygraph examiner is a licensed professional who uses his skills and training to read, interpret, and score the responses to the examination. *Lewis v. Rodriguez*, 107 N.M. 430, 759 P.2d 1012 (Ct. App. 1988). Therefore, the specific rule concerns itself with the admission of the results of the polygraph examination, which requires the professional skill of a trained polygraph examiner. See SCRA 1986, 11-707(C). In light of this, we cannot say the trial court erred in refusing to allow the tape of the examination to be played.

[12] Plaintiff's seventh issue is whether the trial court erred in allowing Defendant's counsel to make conclusory arguments in his opening statement. "The burden is on the plaintiff to establish that the opening statements made by defendant, in all probability, must have produced some effect upon the final results of the trial." *Proper v. Mowry*, 90 N.M. 710, 716, 568 P.2d 236 252 (Ct. App. 1977). Our examination of the record shows Plaintiff failed to make such a showing to the trial court or this court.

Plaintiff's eighth issue is whether the trial court erred in refusing to instruct the jury on assault. Having previously decided that the trial court did not err in granting summary judgment on the assault issue, the jury did not need to be instructed on the assault, because that claim was not properly before them. We affirm.

IT IS SO ORDERED.

case, this opinion section outlines eight grounds of appeal and the final decision of the court. Here the previous court decision was upheld.

4. All cases begin with a review of the facts of the case. The more elaborate and complicated the fact situation, the more developed is this first section. It is crucial that the specific facts be understood, since even a slight variation in facts may lead to wide discrepancies in the rulings. This sample case has a fairly simple fact pattern, and those facts are stated in a single paragraph.

5. Usually the court next considers a legal question. This specific question is the issue of the case. The issue will never be a global question, such as "Is the defendant at fault?" Instead the issue will be more narrow and specific to the case at hand. The legal issue in the sample case could be phrased as "Could there be significant apprehension to warrant a finding of an assault when the injured party is struck from behind?"

6. The court then answers the question. This is the substance of the case. Included in this section are cites to other cases, quotations from recognized authorities in various fields of law, and an analysis of the issue. The reporters divide this section according to the headnotes used at the beginning of the case. This is done for the convenience of a reader who may be scanning for a particular concept. In the sample case, the court addressed some headnotes in a single section, while addressing others singularly.

7. The ruling of the court follows the analysis of the case. The court may affirm, abandon, or partially concur with the lower court findings.

8. Sometimes a dissent section follows the court's findings and is included with the case. This section allows justices who do not concur (either totally or in part) to express their individual views. While absent in the sample case, such a dissent section allows for equally important opinions on the same issues, and dissents may give insight into future arguments and serve as the basis for future landmark decisions.

EXERCISE 2-2

Which district court and federal court of appeals have jurisdiction over your city and state? What types of nursing malpractice cases have these courts heard in the past? How did the courts rule on the issues? How did their decisions affect the professional practice of nursing in your state?

NURSING CONSIDERATIONS

To fully appreciate and incorporate legal principles into individual nurses' practices, nurses must know how to analyze court determinations and be able to base future nursing actions on that analysis. Several benefits may be derived from a critical analysis of a crucial lawsuit.

1. The profession of nursing is forced to examine its practice through impartial and presumably unbiased eyes.
2. The profession is given tested legal principles on which to base future nursing actions and interventions.
3. Nurses and their employers are given an acceptable standard of care that must be matched or exceeded to avoid future litigation.
4. Nursing faculty and hospital instructors are provided a core of legal content for integration through their various programs.
5. The health care consumers' rights to quality and competent health care delivery is defined for the practitioner.

A caveat to nurses: Do not rely on your analysis of a case completely. The intent of this chapter is to aid nurses in interpreting case law. However, it is important that individuals seek further assistance in understanding all the pertinent ramifications of a case. Before acting on one's own interpretation of a case, consult a legal expert or a practicing attorney for an interpretation. This is especially true if the facts of the case are complicated or if the decision is lengthy and complicated by numerous legal doctrines and procedural issues.

It is also important to recognize that judicial rules and holdings vary greatly from one jurisdiction to another. What constitutes the law in one state may be different from what constitutes the law in a different state.

Here are some practical suggestions on how to consult with an attorney and use case-law analysis to improve quality nursing practice:

1. Ask the hospital attorney to meet with a concerned group of hospital nurses to discuss the legal implications of a specific case.
2. Request that a professional organization (either general, such as the State Nurses' Association, or specific, such as the American Association of Critical-care Nurses) present an in-depth program on a case of interest to the membership.
3. Form an interest group and ask for legal assistance from attorneys within the geographic area. This latter suggestion is a good opportunity to involve the nurse attorneys within the area.

EXERCISE 2-3

Invite a hospital staff attorney, or an attorney familiar with the health care industry, to a staff meeting.

Prepare two lists of questions to ask the attorney:

1. Those concerning practice in an acute care setting.
2. Those concerning a home health or community setting.

GUIDELINES: HOW TO READ REPORTED CASES

1. Recognize that you cannot answer all the questions surrounding a case for yourself; consult a licensed attorney, as needed, for clarification.

2. Read the case carefully, especially the facts of the case. Make sure that you are clear on the sequence of events and pertinent fact situations.

3. Identify the issue(s) as addressed by the case. Read the court's decision and analyze how the court answers the issue(s) and how the court gives its reasoning. This is one instance in which a yes or no answer is not sufficient; the reasoning behind the answer is crucial for understanding the law.

4. Research doctrines that are used by the court, especially if you are unfamiliar with the quoted doctrines.

5. Read any dissent very carefully. Dissents often help to clarify the majority opinion by recanting significant facts and applicable doctrines.

6. Incorporate lessons learned from the case into your nursing practice.

SUMMARY

Understanding the court system allows nurses to appreciate which decisions affect nursing practice. Federal cases impact nursing in a variety of states, while local trial court decisions may impact nurses in only a small portion of a state. Likewise, being able to appreciate case law also allows nurses a greater appreciation of legal issues that impact the professional practice of nursing.

AFTER COMPLETING THIS CHAPTER, YOU SHOULD BE ABLE TO

- Differentiate between questions of law and questions of fact in trial settings, and give examples of both.
- List two types of jurisdictions, and give definitions and examples of both.
- Explain the functions of the trial courts, appellate courts, and supreme courts at both the state and federal levels.
- Describe statutes of limitation, their significance, and their purpose in law.
- Describe the process and significance of analyzing a court case.

APPLY YOUR LEGAL KNOWLEDGE

- Does the court in which a case is filed affect the ability of the injured party to have a more or less favorable verdict?
- How do statutes of limitation favor defendants in a lawsuit?
- How does being able to analyze a court case enhance the professional practice of nursing?

REFERENCES

Baca v. Velez, 833 P.2d 1194, 114 N.M. 13 (Ct. App. N.M., 1992).

Black, H. C. (1990). *Law dictionary* (6th ed.). St. Paul, MN: West Publishing Company.

Fiesta, J. (1994). Legal aspects standards of care: Part II. *Nursing Management.* 24(8), 16–17.

Kubrick v. United States, 581 F.2d 1092 (1978).

Noll v. City of Bozeman, 534 P.2d 880, 166 Mont. 504 (Montana, 1975).

Sermchief v. Gonzales, 600 S.W.2d 683 (Mo en banc 1983).

United States Constitution, Article III, Section 2 (1787).

· three

Anatomy of a Lawsuit

PREVIEW

The ultimate goal of any court system is to resolve, in an orderly and fair process, a controversy that exists between two or more parties. To reach this orderly and fair conclusion, the trial process has evolved. This chapter presents all aspects of the trial process, from initiation of the complaint to appeals, and highlights nursing's role in the process.

complaint	interrogatories	opening statements
default judgment	deposition	cross-examination
prelitigation panel	pretrial conference (or hearing)	verdict (or decision)
pleadings		injunction
motion to dismiss	settlement	lay witness
counterclaim	trial	expert witness
right of discovery	voir dire	legal consultant

THE TRIAL PROCESS

Essentially there are six procedural steps to any lawsuit. (See Table 3–1.) Each step, with its special application to nursing, is discussed in the following sections.

Step One: Initiation of the Lawsuit

A party, the plaintiff, who believes he or she may have a valid cause of action against another person initiates a lawsuit. The answering party or parties, the defendant(s) in the lawsuit, may then respond. (In reality, the attorneys carry out the intentions of their clients, but the parties to the suit are always referenced since they are the ones controlling and instigating the proper motions, claims, forms, and the like.)

In most instances it is rare to have a single plaintiff versus a single defendant. More commonly, there are multiple parties on either or both sides to the lawsuit. In medical malpractice suits, a single plaintiff sues multiple defendants, including physicians, the hospital's board of directors, and various members of the nursing staff. Naming as defendants all possible persons or entities involved in the cause of action may be a wise strategy for the plaintiffs, since they could be barred by the statute of limitations from later adding defendants to the lawsuit. Should plaintiffs subsequently discover that a named defendant has been incorrectly named as a party to the suit, that defendant may be *nonsuited* and removed from the case.

Once the plaintiff's cause of action is identified, a *complaint* is filed in a court with competent jurisdiction to hear the case. Upon filing the complaint, the court serves the defendant(s) with a summons to appear before the court

TABLE 3–1. PROCEDURAL STEPS IN THE TRIAL PROCESS

Initiation of the Lawsuit
1. Complaint or summons is initiated by the plaintiff.
2. Service of the complaint is made to the defendant.
3. Health care provider contacts insurance carrier for attorney or provider attains independent attorney.
4. Answer or response is filed by the defendant.
5. If no response comes within the legal time frame, a default judgment is entered by the court against the defendant.
6. Prelitigation panel is held if the state has such a medical review panel.

Pleadings and Pretrial Motions
1. Plaintiff makes initial complaint.
2. Defendant makes original pleadings or answer.
3. Motion to dismiss is initiated by either plaintiff or defendant.
4. Counterclaims are filed with the court.
5. Amended and/or supplemental pleadings are entered.
6. Motion for judgment is based on the pleadings.

Discovery of Evidence
1. Interrogatories are served to plaintiff and defendant.
2. Depositions of witness and named parties are taken.
3. Request to produce documents is made.
4. Requests for an independent medical examination of the plaintiff are made.
5. Subpoena of witnesses are issued as needed.
6. Pretrial conference or hearing is held.
7. Settlements initiated and may be accepted.

Trial Process
1. Jury is selected (voir dire).
2. Opening statements are made, first by plaintiff, then by defendant.
3. Plaintiff's case is presented with cross-examination by defendant.
4. Defendant's case is presented with cross-examination by plaintiff.
5. Motion is made by defendant for directed verdict against plaintiff.
6. Closing statements are made, first by defendant, then by plaintiff.
7. Jury instructions are given.
8. Jury deliberates.
9. Verdict is brought in.

Appeals
1. Appellate level or state intermediate level court
2. State supreme court or highest state court
3. Federal court

Execution of Judgment
1. Payment of damages
2. Specific performance or injunction
3. Imprisonment or fining of defaulting party

at a specified time. This process, known as *service* in both state and federal court systems, alerts the named defendants that a lawsuit is now pending against them. The complaint outlines the names of the parties to the suit, the allegations of the breaches of standards of care, injuries or damages, and the demand for an award. In some states, the demand for damages is a specified amount, while other states determine the amount of the award based on the evidence as presented at court.

Once served, the defendants must respond to the complaint within a specified period of time or forfeit their right to defend the suit. The time frame for answering, determined by state or federal law, may vary according to the jurisdiction. When served, each defendant should promptly notify his or her liability insurance carrier for representation by one of the retained attorneys or procure a personal attorney. Never ignore the complaint because complaints do not just go away when ignored. If the complaint is not answered within the time period allotted by law, a default judgment is entered in the court against the defendant. A *default judgment* means that the defendants automatically lose the lawsuit, whether they had any liability or not. Each defendant should act promptly, since the law sets specific time periods for each phase of the pretrial procedures and motions.

Nurse-defendants should remember the following two points: First after notifying their insurance carrier and arranging to be represented by an attorney in the impending suit, they should also notify the hospital administrative staff of the lawsuit (assuming that they are still employed at the institution named in the lawsuit and their own attorney recommends such notification). This notification allows the hospital attorney to better represent the hospital's interests and the nurses'. Second, nurse-defendants should not discuss the impending suit with anyone except their attorneys and the hospital attorney. The less said, the less likely are nurse-defendants to be misquoted, and the less likely are their comments to be introduced into evidence against them.

In some states, screening panels or medical malpractice tribunals hear the allegations before proceeding to actual court litigation. These *prelitigation panels* ensure that there is an actual controversy or fact question before the case is presented at court. At the prelitigation hearings, evidence concerning the injury, its cause, and its extent are reviewed by a panel of medical and legal experts. The evidence presented may include medical records, expert reports, photographs, x-rays, authoritarian texts, medical journal articles, and medical or legal memoranda.

Not all states have prelitigation panels since arguments abound as to whether they should exist. Defendants' attorneys argue that such panels reduce frivolous lawsuits and expedite the trial process, while plaintiffs' attorneys contend that they merely prolong the legal process and increase the overall expense of the trial. Most malpractice cases take three to six years from the time of injury to a decision, and in states with prelitigation panels the time is increased by six to twelve months.

EXERCISE 3-1

Imagine that you are a staff nurse at ABC General Hospital and have just been named codefendant in a civil suit. Give four reasons for seeking legal representation from a staff attorney at your institution. Why might you consider acquiring independent legal representation?

Step Two: Pleadings and Pretrial Motions

Pleadings, which are written documents setting forth the contentions of the parties, are statements of fact as perceived by the opposing sides to the lawsuit. Pleadings give the basis of the legal claim to opposing parties and prevent unfair surprise to either side. In actuality, the *initial complaint* or *petition* is also a pleading to the court setting out the plaintiff's facts and declaring that an injustice or wrong had been done. Each defendant responds with a pleading giving his or her version of the facts to the court. In the defendants' *original pleadings,* the defendants set forth objections to the plaintiff's complaint. These objections cite *possible errors* in the plaintiff's case. Possible errors may be *procedural;* for example, perhaps the process of service is incorrectly performed or the lawsuit is filed in a court that lacks personal jurisdiction over the defendant. Possible errors may also be *factual;* maybe the defendant named in the suit was in reality on vacation or scheduled to be off at the time of the occurrence and thus has no liability in the matter before the court.

The defendant may also file a ***motion to dismiss,*** stating that there is no valid cause of action on which a claim may be made. The judge may either dismiss the suit upon such a filing or decline to dismiss. If the case is dismissed, the plaintiff may appeal the dismissal. If the motion to dismiss is declined, the defendant must answer the complaint.

A third alternative for the defendant is to file a counterclaim. A ***counterclaim*** states a cause of action that the defendant has against the plaintiff, such as failure to pay a hospital bill on time or negligence on the part of the injured party. For example, if the plaintiff is suing for the improper casting of a broken arm but failed to keep scheduled appointments to check the alignment of the fracture, the plaintiff could have contributed to the purported negligence.

Either side may then file amended or supplemental pleadings as needed. *Amended pleadings* correct or add new material to the original pleadings before the court. For example, an amended pleading would be filed to correct a deficiency in the original pleading. Instead of stating that one injection had been negligently given to the plaintiff by the nurse-defendant, the amended pleading might state that two injections, at two separate times, were administered by the nurse-defendant and that both injections resulted in injury to the plaintiff. *Supplemental pleadings* add to the statement of facts already before the court; they allow the original pleading to stand while supplying additional facts. For example, a supplemental pleading might be filed to bring a third party into the lawsuit.

Pleadings may raise questions of fact or law. If there are no questions of fact, the case may be decided by the judge merely on the pleadings. Usually there are a variety of questions of fact and law, necessitating a full trial with or without a jury.

Once the pleadings have been completed, either or both parties may move for a judgment based on the pleadings. Some state courts allow the party seeking a judgment based on the pleadings to introduce sworn statements as evidence showing that the claim or defense is false. Normally a substantial controversy is involved, and the motion for a judgment based on the pleadings is denied.

Motions, formal requests by one of the parties asking the court to grant its request, may also be filed. Motions may include the need for a speedy trial date owing to the elderly status of the plaintiff or a major witness, the need for a later trial date owing to the length of time needed to obtain necessary documents, or the need for additional documents. Motions are supported with a written narrative, known as a *brief*, which contains legal arguments for the granting of the motion. Motions are then argued before the judge, who issues a ruling regarding the motion.

Step Three: Pretrial Discovery of Evidence

Many state courts and the federal courts allow parties the *right of discovery*, which permits:

1. Witnesses to be questioned by the opposing side prior to the trial itself.
2. The uncovering of relevant written materials.
3. Possible additional examinations of the plaintiff.

Because of the right of discovery, this step of the trial process may take up to two or three years to complete.

There are several methods of allowable pretrial questioning of witnesses. *Interrogatories* are written questionnaires mailed to opposing parties that ask specific questions concerning the facts of the case. Most states limit the number of questions on the questionnaire that a party may be required to complete. Interrogatories must be answered within a time period set by state law and under oath.

Parties should not attempt to answer interrogatories on their own. Most attorneys instruct their clients to answer the questions as completely as possible on a separate sheet of paper. The attorneys then complete the interrogatories for their clients, objecting to objectionable questions and wording answers so as not to suggest or admit liability. Clients should read the answers as completed carefully before signing them and, given that they are under oath, make sure that the answers are true as stated.

A second means of obtaining witness testimony is through *deposition,* which is a witness's sworn statement, made outside the court, that is admissible as evidence in a court of law. Depositions are taken of a witness, who is questioned by the attorney representing the opposing side of the controversy. The deposition's purpose is to assist opposing counsel in preparing for the court case by revealing potential testimony from witnesses before the actual trial.

One must not be fooled by the fact that a deposition is taken at an attorney's office and that few persons are present. A deposition is a crucial part of the discovery phase, and one must be alert to the questions being asked and their answers. The deposing witness is under oath during the entire deposition. The attorney representing the person deposed normally does not ask any questions during the deposition or take an active part in the deposition. The attorney for the deposing party already knows the extent of the testimony and does not need to reveal strategy to the opposing side.

Also present at the deposition is a court reporter who records all questions and answers verbatim. The deposing party is allowed to see and read the final written document before signing it, and the deposition becomes sworn testimony.

Deposing witnesses should give their attorneys sufficient time to object to the various questions, and time should be taken when answering each question. The witness may bring medical records, notes, and literature sources to the deposition, and may refer to them as needed during the deposition. Information should not be guessed at, but the witness should ensure its accuracy before responding. This same information will be given in court.

An error that physicians and nurses frequently make during depositions is in giving too much information. Often health care providers give too much information because they know the right questions to ask and the essential information to elicit, while opposing counsel may not and may ignore an entire area of pertinent information. Do not assist opposing counsels by giving them the answers needed to pursue the case. That is the domain of attorneys, who have the ultimate responsibility to their clients.

A newer concept in taking depositions is to videotape the witness during the entire deposition rather than to record the deposition through a court reporter. If the witness giving the deposition has a pleasing personality and comes across well on tape, playing this type of deposition in court mimics the personal effect of a live appearance. It is the option of deposing parties (and their counsels) to choose this type of deposition.

Taped depositions are frequently reserved for witnesses who will not be present for the actual trial. For example, witnesses who are outside the jurisdiction of the court or those who may be unavailable during the time of the trial hearing may chose to have their depositions videotaped.

Depositions serve to uncover facts for the opposing side and to perpetuate the testimony of witnesses. Near-death witnesses may actually have their testimony preserved for trial through pretrial depositions.

Either side in the controversy may also obtain and examine copies of the medical records, business records, x-ray films, and the like through a *request to produce documents.* The court may also require a physical or mental examination of a party through a *request for an independent medical examination of the plaintiff,* if the medical information so obtained is pertinent to the case. Either party may object to these requests based on grounds that they are unduly burdensome, seek confidential or privileged information, or are protected as part of the attorney's work product. Generally, the scope of discovery is large and parties are allowed to discover all relevant materials that would be admissible in the subsequent trial.

During the discovery phase, both sides are deciding on their strategy for the ensuing trial and are interviewing the witnesses they need to testify in court. Both sides are also obtaining evidence to submit at trial in the form of x-ray films, medical records, consultation reports, and other tangible items that affect the case.

The final phase of the pretrial procurement of evidence is a **pretrial conference,** or **pretrial hearing.** This is a fairly informal session during which the judge and the representing attorneys agree on the issues to be decided and settle procedural matters. The pretrial conference may result in the finalization of a *settlement,* which is favored by the judicial system because it allows for a quick resolution. A settlement is not synonymous with the admission of guilt or of liability, but is a means of allowing the parties to forgo the trial process and to settle for an agreed-on dollar figure. Included among the many reasons for settling a case prior to trial are the expense of the trial process, the lengthy delays in reaching a trial date, the emotional and physical drain on an already injured plaintiff, the uncertainty of the jury trial process, and the nature of the harm complained of and its potential ability to shock a jury.

Step Four: The Trial

At the *trial,* the evidence is presented, facts are determined by the jury, principles of law are applied to determined facts, and a solution is formally reached. Evidence is usually presented through various witnesses' answers to specific questions. The jury relies on the testimony and credibility of the witness in determining the facts of the case.

If a jury trial has been requested, the trial begins with the selection of the jury, or *voir dire.* A panel of qualified persons is questioned by the attorneys representing both sides, and a four-, six-, or twelve-person jury is selected and sworn in by the judge. In some jurisdictions, a panel of six may be stipulated by the parties to the lawsuit. If no jury is requested or mandated by law, the judge serves as both judge and jury.

After jury selection, both sides make their opening statements. The *opening statements* generally indicate for the jury what both sides intend to show by the evidence to be presented. Since the plaintiff has the legal burden of proof to show not only that an incident occurred but that the incident in fact caused the plaintiff's injury, the plaintiff's attorney has the first opening statement.

Witnesses are then called, one by one, to answer specific questions. The witnesses are directly questioned first by the attorney calling the witness. The opposing side then has the opportunity for *cross-examination,* during which the questioning attorney attempts to discredit or negate the witness's testimony. The attorney originally calling the witness may then ask additional questions in an attempt to reestablish the credibility of the witness.

The plaintiff calls all his or her witnesses in presenting the entire case. The plaintiff's side then *rests the case,* meaning that they have attempted to meet the burden of proof and have legally established their cause of action. At that point the defendants' attorneys may *petition for a directed verdict,* indicating from their perspective that the plaintiff has failed to present sufficient facts on which to decide the case in the plaintiff's favor. This motion for a directed verdict is typically overruled, and the defendants then call their witnesses one by one to present their case to the jury.

At the conclusion of the defendant's entire case, both sides or either side may again move for a directed verdict. If these attempts are overruled (and they traditionally are), the attorneys make their final arguments, and the judge instructs the jury as to their charge and the principles of law involved. This last step varies greatly from jurisdiction to jurisdiction. The jury then retires to deliberate and to reach a *verdict* (or *decision*).

Once the verdict is known, the losing side may move for a new trial. If the motion is granted, the entire trial is repeated before a new jury panel. If it is denied, the judgment becomes final, and the losing side may appeal to the proper appellate court if there are legal grounds for such an appeal.

EXERCISE 3-2

Plaintiff P has sued Nurse N for malpractice, stating that she was given an oral medication by Nurse N and that she then suffered a severe allergic reaction to the medication. What additional information is necessary for the court to enter a directed verdict for Plaintiff P? Clues: Think about the patient's role in receiving the medication and the nurse's responsibilities in administering medications.

Step Five: Appeals

The appropriate appellate court reviews the case based on (1) the trial record, (2) written summaries of the principles of law applied, and, in many states, (3) short oral arguments by the representing attorneys. The case, depending on the outcome at the intermediate appellate level, may eventually be appealed to the state supreme court. Once decided at this highest level, the judgment typically becomes final, and the matter is closed. A few cases may be appealed to the U.S. Supreme Court, but this is a rarity in medical malpractice cases today.

Step Six: Execution of Judgment

Most lawsuits involving nurse-defendants result in one of two possible conclusions: the awarding of money damages against them or the dismissal of all causes of action against them. Nothing can return plaintiffs to their original, pretrial status, and the American judicial system attempts to compensate the plaintiff (if the evidence supports compensation) with money damages. Other forms of conclusion include an *injunction* requiring the nurse-defendant either to perform or to refrain from performing a certain action.

After all appeals, the plaintiff asks that the judgment as provided for by the court be executed. This procedure gives legal relief to the plaintiff if a losing defendant chooses to ignore a court order. If an injunction has been mandated by the court, the defendant may be fined or imprisoned. For a default judgment or money damages award, the defendant's wages may be garnished (ie, a certain amount of money is taken from the defendant's earnings and given to the winning plaintiff on a weekly or monthly basis), or property may be confiscated and sold to pay the amount of the award. Since not all states apply garnishment laws in the same manner and some states restrict the type of property that may be confiscated, there will be some differences from state to state in the *execution of judgment.*

EXPERT AND LAY WITNESSES

Lay Witness

Most nurses are aware of the expert witness status. Equally important in the judicial system is the *lay witness,* who establishes facts at the trial level, stating for the judge and jury exactly what transpired. The lay witness is allowed to testify only to facts and may not draw conclusions or form opinions; they define for the jury what happened. Both sides to the controversy have lay witnesses who attempt to describe for the jury what, when, and how a particular event occurred. The lay witness thus has a direct connection with the case in controversy. Lay witnesses at the trial may be the patient, the patient's family members, nurses not named in the lawsuit, or other staff members.

Expert Witness

The second type of witness, the *expert witness,* explains highly specialized technology or skilled nursing care to the jurors, who usually have little or no exposure to medicine and nursing. Expert testimony is admissible when conclusions by a jury depend on factual and scientific information that is more than common knowledge.

The use of nurses as expert witnesses has evolved since the late 1970s and early 1980s. Before then, physicians served as nursing's voice and testified at court regarding the role and accountability of professional nurses. Two court cases in 1980, one in North Carolina and one in Georgia, set the stage for acceptance by the court of nurses serving as expert witnesses in defining the role of nursing (*Maloney v. Wake Hospital Systems* and *Avet v. McCormick*). In *Maloney*, the court held that "the role of the nurse is critical to providing a high standard of health care in modern medicine. Her expertise is different from, but no less exalted, than that of the physician" (1980, at 683). Other courts have concluded that physicians may not establish the nursing standards of care. In *Young v. Board of Hospital Directors, Lee County* (1984), the court held that a psychiatrist was not familiar with the daily practices of psychiatric nursing and therefore could not testify to a deviation from nursing standards.

The minimum credential for a nurse expert witness is current licensure to practice professional nursing within a state. Other criteria for selection include the total lack of involvement with the defendants, either as an employee or consultant, clinical expertise in the area of nursing at issue, certification in the clinical area if possible, and recent continuing or formal education relevant to the specialty of nursing at issue. If possible, the expert witness should also have earned graduate degrees and authored publications in nursing. Some attorneys will substitute status as a nurse manager, nurse educator, or preceptor for advanced degrees.

The purpose of these criteria for the nurse expert witness is to display for the jury that the nurse is well qualified to be an expert witness. Therefore, credentials that speak to the highest level of nursing expertise and knowledge of the appropriate standard of care weigh favorably with judges and jurors. Such criteria also further ensure the objectivity of the nurse expert. Expert witnesses who have either worked for the defendant institution or who are associated with nurse-defendants on a personal level may be seen as giving subjective testimony. Such subjective testimony is most likely to be seen as a verdict for the plaintiff and against the defendants.

When nurses are first contacted about the possibility of serving as expert witnesses, they should consider certain guidelines. First, is the case of interest to them and is it in the area of their expertise? Second, all materials sent should be reviewed carefully and a determination made whether a standard of care has been upheld or breached. Do not put thoughts and opinions in writing at this stage since such writings may be viewed by both sides to the controversy. Formal writings can be done once the position of expert witness has been confirmed. Third, decide on the fee schedule before proceeding. Acceptable fee schedules can be determined by the geographic area and whether the nurse will appear at trial. Finally, know the time frames for discovery and the actual court trial, so that the expert witness can be available for an extended period of time, if that is foreseen.

An expert may also serve as a *legal consultant,* whose name is not provided to the opposing side and whose reports or comments are not disclosed. When nurses are named as expert witnesses, their reports and comments are discoverable by opposing counsel on request (Quigley, 1991).

When the need for an expert witness arises, both sides in the controversy retain their own. Testimony is generally in the form of opinions and answers to hypothetical questions. This practice has evolved because expert witnesses have the ability to analyze facts presented and to draw inferences from those facts, something the lay witness is not allowed to do.

Once selected as an expert witness, the nurse is prepared for this role by the attorney. Legal doctrine or state procedural rules that pertain to the individual case are discussed. The following should also be reviewed:

1. The facility or area where the incident occurred, to identify special environmental factors and the location of the patient in relation to needed equipment, medications, and staff.
2. The state nurse practice act and any relevant rules that the board of nursing may have promulgated.
3. Relevant nursing literature to ensure the status of acceptable practice at the time of the occurrence.
4. The applicable nursing process of the institution during the time of the occurrence.
5. All written records that pertain to the incident or that may have implications for assessment, planned actions, implementation, and evaluation of the incident.
6. Supportive management records and/or patient classification acuity records.
7. Support functions provided by the institution for nursing.

Each of these has implications for the applicable standard of care during the incident.

Unfortunately, the number of lawsuits naming nurses as defendants is currently on the rise. The role of expert nurses is therefore more vital. Some experts estimate that the role of expert nurse witnesses will increase in importance as nurses are expected to testify not only in malpractice cases, but in custody and criminal cases, especially where nurses have been managing the care of either defendants or plaintiffs (Josberger and Ries, 1995).

Nurses are the only professionals with the competency, credentials, and right to define nursing or to judge whether the appropriate standard of care has been delivered. As nurses come forward to assume this role, the system will adjust not only to incorporate them, but to actively solicit their professional testimonies.

EXERCISE 3-3

List three possible instances in which no expert witness testimony is needed to assist the jury in their deliberations. Here is an example: Patient P is an elderly man, admitted 30 minutes previously from the postanesthesia care unit. Earlier in the day, he had surgery to remove his gallbladder. Patient P fell out of bed, breaking his knee and wrist. Nurse N admits leaving both siderails down and the bed in its highest position.

GUIDELINES FOR TESTIFYING AS AN EXPERT WITNESS

1. Time must be taken when considering an answer to each question. Once spoken, an answer cannot be retracted. Understand the question or ask that it be repeated or rephrased. Also, give your attorney time to object to the question. Objections after an answer is given serve little value in jurors' minds.

2. A favorite ploy of opposing counsel is to either fluster, confuse, or anger an expert witness. Such ploys may prevent a clear and concise answer, and may cause you to blurt out the first thought that enters your mind. All answers must be carefully considered, giving only the information that answers the questions. The battle being played out in court is about the facts of the case, not about people and personalities. Remain as objective as possible, take a deep breath if needed, and answer objectively, not defensively.

3. Remember that any intervention can be accomplished in several ways. The fact that an alternative approach has been selected does not equate with substandard care. Do not allow yourself to be backed into a corner where only one means of implementing an intervention is correct. Keep your options open and reiterate that any of these approaches could have been selected.

4. Ensure that interventions as presented were appropriate at the time of the occurrence, not at the time of the court case. The expert witness should not be manipulated into discussing current practice standards, because they most likely do not reflect the standard at the time the incident occurred.

5. Testimony previously given during a deposition is sworn testimony and cannot be changed at trial. If you are unsure of your previous testimony, such as quoting the patient's blood pressure or wedge pressure, verify the information before speaking. You may refer to your deposition or to the patient record before responding. If the answers are different, the next question by opposing counsel will inevitably be "Tell me, nurse, are you lying now or were you lying before?" Either answer destroys all credibility with the jury.

6. The expert witness should answer only what pertains to nursing, a nursing role, or standards of nursing care. If you cannot answer the attorney's questions without testifying to medical standards, then say that it is outside of the scope of nursing and that you cannot answer. The attorney can also be asked to rephrase the question so that it pertains to nursing standards of care.

7. Remember to dress appropriately, in a suit or other conservative dress, since appearance makes a valuable first impression with the jury. Look at the jury as you give your answers, thus showing your sincerity and knowledge.

8. Give only enough information to answer the question. If a simple yes or no will suffice, stop after stating yes or no. Frequently, nursing experts damage their credibility by trying too hard to ensure that the jury is aware of their knowledge base. The jury will already know that you are knowledgeable by the introduction of your credentials.

9. If opposing counsel asks if you are being paid to appear and to testify, the answer is yes. Stress, though, that the payment is not for testimony, but for any provisions or inconveniences you had to make to be in court, such as travel to a distant court, lost work hours, child care, and review of pertinent facts and standards. The difference is subtle, but extremely important.

10. Expect opposing counsels to question your credentials. Remember that they are trying in every way possible to lessen the weight of your testimony in the eyes of the jurors. Rather than credentials, your ethics may be attacked, such as with a question asking if you had solicited the attorney of record for the opportunity to testify.

SUMMARY

To resolve disputes between two or more parties in an orderly and fair manner, the court system and the trial process have evolved. There are essentially six steps to the trial process, all of which are important in the final outcome of the case. Nurses may be most involved as expert witnesses, presenting complicated facts and explaining standards of nursing care to the judge and jury.

AFTER COMPLETING THIS CHAPTER, YOU SHOULD BE ABLE TO

- List and explain the purpose of the six procedural steps in the trial process.
- Distinguish between traditional depositions, recorded by a court reporter, and the more modern videotaped depositions, stating the pros and cons of both methods.
- Distinguish between lay and expert witnesses, as well as their roles in the trial process.

APPLY YOUR LEGAL KNOWLEDGE

- Does the trial process ensure that both plaintiffs and defendants have equal opportunity to present their cases?
- When is it advisable to settle a case rather than persist with a long and lengthy trial?
- How does understanding the trial process aid the professional nurse?

REFERENCES

Aiken, T. D. with Catalano, J. T. (1994). *Legal, ethical, and political issues in nursing.* Philadelphia: F. A. Davis, Company.

Avet v. McCormick, 271 S.E. 2d 833 (Georgia, 1980).

Josberger, M. C. and Ries, D. T. (1995). Nurse experts. *Trial, 21*(6), 68–71.

Maloney v. Wake Hospital Systems, 262 S.E. 2d 680 (North Carolina, 1980).

Quigley, F. M. (1991). Responsibilities of the consultant and expert witness. *Focus on Critical Care, 18,* 238–239.

Young v. Board of Hospital Directors, Lee County, #82-429 (Florida, 1984).

II

LIABILITY
ISSUES

· four·

Standards of Care

PREVIEW

Standards of care are implemented daily in all aspects of health care delivery, forming the basis for quality, competent health care. Standards of care are the criteria for determining if less than adequate care was delivered to health care consumers. This chapter explores the foundations of standards of care, describing how they are derived and defined within courts of law.

standards of care	the Joint Commission for Accreditation of Healthcare Organizations (JCAHO)	error in judgment rule
internal standards		two schools of thought doctrine
external standards	locality rule	

DEFINITION OF STANDARDS OF CARE

Standards of care may be viewed as the level or degree of quality considered adequate by a profession. Standards of care are the skills and learning commonly possessed by members of a profession. Created by the duty undertaken, they describe the minimal requirements that define an acceptable level of care, that is, to exercise ordinary and reasonable care to see that no unnecessary harm comes to the patient.

The basic purposes of standards of care are to protect and safeguard the public as a whole. Were there no standards of care, consumers would be open to varying levels of care and varying degrees of quality of care, and they would eventually suffer. Standards of care have evolved to help health care recipients avoid substandard health care and to give guidance to health care providers.

Standards of care may easily be differentiated from objectives, philosophies, and guidelines. *Objectives* are goals that give direction to what must be accomplished. For example, a goal may be to ambulate the patient 20 steps. *Philosophies* state why an action is performed. Ambulation of the postoperative patient helps to prevent complications due to thrombus formation and orthostatic hypotension. *Guidelines* describe recommended courses of action. Patients should be ambulated more than once per day, preferably when they are most rested and steady on their feet.

Standards are authoritative statements promulgated by a profession by which the quality of practice, service, or education can be evaluated (American Nurses Association, 1991). A standard of care may be written as "The early postoperative patient must be ambulated pursuant to a valid order with two nurses or assistants in attendance, and vital signs will be taken and recorded both before and after ambulation."

ESTABLISHMENT OF NURSING STANDARDS OF CARE

Nursing standards of care may be established in a variety of ways and are often classified into two broad categories: internal and external standards.

Internal Standards

Internal standards are those set by the role and education of the nurse or by individual institutions. These include the professional nurse's job description, education, and expertise as well as the individual institution's policies and procedures.

In court cases, institutional policies and procedures are presented and evaluated to determine if a nurse defendant has met the standards of care for the institution. In *Schneider v. Kings Highway Hospital Center* (1986), a clearly written policy existed: Bed siderails were to be in the raised position for all patients over the age of 70. When Mrs. Schneider was found on the floor next to her bed and the siderails down, the court concluded that a staff member had either lowered the rails or had never placed the rails in the raised position. Either conclusion fell below the stated institution policy and thus fell below an acceptable standard of care. *Santa Rose Medical Center v. Robinson* (1977) extended internal standards to include hospital in-service films as policy and procedure. In that case, the standard of care for closed-head injuries was reduced to an in-service film, and the viewing of the film was mandatory for all staff members. When members of the staff violated the standard of care as outlined in the film, the court allowed the jury to view the film to show what the hospital's standard of care should have been.

Courts have routinely allowed policy and procedure manuals to be introduced as criteria for the acceptable standard of care. Policies and procedures need not be in writing to be considered legally enforceable. Unwritten policies may potentiate liability because not all employees are aware of the policy's existence. In *Hartman v. Riverside Methodist Hospital* (1989), the patient had undergone emergency surgery after eating a full meal. The nurses in the postanesthesia care unit were informed that the patient had received Fentanyl and that she "had a full stomach." Precautions should have been taken to ensure that Mrs. Hartman did not aspirate. Instead, the patient was given a pain medication and died of aspiration. The unwritten policy of the attending anesthesiologist was that no medications were to be given his patients unless he was first consulted and ordered such medication directly. The other attending anesthesiologists had no such unwritten policy, and nurses could give pain medications without prior approval. Since not all of the nurses knew this unwritten policy, this patient was medicated and the court found in favor of her family and against the hospital and employees.

External Standards

External standards are those set by the state boards of nursing, professional organizations, specialty nursing organizations, federal organizations, and federal guidelines. These standards are seen as external because they transcend individual practitioners and single institutions. In many instances, external standards are synonymous with national standards.

State boards of nursing publish acceptable standards in the state nurse practice act or in rules and regulations promulgated to enforce the state nurse practice act. These rules and regulations have the force of law because they are created to carry out the law. Courts consider whether standards of care were met or violated based on the evidence presented.

Professional organizations add to the body of acceptable standards of care for professional nursing. The profession has the inherent right to direct and control its activities. The most active professional organization in this area is the American Nurses Association (ANA) with its state components. The ANA Congress for Nursing Practice set eight basic standards of care in 1973. Based on the nursing process, these eight standards are applicable to all nurses, regardless of clinical specialty. These standards of care for nursing practice represent the first step in unifying standards of care throughout all jurisdictions.

The ANA and the state nurses associations have lobbied to encourage the enactment of generic standards of care through state legislative processes. One of the basic arguments for such generalized standards of care is to upgrade the standards set by individual hospitals and institutions that were traditionally based on a local standard of acceptability. In 1974, the ANA's specialty standards of care were first published. These specialty standards of care were published for various clinical specialties, including (1) community health nursing, (2) geriatric nursing, (3) maternal-child health nursing, (4) mental health nursing, and (5) medical-surgical nursing. Today ANA publishes some 20 standards that pertain to specialty practice areas (American Nurses Association, 1995).

The ANA also publishes a *Code of Ethics* (1976) for nurses. This *Code of Ethics* addresses both standards and ethics, particularly in the areas of professionalism and quality nursing performance.

In 1991, the ANA Congress of Nursing Practice adopted the Standards of Clinical Nursing Practice. This document is divided into standards of care and standards of professional performance. The standards of performance section outlines professional activities such as formal and continuing education, research, ethics, peer review, and continuous quality improvement. The language of this document has been broadened so that standards of care and standards of performance are described in terms of competency as opposed to reasonable or acceptable level of performance (American Nurses Association, 1991). This broadened language has been incorporated so that criteria used to measure compliance may change as needed with technological advances and alternative delivery sites.

Standards of care are also set by the National League for Nursing (NLN). The NLN looks to the quality of nursing education and accredits schools of nursing on both the undergraduate and graduate levels. Directly and indirectly, these standards of education influence the quality of acceptable nursing standards within a community.

Individual nursing specialty practice organizations also publish standards of care to upgrade and generalize the standards for patients within a clinical setting or within a category. For example:

1. The American Association of Critical-care Nurses (AACN) publishes standards of care for the critically ill patient.
2. The Emergency Nurses Association (ENA) publishes standards of care for trauma and urgent care patients.
3. The Oncology Nursing Society (ONS) issues standards for cancer patients.
4. The Association of Operating Room Nurses (AORN) publishes standards of care for patients in the perioperative setting.
5. On an international perspective, the International Council of Nursing (ICN) has published its standards through an ethical code (1973).

Federal organizations and federal guidelines are other examples of external standards. The *Joint Commission for Accreditation of Healthcare Organizations (JCAHO)* sets nursing standards by publishing the *Accreditation Manual for Hospitals* on a yearly basis (1995). Their requirements for individualized nursing care plans set a standard of care. For example, one of their standards states that patients must be assessed and individualized care plans written. Such a requirement may actually assist nurses if a lawsuit is filed. The individualized care plan may indeed show that the nursing staff met the standard of care for safety by innovative measures aimed at preventing an individual patient's fall. Other federal agencies, such as the Social Security Administration (overseeing Medicare and Medicaid funding, nursing home qualifications, and maternal and child health programs), also are directly responsible for setting nursing standards of care.

EXERCISE 4-1

Review your current institution's policy and procedure manual. Randomly select a policy and procedure. Show how the language used makes this a standard as opposed to an objective, philosophy, or guideline. Rewrite the policy three times so that it is (1) an objective, (2) a philosophy, and (3) a guideline. Why do standards give the most guidance to nurses for effective patient care?

EXERCISE 4-2

Obtain copies of standards of care from at least two specialty organizations, such as AACN, AORN, ENA, or ONS. Compare and contrast the written standards against your institution's policies and procedures. How do your internal standards compare with the national standards? If your internal standards need upgrading, how would you begin to rewrite them?

NATIONAL AND LOCAL STANDARDS OF CARE

Appropriate standards of care may be based on a national versus local standard. *National standards* are based on reasonableness and are the average degree of skill, care, and diligence exercised by members of the same profession. A national standard means that nurses in rural settings must meet the same standards as members of the profession practicing in large urban areas.

In areas of specialty practice, courts are almost universally holding health care providers to a national standard of care (*Brune v. Belinkoff*, 1968). In that case it was ruled that a person holding himself out as a specialist should be held to the same standard of skill and care of the average member of that specialty, not merely the skill and ability of specialists practicing in a particular city.

There are two important reasons for national standards of care, and both are fairly obvious. With the advent of educational programs, educational videos, and the ability to transport specialists across the nation, all areas with health care delivery systems have access to the same information and educational opportunities. This is increasingly true today as advancing technology allows patient data and test results to be reviewed by consultants worldwide. A second reason is that all patients have the right to quality health care, whether hospitalized in a small community or in a large university institution.

Some states still follow a *locality rule,* which allows standards of care to be viewed from the perspective of care within a given geographic area or a "similar community." Under this perspective, health care is judged by the skill, care, and diligence of members of the profession within that geographic area. The trend today, however, is toward a total national standard.

IMPORTANCE OF STANDARDS OF CARE TO INDIVIDUAL NURSES

Standards of care are referenced in medical malpractice cases against nurses to prove that they breached the duty of care owed the patient. *Duty of care* has frequently been defined to mean the applicable standard of care. The test for the court to apply is what a reasonable, prudent nurse, with like experience and education, would do under similar conditions in the same community (*Fraijo v. Hartland Hospital*, 1979).

When deciding which standards of care to apply, courts also consider two other doctrines. The honest *error in judgment rule* allows the court to evaluate the standards of care given a patient even if there was an honest error in judgment, including an error in the diagnosis. What the court evaluates is the care given and whether that care met the prevailing standards, not whether the judgment was correct. *Fraijo v. Hartland* (1979) is the landmark case in this matter. The court stated that a nurse is not bound to do exactly what another nurse would do, only to select one approach among several that exists at the time and is reasonable.

GUIDELINES: STANDARDS OF CARE

1. Recognize that all professions have standards of care. Standards are the minimal level of expertise that must be delivered to the patient and are the starting point for greater expectations.

2. Standards of care may be either externally or internally set. Nurses are responsible for both categories of standards: those set on a national basis and those set by the role of nursing.

3. Standards of care may be found in:
   a. The state nurse practice act.
   b. Published standards of professional organizations and specialty practice groups, such as the American Association of Critical-Care Nurses or the Association of Operating Room Nurses.
   c. Federal agency guidelines and regulations.
   d. Hospital policy and procedure manuals.
   e. The individual nurse's job description.

4. Nurses are accountable for all standards of care as they pertain to their professions. To remain competent and skillful, nurses are encouraged to read professional journals and to attend pertinent continuing education and in-service programs.

5. Standards of care are determined for the judicial system by expert witnesses. Such persons testify to the prevailing standards in the community—a standard that all nurses are accountable for matching and exceeding. The adherence to such standards states that patients are ensured quality, competent nursing care.

The second consideration by courts is the *two schools of thought doctrine,* which supports the nurse who chooses among alternative means of delivering quality health care. In this instance, the court evaluates the standards of care given when the nurse chooses among the alternative modes of treatment. Were standards of care met in the chosen mode of treatment? If the answer is yes, courts support the quality of care as delivered, even though other nurses would choose a different course of action (*Fury v. Thomas Jefferson University,* 1984).

Standards of care provide the criterion for determining if a nurse has violated the state nurse practice act. The court in *Botehlo v. Bycura* (1984) held that when patients choose a practitioner of a recognized branch of the health care professions, they elect to undergo the care and treatment common to that pro-

Guidelines: Standards of Nursing Practice

Registered professional nurses shall:

1. Be responsible for knowing and conforming to the law governing the practice of professional nursing.
2. Be responsible and accountable for their actions commensurate with educational preparation and experience in nursing.
3. Assess and evaluate the health status of patients or clients based on objective and subjective data as it relates to their individual physiological, psychological, and social processes.
4. Make nursing judgments and decisions about the nursing care for patients or clients by using assessment data to formulate and implement a plan of goals and objectives, and to evaluate patients' or clients' responses to the nursing care.
5. Be responsible for accurate reporting and documentation of patients' or clients' symptoms, responses, and progress.
6. Evaluate patients' or clients' status and institute appropriate nursing intervention that might be required to stabilize their condition or prevent complications.
7. Promote and participate in patient or client education and counseling based on the individual's health needs and illness status, and involve the individual and significant others for a better understanding and implementation of immediate and long-term health goals.
8. Provide patients or clients and their significant others with the information they need to make decisions and choices about promoting, maintaining, and restoring health.
9. Collaborate with members of related health disciplines in the interest of patients' or clients' health care.
10. Consult and utilize community agencies as resources for the continuity of patient or client care.
11. Be aware of the rationale for the effects of the administration of medications or treatments as prescribed by a licensed physician or dentist.
12. Be responsible and accountable for the quality and the quantity of nursing care rendered under their supervision. Assignment and delegation of duties to other nursing personnel shall be commensurate with their educational preparation and demonstrated proficiency.
13. Assist personnel under their supervision to develop the necessary skills needed for continued competence in providing patient or client care, comfort, and safety.
14. Be responsible for individual professional growth.

Source: Texas Register. Licensure and Practice. Rule 217.13

fession. Thus nurses must meet the standards of care of the profession. Each state publishes acceptable standards of care as part of the nurse practice act or through the rules and regulations promulgated by the state board of nursing. Violations of those standards open the nurse to possible disciplinary action by the board. See Chapter 11 for a full explanation of nurse practice acts and the board of nursing.

Standards of care may be used by the state criminal system to decide if the nurse has violated the state or city criminal codes. In *State of Louisiana v. Brenner* (1986), standards of care were examined to show that the nursing home staff had failed to properly train staff members, to supply an adequate staff, and to adequately maintain patients' records, among other charges of cruelty, neglect, and mistreatment of the infirm.

Finally, standards of care provide the criterion for placing nursing practice on a professional level. Standards of care both increase the status of the nursing profession and set minimal standards for nursing practice. National standards of care have further increased this acceptance of professional status. National standards dictate that all patients receive the same expert nursing care, whether they are cared for in a major medical center or in a small community hospital. The ANA, through its many publications regarding standards and its *Code for Ethics* (see Appendix A), has delineated standards promoting professionalism and quality nursing care.

EXPERT TESTIMONY

In courts of law, the deviation of the standard of care is proven through the use of expert witnesses. See Chapter 3 for a review of this concept.

EXPANDED NURSING ROLES

With the advent of expanded roles in nursing and the rewriting of several state nurse practice acts to accommodate these expanded roles, the standard of care owed the patient by advanced nurse practitioners is frequently that of a medical (physician) standard of care or a "nurse practitioner" standard of care. Chapter 12 discusses the expanded nursing role and further clarifies this concept.

EXERCISE 4-3

Reread "Guidelines: Standards of Nursing Practice" in this chapter. How do these standards support the standards of care of your institution? Give examples of how they do or do not meet the standards of nursing practice.

SUMMARY

Standards of care, derived from a variety of sources, are crucial in ensuring that patients are provided quality, competent nursing care. Standards of care form the basis of the professional duty owed to patients.

- Define standards of care from both a legal and a nursing perspective.
- Compare and contrast internal versus external standards of care.
- Discuss the concept of the reasonably prudent nurse in defining standards of care.

APPLY YOUR LEGAL KNOWLEDGE

- How do standards differ from objectives, philosophies, and guidelines?
- How can professional nurses ensure that they are practicing according to the appropriate standards of care?
- How would you prepare to be an expert witness for the purpose of defining standards of care?

REFERENCES

American Nurses' Association. (1995). *Catalogue of Publications.* Washington, DC: Author.

American Nurses' Association. (1973). *Standards of Nursing Practice.* Kansas City, MO: Author.

American Nurses' Association. (1991). *Standards of Clinical Nursing Practice.* Washington, DC: Author.

Botehlo v. Bycura, 320 S.E. 2d 59 (Pennsylvania, Supp. 1984)

Brune v. Belinkoff, 354 Mass. 102, 235 N.E. 2d 793 (1968).

Fraijo v. Hartland Hospital, 99 Cal. Rept. 3d 331, 160 Cal. Rept. 848 (1979).

Fury v. Thomas Jefferson University, 472 A. 2d 101 (Louisiana, 1984).

Hartman v. Riverside Methodist Hospital, 577 N.E. 2d 112 (Ohio, 1989).

Hiatt v. Groce, 215 Kan. 14, 523 P.2d 320 (1974).

International Council of Nursing (1973). *Code for Nurses.* Geneva: Author.

Joint Commission for Accreditation of Healthcare Organizations (1995). *Accreditation manual for hospitals.* Oakbrook Terrace, IL: Author.

Santa Rosa Medical Center v. Robinson, 560 S.W.2d 751 (Tex. Civ. App.-San Antonio, 1977).

Schneider v. Kings Highway Hospital Center, 490 N.E.2d 1221 (New York, 1986).

State of Louisiana v. Brenner, 486 S.O.2d 101 (Louisiana, 1986).

Texas Register. *Licensure and practice.* Rule 217.13.

• five

Negligence and Malpractice

PREVIEW

Health care providers and the general public frequently interchange the terms "malpractice" and "negligence." While the distinction is technical, nurses should be able to distinguish between the two terms and to apply both in providing quality nursing care. This chapter discusses the elements of negligence and malpractice, and presents guidelines for preventing potential lawsuits in this area of the law.

tort law	duty of care	injury or harm
negligence	breach of duty	damages
malpractice	forseeability	res ipsa loquitor
tortfeasor	causation	locality rule

NEGLIGENCE AND MALPRACTICE: APPLICATION OF TORT LAW

Both negligence and malpractice fall into the classification of *tort law,* which is a branch of civil law that concerns legal wrongs committed by one person against another person or against the property of another person. (Review Chapter 1 for a more thorough discussion of tort law.)

NEGLIGENCE VERSUS MALPRACTICE

Of primary importance to health care providers is the area of negligence or malpractice. Used interchangeably, these two terms enjoy a fine distinction.

Negligence is a general term that denotes conduct lacking in due care. Thus, negligence, equated with carelessness, is a deviation from the standard of care that a reasonable person would use in a set of circumstances. Negligence may also include doing something that the reasonable and prudent person would not do. As such, anyone, including nonmedical persons, can be liable for negligence. An example is the fall by an elderly person who is being cared for by a sitter. The reasonable person in the place of the sitter has a standard of care to prevent such a fall.

Malpractice is a more specific term and looks at a professional standard of care as well as the professional status of the care giver. To be liable for malpractice, the *tortfeasor* (the person committing the civil wrong) must be a professional—a physician, nurse, accountant, lawyer, or other type of professional. Courts have continually defined malpractice as any professional misconduct or unreasonable lack of skill or fidelity in professional or judiciary duties. Moreover, the wrong or injudicious treatment must result in injury, unnecessary suffering, or death to the patient, and it proceeds from ignorance, carelessness, the want of proper professional skill, the disregard of established rules and principles, neglect, or a malicious or criminal intent. In a more modern definition, malpractice is the failure of a professional person to act in accordance with the prevailing professional standards or the failure to foresee consequences that a professional person, having the necessary skills and education, should foresee.

The same types of acts may form the basis for negligence or malpractice. If the action is performed by a nonprofessional person, the result is negligence. When the same action is performed by a professional person, the act forms the basis for a malpractice lawsuit. In the preceding example, an elderly person fell while being watched by a sitter. The result was negligence on the part of the sitter. Had a professional nurse failed to raise the siderails and the elderly patient had then fallen, the nurse could have been liable for malpractice. Some actions will almost always constitute malpractice because only a professional person would be performing the actions. These include drawing arterial blood gases via a direct arterial stick or initiating blood transfusions.

Is the distinction important? Many authorities have concluded that the general public has a right to expect and receive a higher standard of care from a professional person than from a nonprofessional worker. Courts have likewise concluded that this increased expectation of duty exists, and as a result substantially higher awards have been given to injured parties.

EXERCISE 5-1

List the types of nursing actions that you perform daily in your clinical setting. Could all types of nursing actions be the basis for both negligence and malpractice? Why or why not?

ELEMENTS OF MALPRACTICE OR NEGLIGENCE

To be successful in either a malpractice or negligence cause of action in court, in most jurisdictions the plaintiff must prove the following elements to establish liability on the part of the defendant(s):

1. Duty owed the patient.
2. Breach of the duty owed the patient.
3. Foreseeability.
4. Causation.
5. Injury.
6. Damages.

Remember that malpractice is negligence on the part of a professional person. Therefore the elements are the same. The only difference is the status of the person committing the action or failing to act when legally required to act.

TABLE 5–1. NEGLIGENT TORTS

Elements	Examples of Nursing Actions
Duty owed	Failing to monitor the patient
Breach of duty owed the patient	Failing to report a change in patient status
Foreseeability	Failing to report another health care provider's incompetence
Causation	Failing to provide for the patient's safety
Cause-in-fact	Improper medication administration
Proximate cause	Allowing a patient to be burned
Injury	Failing to question an inappropriate medical order
Damages	Failing to provide patient education
General	and discharge instructions
Emotional	
Punitive/exemplary	

Duty Owed the Patient

Duty of care is owed to others and involves how one conducts oneself. When engaging in an activity, an individual is under a legal duty to act as an ordinary, prudent, reasonable person would act. The ordinary, prudent, reasonable person will take precautions against creating unreasonable risks of injury to other persons. The duty of care that is owed has two distinct aspects: (1) It must first be shown that a duty was indeed owed the patient, and (2) the scope of that duty must be proven. The first aspect may be the easier to prove.

The duty of care owed to a given patient is usually fairly easily established, especially if the nurse is employed by a hospital or clinic. Once the nurse–employer and patient–hospital relationships are established, the doctrine of reliance arises: The patient has a right to rely on the fact that the nursing staff has a clear-cut duty to act in the patient's best interest.

Duty, however, is created by a relationship and not merely by employment status. More important than employment is the concept of a nurse–patient relationship or a provider–patient relationship. This *reliance relationship*—of one person depending on another for quality, competent care—actually forms the basis of the duty owed concept.

Today's primary nursing easily creates a concept of reliance in that the nurse is assigned the entire nursing care of a patient. Thus the duty of care and the establishment of a nurse–patient relationship are readily seen. But even the more traditional, team nursing approach creates such a duty of care. In that functional mode, several nurses were assigned a group of patients, and both reliance and a nurse–patient relationship existed.

Even if the nurse was not assigned to a particular patient, a general duty of care quickly arises if the patient presents with an emergency or is in need of instant help. For example, a general duty of care exists if the nurse is on the way to another part of the hospital and happens to pass the open door of a patient about to fall out of bed. Although not assigned to that patient or even to the nursing unit, the nurse has a limited duty to assist all patients in times of crisis and imminent harm.

Most cases have not concerned themselves with this portion of the nursing duty element because a showing of hospital employment is usually considered sufficient in proving that a duty is owed to the patient. An exception to this rule is *Lunsford v. Board of Nurse Examiners* (1983), a landmark decision concerning when the nurse–patient relationship arises. There the nurse attempted to show that, as the patient was never formally admitted to the hospital and there was no physician–patient relationship, a nurse–patient relationship had never been formed. Thus there was no duty owed the patient. The court refused this argument, stating that, by virtue of licensure, a nurse–patient relationship automatically existed when the patient presented at the hospital's admitting office for emergency care and was met by the nurse.

The second aspect of duty is the *standard of care* that must be delivered. The standard of care owed is that of the reasonably prudent nurse under similar circumstances as determined by expert testimony, published standards, and common sense. The test for the court to apply is what a reasonable, prudent nurse, with like experience and education, would do under similar conditions in the same community (*Fraijo v. Hartland Hospital,* 1979). See Chapter 4 for a more extensive discussion of the standards of care that must be delivered to a patient.

Breach of Duty Owed the Patient

Naturally following is the second element of malpractice and negligence, **breach of duty**, which involves showing a deviation from the standard of care owed the patient, that is, something was done that should not have been done or that nothing was done when something should have been done. For example, an incorrect medication was administered to a patient or a scheduled medication was omitted. Omissions entail as much potential liability as commissions.

Foreseeability

Foreseeability means that certain events may reasonably be expected to cause specific results. For example, the omission of an ordered insulin injection to a known diabetic patient will foreseeably result in an abnormally high serum glucose level. The challenge is to show that one could reasonably foresee a certain result based on the facts as they existed at the time of the occurrence rather than what could be said based on retrospective thinking and results. In the insulin example, could one foresee, at the time ordered insulin was omitted, that the patient would lapse into a diabetic coma and arrest?

Some of the more common cases concerning foreseeability include those involving medication errors and patient falls. The questions of when and how to provide siderails, restraints, and other protections have been addressed by most jurisdictions in the United States (*Landes v. Women's Christian Association,* 1993; *Pierce v. Mercy Medical Health Center, Inc.,* 1992; *Atkins v. Pottstown Medical Center,* 1993; and *Ciarlo v. St. Francis Hospital,* 1994). In *Landes,* a postoperative patient fell when he was escorted to the bathroom and left there unattended. In *Pierce,* a similar occurrence happened when, soon after administering Tigan to a patient, the nurse helped the patient to the shower where she was left unattended and subsequently fell. The *Atkins* case presents a similar conclusion, although in this case a preoperative patient was allowed to use the bathroom unaided after he had received his preoperative sedation. In *Ciarlo,* the nurse inadvertently gave IV KCL rather than the IV Lasix that had been ordered for the patient.

Note that none of these cases involved any high technology or advanced nursing skills. These cases represent the most commonly occurring injuries to patients: injuries that occur because of lack of foresight, common sense, and adherence to standards of care. In *Kadyszeweki v. Ellis Hospital Association* (1993), the court found liability when a 67-year-old patient, having received a combination of Demerol, Phenobarbital, Vistaril, and Motrin fell when she attempted to get to the bathroom. At court, she stated that she had been trying unsuccessfully for over 30 minutes to get someone to help her to the bathroom and that she had no trouble getting out of bed as the siderails were not raised. The court focused their conclusion more on the lack of siderails (a direct violation of the hospital policy and procedure manual) than on the failure of staff to respond to the patient's bell.

Causation

Somewhat more difficult to prove is *causation,* which means that the injury must have been incurred directly by the breach of duty owed the patient. Causation is frequently subdivided into (1) cause-in-fact and (2) proximate cause.

Cause-in-fact denotes that the breach of duty owed caused the injury. If it were not for the breach of duty, no injury would have resulted. For example, a medication is incorrectly administered in the wrong dosage, and the patient subsequently suffers direct consequences due to the medication. In *Nicole Adams v. Childrens Mercy Hospital* (1992), a child was given three times the amount of saline solution indicated during skin graft surgery for burns. She subsequently sustained permanent brain injury and was awarded $20 million in compensation.

Several tests have been established to determine cause-in-fact.

1. The *but for* test answers the question if the act or omission is a direct cause of the injury or harm sustained. Would the injury have occurred but for the act or omission by the defendant? Would the patient have developed complications, such as an abscess, but for the sponge that was inadvertently left in the abdomen during surgery?
2. The *substantial factor* test has been developed to aid in pinpointing liability when several causes occur to bring about a given injury. With several possible causes, the but for test is inadequate because the answer to each defendant's liability would be that no defendant caused the entire set of circumstances, and therefore the entire result could not have been foreseen. Rather than allow such a result, the substan-

tial factor test is used, not to determine certainty but to establish a causal link between actions and injury. This test asks if the defendant's act or omission was a substantial factor in causing the ultimate harm or injury. If the answer is yes, there is cause-in-fact. For example, in *Barton v. AMI Park Place Hospital, et al.* (1992), a high school student was injured in an automobile accident and admitted to the hospital with right upper quadrant pain. While in the emergency room and later the intensive care unit (ICU), nurses and physicians failed to properly monitor blood pressure, respirations, and bleeding; he died seven hours after admission. His parents asserted that the staff had failed to stop his bleeding, monitor vital signs, transfer him to an ICU early enough, and transfer him to a better equipped hospital in time to save his life. Obviously, all staff concerned with his care could be reasonably said to have been a substantial factor in his demise.

3. The *alternate causes* approach also addresses the problem in which two or more persons have been accused of negligence. Under this test, the plaintiff must show that the harm or injury was caused by one of the multiple defendants, and the burden of proof then shifts to the defendants to show who actually caused the harm or injury at issue. In *Donahue v. Port* (1994), a 32-year-old male lost his leg due to failure to diagnose vascular problems associated with a dislocated knee. At trial, the defendant orthopedic surgeon claimed that the nurses were negligent in not reporting vascular problems until it was too late to save the leg. An expert witness for the nurses testified that, if there was an initial popliteal artery injury, there was only a 12-hour window in which to successfully repair the artery and that the 12-hour window had expired before the patient was treated. The patient has the burden of proof to show that the harm was caused by one of the defendants, and the defendants have to show which one of them did (or did not) cause the harm. If neither defendant could establish his or her own innocence or the other's negligence, they may both be liable.

The alternate causes approach is frequently seen in a negative light by juries. Defendants blaming each other have often resulted in large malpractice awards for the injured plaintiff (Fiesta, 1994), and thus is not often used at trial.

Proximate cause attempts to determine how far the liability of the defendant extends for consequences following negligent activity. Thus proximate cause builds on foreseeability. Could one foresee the extent to which consequences will follow a negligent action? For example, in *Crosby v. Sultz* (1991), the court held that a doctor was not responsible for a patient's driving habits, and found that the physician had no duty to protect third parties from injuries received in unforeseeable accidents. In that case, a diabetic patient temporarily lost consciousness while driving and harmed Mrs. Crosby and her three children. The plaintiffs were unable to show that diabetes made it impossible for Sultz to drive safely and therefore could not show that the physician's failure to prevent his patient from driving was a proximal cause of the harm done.

Nursing cases that illustrate proximate cause include *Gallimore v. Children's Hospital Medical Center* (1992) and *Flores v. Cyborski* (1993). In the first case, the nurse administered 200 mg of gentamicin IV rather than the ordered dose of 30 mg. The court found the nurse liable for the child's subsequent hearing loss. The issue in *Flores* concerned whether the failure of the nurse to recognize and respond to changes in a patient's condition was the proximate cause of the patient's death. Mrs. Cyborski had been admitted to a medical center with an initial diagnosis of respiratory insufficiency and pneumonia. By the fourth day of admission, she was pain-free, afebrile, and had adequate blood gases. Early on the morning of the fourth day after admission, at 4:20 AM, she developed sharp chest pains, had a heart rate of 180, and was extremely short of breath. The physician was not notified of the changes in her condition until the nurse called him at 6:15 AM to notify him that resuscitation of his patient was currently being administered. On autopsy, it was found that the patient had sustained a large pulmonary embolism. The court found that the nurses had deviated from standards of care and that the failure to notify the physician promptly was the sole proximate cause for the patient's demise. The court also found that the directed verdict for the defendant's affirmative defense at trial level was correct.

Proximate cause is fairly clear as long as the result is directly related. Proximate cause becomes less clear when intervening variables are present. Intervening forces may combine with the original negligent action to cause injury to the patient. As a rule of thumb, in medical malpractice cases, the health care provider is frequently liable for intervening forces when they are foreseeable. For example, a patient, hurt in an automobile accident, sued the driver's physician, alleging that the driver was given an excessive amount of Valium by the physician and that the physician failed to adequately evaluate his patient's psychiatric and drinking history before prescribing Valium. The court could conclude that a foreseeable consequence of prescribing Valium under such circumstances is that the patient with psychiatric problems will drink, and such a patient, high on alcohol and Valium, may injure others.

Injury

The fifth element that must be shown is an actual *injury* or *harm*. The plaintiff must demonstrate that some type of physical, financial, or emotional injury resulted from the breach of duty owed the patient. Generally speaking, courts do not allow lawsuits based solely on negligently inflicted emotional injuries. Such emotional injuries are actionable only when they accompany physical injuries.

In *Armstrong* (1993), the emergency room patient was unconscious and a mistake was made in notifying his next of kin. The nurse called information for the phone number of Thomas Armstrong and was given the number of Thomas J. Armstrong, not the patient Thomas H. Armstrong. Thus the wrong wife was called, came to the emergency center, and was shown x-rays of the patient's crushed cranium before discovering that it was not her husband that was injured. She sued for negligent infliction of emotional damages and was awarded $1,000 by the jury. On appeal, the decision was overturned and the court stated that the purpose of the judicial system is not to compensate for "every minor psychic shock incurred in the course of everyday living. The law is not the guarantor of an emotionally peaceful life and cannot protect any of us from the emotional slings and arrows of daily living" (1993, p. 17).

Pain and suffering are allowed if they accompany a physical injury but not by themselves. This contrasts with intentional infliction of emotional harm, an intentional tort (see Chapter 6).

An exception to the nonrecovery for emotional harm concerns instances in which parents view an injury to their children. The courts in these type of cases have frequently allowed damages for a purely emotional injury.

Damages

Unlike intentional torts, *damages* are not presumed. Nominal damages (such as a $1 or $2 award) do not exist for negligent torts. The basic purpose of awarding damages is compensatory, with the law attempting to restore injured parties to their original position as far as is financially possible. The goal of awarding damages is not to punish defendants, but to assist the injured parties.

Essentially four types of damages may be compensated:

1. *General damages* are those that are inherent to the injury itself. Included in general damages are pain and suffering (past, present, and future) and any permanent disability or disfigurement because of the injury.
2. *Special damages* account for all losses and expenses incurred as a result of the injury. These include medical bills, lost wages (past, present, and future), cost of future medical care, and cost of converting current living areas to more easily accommodate the injured party.
3. *Emotional damages* may be compensated if there is apparent physical harm as well. A very limited number of cases, such as *Bond v. Sacred Heart Medical Center* (1991), allowed an award for a mother's mental distress when her 3-day-old infant was dropped on his head. The baby had somehow become entangled in his IV tubings and was thrown to the floor when the door of his incubator was opened, resulting in permanent brain damage.
4. *Punitive* or *exemplary damages* may be awarded if there is malicious, willful, or wanton misconduct. Plaintiffs must show that the defendant acted with conscious disregard for their safety. In this instance the damages are usually considerable and are awarded to deter similar conduct in the future. This type of damage award is usually not covered by professional liability insurance coverage, since the harm is with malice and forethought. In one of the few cases in which punitive damages were awarded against nurse defendants, a decision was made to move a patient to another room on the same unit, without supplemental oxygen. The patient was terminal, with less than 24

hours to live, and the family begged that supplemental oxygen be given during the move. The nurses declined, and the patient—a "no-code" patient—arrested about 15 feet from his original room and was pronounced dead by the attending physician. The court found that punitive damages were appropriate because the nurses' action was extreme deviation from the standard of care (*Manning v. Twin Falls Clinic and Hospital,* 1992).

Sometimes general and special damages are grouped into one category called *compensatory damages.* The last two classifications are retained, and thus there are three categories for damage awards.

EXERCISE 5-2

A nurse administers a medication to a patient as ordered by the patient's physician. Can the nurse be found liable if the patient suffers an allergic reaction? Does liability depend on whether it was a fatal allergic response or merely a mild allergic response to the medication?

DOCTRINE OF RES IPSA LOQUITOR

The doctrine of *res ipsa loquitor* allows a negligence cause-of-action without requiring that all six elements of malpractice or negligence be proven. Essentially res ipsa loquitor allows the jury to find the defendant negligent without any showing of expert testimony on the plaintiff's part.

Res ipsa loquitor, meaning "the thing speaks for itself," is a rule of evidence that emerges when plaintiffs are injured in such a way that they cannot prove how the injury occurred or who was responsible for its occurrence. The negligence of the alleged wrongdoer may be inferred from the mere fact that an accident or incident happened. The proviso is that the nature of the incident and the circumstances surrounding the incident lead reasonably to the belief that, in the absence of negligence, it would not have occurred. The instrument that caused the injury must be shown to have been under the management and control of the alleged wrongdoer, not the injured party.

This doctrine is used by the courts when the person injured has an insurmountable burden in proving the facts of the case. For example, the landmark case for this doctrine is a California case in which the injured party underwent a routine appendectomy and suffered a permanent loss of neuromuscular control of the right shoulder and arm as a result of the surgery (*Ybarra v. Spangard,* 1944). The injured party had no means of accurately showing how or when this permanent injury occurred. All the patient could show was that this was not the type of complication normally incurred with an appendectomy and that he had full range and movement of the affected arm prior to the surgical procedure.

Guidelines: Avoiding Negligent Torts

1. Treat patients and their families with respect and honesty. Communications done in a truthful, open, and professional manner may well prevent a negligence cause-of-action.

2. Use your nursing knowledge to make appropriate nursing diagnoses and to implement necessary nursing interventions. You have an affirmative duty not only to make correct nursing diagnoses, but also to take the actions required to implement your diagnoses.

3. Remember that the first line of duty is to the patient. If the physician is hesitant to order the necessary therapy or to respond to a change in the patient condition, call your supervisor or another physician. Question orders if they are (1) ambiguous or unclear, (2) questioned or refused by the patient, (3) telephone orders, and/or (4) inappropriate, such as when a major change occurs in the patient's status and the orders remain unchanged. For telephone orders, reread the orders to the physician and clarify them prior to hanging up the phone.

4. Remain current and up-to-date in your skills and education. Take advantage of continuing education programs and in-service programs on a regular basis. Read your professional journals. Refuse to perform skills and procedures if you are unfamiliar with them, have never performed them, or lack the necessary materials and equipment to perform them safely.

5. Base your nursing care on the nursing process model. Using all steps of the model prevents the inadvertent overlooking of vital parts of required nursing care for a patient.

6. Document completely every step of the nursing care plan and the patient's responses to interventions. Express yourself clearly and completely. Chart all entries as soon as possible while the facts and observations are still clear in your mind.

7. Respect patients' rights to education about their illnesses, and ensure that patients and their families are taught about the disease entity, therapy, and possible complications prior to discharge.

8. Delegate patient care wisely, and know the scope of practice for yourself and those whom you supervise. Never accept or allow others to accept more responsibility than they can handle or than they are allowed to accept by law.

9. Know and adhere to your hospital policies and procedures. Help to update those that are outdated, and ensure that the personnel you supervise are also aware of hospital policies and procedures. All personnel should reread the manual periodically.

10. Keep your malpractice liability insurance policy current, and know the limits of its coverage. This may not help you give better care, but it will help you if a patient should name you in a malpractice cause-of-action.

To prevent injured parties from an unfair disadvantage and to prevent wrong-doers from benefiting by their silence, the court enacted the doctrine of res ipsa loquitor. The injured party must prove three elements for this doctrine to apply:

1. The accident must be the kind that ordinarily does not occur in the absence of someone's negligence.
2. The accident must be caused by an agency or instrumentality within exclusive control of the defendant.
3. The accident must not have been due to any voluntary action or contribution on the part of the plaintiff (*Ybarra v. Spangard,* 1944, at 687).

Once these three elements are shown, the defendant must disprove them. The courts view the defendants as being in a better position to actually explain what happened, since they had exclusive control during the time the incident occurred.

The doctrine of res ipsa loquitor is normally applied in medical malpractice cases in which the injured party was unconscious, in surgery, or an infant. Typical examples of cases for which the courts have allowed the doctrine of res ipsa loquitor to be applied include those in which a foreign object has been left in the patient during surgery, infection was caused by unsterile instruments, neuromuscular injury occurred due to the improper positioning of an unconscious patient, burns occurred during surgery, or a surgical procedure was performed on the wrong limb or part of the body.

Not all states apply the doctrine of res ipsa loquitor in the same manner. Some states have actually expanded the doctrine through recent court cases. Other states have tended to limit the application of the doctrine, especially in areas where more than common knowledge is needed to ensure the jury's understanding of the facts, such as in the area of secondary infections. A third trend by states is to deny the injured party the use of the doctrine through statutory or decisional law. This latter denial of the doctrine is based on the fact that negligence must be proven, not presumed (*Annotations,* 1989).

LOCALITY RULE

Whenever the legal system refers to the reasonable, prudent practitioner, there is a statement to the effect that the professional is viewed in the context of a prevailing community standard, "in a similar community," or "under the same circumstances." Known as the *locality rule,* such a statement attempts to hold the standard of the professional to that of other professionals practicing in the same geographic area of the country.

The locality rule arose because there were wide variations in the care that a patient received, depending on the setting of the hospital—rural or urban. Rural hospitals and health care providers did not have the same sophistication and means of technology that were available in large medical centers.

In most jurisdictions the locality rule has been abolished either by statute or by judicial rulings. Today a *national standard* is emerging that offers to all persons an acceptable minimal standard of care.

Several factors arose to help abolish the locality rule. First, because of mass media, national conferences, and improved transportation, health care providers were no longer able to defend the acceptance of a lower standard for rural areas. The practitioner has available all the teaching aids and continuing education programs needed to stay on top of new and innovative therapeutic approaches, as well as to understand new technological advances. The patient may, fairly readily, be transported to a larger, metropolitan area, or the needed equipment and personnel can be transported to the patient.

Second, professional organizations (eg, the Joint Commission for the Accreditation of Healthcare Organizations or the American Association of Critical Care Nurses) have moved toward the creation of an acceptable standard for given patients by publishing national standards of care. Additionally, state nurse practice acts have enacted standards of nursing practice for all nurses within the jurisdiction, not just for nurses in large medical centers.

Third, standards for the accreditation of hospitals should be the same no matter where the hospital is located geographically.

AVOIDING MALPRACTICE CLAIMS

Nurses frequently inquire about the impact that the medical malpractice crisis will have on the professional practice of nursing. This is especially true as more and more nurses are being sued along with physicians or hospitals. Can anything be done to stop the increased litigation? And what should nurses do to protect themselves?

They can limit their potential liability in several ways. Possibly the first and most important concept to remember is that the patient and the patient's family who are treated honestly, openly, and respectfully and who are apprised of all facets of treatment and prognosis are not likely to sue. Communications done in a caring and professional manner have been shown time and time again to be a major reason why more people do not sue, despite adequate grounds for a successful lawsuit. Even given untoward results and a major setback, the patient is less likely to file suit if there has been an open and trusting nurse–patient relationship or physician–patient relationship. Remember that it is people who sue, not the action or event that triggered a bad outcome.

Second, nurses should know relevant law and legal doctrines, and they should combine these concepts with the biological, psychological, and social sciences that form part of the basis of all rational nursing decisions. The law can and should be incorporated into everyday practice as a safeguard for the health care provider as well as the health care recipient.

Third, nurses should stay well within their areas of individual competence. To remain competent, nurses should upgrade technical skills consistently, continuously attend pertinent continuing education and in-service programs on a regular basis, and undertake only those actual skills that they can perform competently.

Fourth, joining and actively supporting professional organizations allow nurses to take advantage of their excellent educational programs and to become active in the organizations' lobbying efforts, especially if it means a stronger nurse practice act or the creation or expansion of advanced nursing roles. Far too many nurses are reluctant to become politically involved. Yet, as a unified profession, nursing could have a very strong voice, particularly in upgrading and strengthening nurse practice acts.

Fifth, recognize the concept of the *suit-prone patient*. This type of patient is more likely than other patients to initiate malpractice action in the event that something untoward happens during the treatment process. Because the psychological make-up of these persons breeds resentment and dissatisfaction in all phases of their lives, they are much more apt to initiate a lawsuit.

Suit-prone patients tend to be immature, overly dependent, hostile, and uncooperative, often failing to follow a designated plan of care. Unable to be self-critical, they shift blame to others as a way of coping with their own inadequacies. Suit-prone patients actually project their fear, insecurity, and anxiety to health care providers, overreacting to any perceived slight in an exaggerated manner.

Recognizing such patients is the first step in avoiding potential lawsuits. The nurse should then attempt to react on a more human, or personal, basis such as expressing satisfaction with these patients' cooperation, showing empathy and concern with their suffering and setbacks, and repeating needed information to keep them less fearful with unknown treatments and procedures. An atmosphere of attentiveness, caring, and patience helps prevent the suit-prone patient from filing future lawsuits.

Sixth, recognize that nurses' personality traits and behaviors may also trigger lawsuits. So-called *suit-prone nurses* (1) have difficulty establishing close relationships with others, (2) are insecure and shift blame to others, (3) tend to be insensitive to patients' complaints or fail to take the complaints seriously, (4) have a tendency to be aloof and more concerned with the mechanics of nursing as opposed to establishing meaningful human interactions with patients, and (5) inappropriately delegate responsibilities to peers to avoid personal contact with patients. These nurses need counseling and education to change these behaviors into more positive attitudes and behaviors toward patients and staff. Such positive changes lessen future potential lawsuits.

Seventh, while it may not prevent lawsuits, nurses are urged to investigate having professional liability insurance. This will better protect them should a lawsuit be filed.

Eighth, it seems inevitable that at some point the consumer of health care must begin to accept responsibility for risks along with the health care providers. One of the reasons cited for high medical malpractice claims against obstetricians is the fact that consumers want total assurance that they will have only healthy, perfectly formed children. Perhaps part of nursing's imminent tasks is in helping to educate consumers. All health care entails some risks, no matter how remote or far-fetched.

EXERCISE 5-3

Recall all the patients that you have cared for in the past seven to ten days. Were any of those patients classifiable as suit-prone? Did all of them fit this classification? Did the ones that you classified as suit-prone meet *all* the criteria in the text? What can nurses do to lessen the potential of future lawsuits?

SUMMARY

Malpractice—negligence as it pertains to professionals—is the leading cause of lawsuits filed today in the medical arena. All six elements of malpractice must be proven in court for the injured party to prevail. There are guidelines to prevent or lessen the possibility of malpractice suits being filed against health care providers.

AFTER COMPLETING THIS CHAPTER, YOU SHOULD BE ABLE TO

- Distinguish negligence from malpractice.
- List the six elements of malpractice, and give an example of each element in professional nursing practice.
- Define the three tests currently used by courts in establishing cause-in-fact.
- Analyze the doctrine of res ipsa loquitor, and give an example of when the doctrine would apply to professional nursing practice.
- Compare and contrast the locality rule to a national standard.
- List eight ways to avoid or lessen the potential for malpractice cases.

APPLY YOUR LEGAL KNOWLEDGE

- What types of patients are more likely to bring nursing malpractice suits?
- When a patient injury occurs, is the nurse or another staff member always legally responsible?
- What are the more common types of nursing malpractice today?
- Why is the distinction between malpractice and negligence important?

REFERENCES

Annotations 67 ALR 4th. Applicability of res ipsa loquitor in cases of multiple medical defendants—modern status, 544–601.

Atkins v. Pottstown Medical Center, 634 A.2d 258 (Pennsylvania, 1993).

Barton v. AMI Park Place Hospital, et. al., No. 909-066318 (Texas, 1992).

Bond v. Sacred Heart Medical Center, No. 86-2-03311 (February, 1991).

Borghese v. Bartley, 402 So.2d 475 (Fla. App. 1981; reh. den. 1981).

Buck v. St. Clair, 702 P.2d 781 (1984).

Ciarlo v. St. Francis Hospital, WL 713864 (Del. Super, 1994).

Crosby v. Sultz, 592 A.2d 1337 (Pa. Super. Ct., 1991).

Donahue v. Port, Case #92-CIV-4477 (Pennsylvania, February 1994).

Fiesta, J. (1994). *20 legal pitfalls for nurses to avoid.* Albany, NY: Delmar Publishers, Inc.

Flores v. Cyborski, 629 N.E.2d 74 (Illinois, 1993).

Forthofer v. Arnold, 60 Ohio App. 436, 21 N.E.2d 869 (1938).

Fraijo v. Hartland Hospital, 99 Cal. Rept. 3d 331, 160 Cal. Rept. 848 (1979).

Hamil v. Bashline, 392 A.2d 1280 (Pennsylvania, 1978).

Gallimore v. Children's Hospital Medical Center, WL 37742 (Ohio App. Dis 1, 1992).

Kadyszewski v. Ellis Hospital Association, 595 N.Y.S.2d 841 (New York, 1993)

Landers v. Women's Christian Association, 504 N.W.2d 139 (Iowa, 1993).

Lunsford v. Board of Nurse Examiners, 648 S.W.2d 391 (Tex. Civ. App.—Austin 1983).

Manning v. Twin Falls Clinic and Hospital, 830 P.2d 1185 (Idaho, 1992)

Medical Malpractice Verdicts, Settlements and Experts 7(6), 6 (1992).

Nicole Adams v. Childrens Mercy Hospital, case #73867 (1992).

Pierce v. Mercy Medical Health Center, Inc., 847 P.2d 822 (Oklahoma, 1992).

Ybarra v. Spangard, 154 P.2d 687 (California, 1944).

· six

Intentional Torts

PREVIEW

Although most cases involving nurses and patients concern negligence, the nurse may also be held accountable for intentional wrongdoings. Both intentional wrongdoings and negligence have their bases in tort law. This chapter differentiates between these two concepts and gives examples of the more commonly encountered intentional torts seen within hospitals and community settings.

KEY CONCEPTS

tort	battery	intentional infliction of emotional distress
intentional torts	false imprisonment	
quasi-intentional torts	conversion of property	invasion of privacy
assault	trespass to land	defamation

DEFINITION OF A TORT

A *tort* is a civil wrong committed against a person or the person's property. Torts, a term derived from French, are "acts or omissions which unlawfully violate a person's rights by law and for which the appropriate remedy is a common law action for damages by the injured party" (Keeton, 1984, p. 2). Tort law is based on fault. The accountable person either failed to meet his or her responsibility or performed an action below the allowable standard of care. Tort law is distinguishable from contract law. Torts are civil wrongs that are not based on contracts. *Tort law* may also be said to be based on personal transgressions in that the responsible person performs an action incorrectly or omits a necessary action.

DEFINITION OF AN INTENTIONAL TORT

An *intentional tort* has three elements:

1. There must be a volitional or willful act by the defendant.
2. The person so acting must intend to bring about the consequences or appear to have intended to bring about the consequences.
3. There must be causation. The act must be a substantial factor in bringing about the injury or consequences.

Intentional torts may be differentiated from negligence in the following manner:

1. Intent is necessary. The nurse must have intended an action. For example, the nurse must intend to hold the patient so that an injection might be given to the patient or so that a nasogastric tube might be inserted into the patient's stomach.
2. There must be a volitional or willful action against the injured person. There cannot be solely the omission of a duty owed as with negligence.

TABLE 6–1. SHARED ELEMENTS OF INTENTIONAL TORTS

1. There must be a volitional (voluntary and willful) act by the defendant.
2. The person so acting must intend to bring about the consequences.
3. There must be causation, ie, the act must be a substantial factor in bringing about the injury or consequences.

In the preceding example, the nurse holds the patient so that the injection can be given or the nasogastric tube inserted.

3. Damages are not an issue. The injured party need not show that damages were incurred. Whether the patient encounters out-of-pocket expenses or not, the patient could still show that an intentional tort had occurred.

The law also recognizes *quasi-intentional torts.* A tort becomes quasi-intentional when intent is lacking but there is a volitional action and direct causation. In other words, more than mere negligence is involved, but the intent that is necessary for an intentional tort is missing in quasi-intentional torts. As with intentional torts, in quasi-intentional torts damages are not an issue.

INTENTIONAL TORTS

The more commonly seen intentional torts within the health care arena are assault, battery, false imprisonment, conversion of property, trespass to land, and intentional infliction of emotional distress. Defamation and invasion of privacy are usually discussed with intentional torts, although these two wrongs are more correctly classified as quasi-intentional torts.

Assault

An *assault* is any action that places another person in apprehension of being touched in a manner that is offensive, insulting, or physically injurious without that person's consent or authority. No actual touching of the person is required. The action or motion must create a "reasonable apprehension in the other person of immediate harmful or offensive contact to the plaintiff-person" (Words and Phrases, 1994).

Usually thought of as a violent, angry, or unwarranted contact with the patient, knowledge is the prerequisite to assault. For example, nurses cannot assault patients who are sleeping or unconscious because, no matter how angry or violent they might be or how irrational their actions, the patient has no knowledge of the potential contact and is therefore not apprehensive of the potential contact. In *Baca v. Valez*, an operating room nurse sued for assault and battery when an orthopedic surgeon struck her on the back with a bone chisel. In finding that there was no assault (although a battery had occurred), the court concluded that since she was struck in the back, there was "no act, threat or menacing conduct that causes another person to reasonably believe that he is in danger of receiving an immediate battery" (1992, at 1197).

Words alone are not enough for assault to occur, although the addition of words may accompany the overt act. For example, the nurse moves toward the patient with a syringe in one hand while telling the patient why the injection is necessary or while telling the patient to "lie still or this will really hurt!" Either example is an assault if the patient is apprehensive of an offensive touching of his or her body.

An assault also requires the present ability to commit harm. For example, if someone is threatened over a telephone, there is no present ability to commit a harm, and thus there is no tort committed.

Two important reminders: (1) The actual touching of the person (battery) does not have to follow an assault, and (2) either the nurse or the patient may be the *tortfeasor* (person committing the tort). Assault is the apprehension of an unwarranted touching, and the apprehension is all that is needed to prove that a tort has occurred. The nurse may approach the patient or the patient may approach the nurse.

Battery

A *battery*, the most common intentional tort within the practice of nursing and medicine, involves a harmful or unwarranted contact with the patient-plaintiff. Liability for such an unwarranted contact is based on the individual's right to be free from unconsented invasions of the person.

The legal system recognizes several factors regarding battery:

1. A single touch, however fleeting and faint, is sufficient for the tort to have occurred. Everyday examples include brushing against another person in a crowded elevator or auditorium, or placing one's hand on the patient's shoulder for reassurance. It is the touching, not the manner of the touch, that creates the tort.

2. No harm, injury, or pain need befall the patient. The unwarranted contact frequently will not harm or physically hurt the patient.

3. The patient need not be aware of the battery for the tort to have occurred. Unlike assault, in which knowledge is a key factor, taking a pulse of a sleeping patient could be considered a battery at law.

4. Causation is an important factor, and the nurse may be liable for direct as well as indirect contact. For example, the nurse, intending to restrain a patient for the purpose of starting an intravenous infusion, accidentally drops the intravenous tray on the patient. Even though the nurse has not directly touched the patient, a battery has occurred because the nurse put the scenario into motion.

5. The nurse may also commit a battery by the unwarranted touching of the patient's clothes or of an article held by the patient, such as a purse or a suitcase. For purposes of a battery, anything that is connected with the patient's person is viewed as part of the person.

Most lawsuits in the health care area have focused on consent for medical or surgical procedures. Lack of consent always sets the stage for a potential assault and battery lawsuit. The classic and landmark case of *Schloendorff v. Society of New York Hospitals* (1914) held that the medical practitioner had committed a battery when he removed a tumor from a patient who had authorized merely an examination. *Mohr v. Williams* (1905) had reached a similar previous conclusion when that court found the practitioner liable for performing surgery without prior consent. That court also limited damages because of the good faith of the practitioner and the beneficial results of the surgery to the patient.

More recent examples of such unwarranted treatment are *Loungbury v. Capal* (1992), *Foflygen v. R. Zemel* (1992), and *Anderson v. St. Francis-St. George Hospital* (1992). Each of these cases held that treatment without prior consent by the patient resulted in a battery.

False Imprisonment

False imprisonment is the unjustifiable detention of a person without legal warrant to confine the person. Nurses falsely imprison the patient when they confine the patient or restrain the patient in a confined, bounded area with the intent to prevent the patient from freedom and nonrestraint. The confined area may be the patient's room or bed. False imprisonment may also occur if the act is directed at the patient's family or possessions. For example, one has effectively been confined if the nurse refuses to give the patient her purse, car keys, or clothing, or refuses to allow the patient to see his family members unless the patient stays in bed.

There must be knowledge of the restraint for false imprisonment to occur. Sedated patients who are incapable of realizing their confinement do not have a suit for false imprisonment. Likewise, future threats are not enough to sustain the tort of false imprisonment. Threatening a patient who is about to leave against medical advice with "if you leave now, no physician will ever take your case in the future" does not constitute false imprisonment, though it may be inadvisable from a nursing perspective. Detaining patients who wish to leave against medical advice until the supervisor can be located or until the patient's physician can be contacted to come and see them is false imprisonment.

Some circumstances, though, justify detainment. Hospitals have a common law duty to detain persons who are confused or disoriented. Most states have laws authorizing the detainment of mentally ill persons or persons with a contagious disease who would be a threat to society. In *Blackman v. Blackman for Rifkin* (1988), the hospital was allowed to detain a highly intoxicated, head trauma patient in the emergency center despite her insistence that she be allowed to leave.

As a rule of thumb, mentally ill persons may be detained only if they are a threat to themselves or are capable of jeopardizing others. The only force that may be used to detain such persons is that necessary under the circumstances, or the patient may be able to show battery and false imprisonment.

Restraints are an interference with the patient's liberty, but relatively few cases exist in which a patient has filed for false imprisonment due to use of restraints. Care, caution, and reasonableness are the prerequisites to use of restraints.

Conversion of Property

The tort of *conversion of property* arises when the health care practitioner interferes with the right to possession of the patient's property, either by intermeddling or by dispossessing the person of the property. Examples include searching a patient's suitcase and removing prescription drugs from the patient's possession or taking the patient's car keys or clothing without just cause. Often this tort is seen in combination with other torts. Taking a patient's car keys to prevent the patient from leaving the hospital could also be termed false imprisonment. But, as with the other intentional torts, the practitioner may be free from liability if there is adequate justification for the action. For example, taking the car keys to prevent confused, disoriented persons from driving their cars is permissible.

Trespass to Land

Trespass to land is the tort of unlawful interference with another's possession of land, and may occur either intentionally or as the result of a negligent action. The tort occurs when a person (1) intrudes onto another's property, (2) fails to leave the property when so requested, (3) throws or places something on the property, or (4) causes a third person to enter the property.

Institutions and health care facilities, including parking areas, are private property and people do not have an absolute right to remain on the property. Trespass to land thus occurs when a patient refuses to leave the institution after having been properly discharged or when visitors refuse to leave the area. Trespass may also occur when protestors enter the health care facility as part of a dispute.

Intentional Infliction of Emotional Distress

Sometimes called *extreme and outrageous conduct,* the tort of *intentional infliction of emotional distress* includes several types of outrageous conduct that cause severe emotional distress. Three conditions must be met to prove this tort:

1. The practitioner's conduct goes beyond behavior that is usually tolerated by society.
2. The conduct is calculated to cause mental distress.
3. The conduct actually causes the mental distress.

Rude and insulting behavior is not sufficient to recover under this tort; the behavior must be beyond all realms of decency. Depending on state law, patients' families who witness the conduct may also recover damages.

TABLE 6–2. INTENTIONAL TORTS

Tort	Shared Elements Plus ...	Examples of Nursing Actions
Assault	Places another in apprehension of being touched in an offensive, insulting, or physically injurious manner	Threatening patients with an injection or with starting an intravenous line
Battery	Actual contacts with another person or the person's clothing without valid consent	Forcing patients to ambulate against their will Holding patients so that a nasogastric tube can be inserted
False Imprisonment	Unjustifiably detains a person without legal warrant to do so	Refusing to allow patients to leave against medical advice Restraining competent patients against their wishes
Conversion of Property	Interferes with the patient's right of possession in his/her property	Searching patients' belongings and taking medications or removing the patient's clothing
Trespass to Land	Unlawfully interferes with another's possession of land	Patient refusing to leave the hospital after being discharged Visitor's refusal to leave the hospital when so requested
Intentional Infliction of Emotional Distress	Displays conduct that goes beyond that allowed by society, conduct that is calculated to cause mental distress	Handing a mother her stillborn child in a gallon jar of formaldehyde

Unless the conduct goes outside the reasonable bounds of decency, courts are reluctant to allow plaintiff recovery for this tort. This tort should be easily avoided by treating patients and their families in the same civil, reasonable manner that one would want for oneself or loved ones.

EXERCISE 6-1

A private duty nurse is hired to care for an alcoholic patient in the patient's residence. While on duty, the nurse argues with the patient, and the patient throws a table lamp at the nurse, striking her on the head and upper torso. If she decides to sue the patient, what grounds would she assert in her case? Does the patient have grounds that he could assert in a court of law? If you were the judge, what would be your verdict?

QUASI-INTENTIONAL TORTS

Invasion of Privacy

The right to protection against unreasonable and unwarranted interferences with the individual's solitude is well recognized. The tort of *invasion of privacy* includes the protection of personality, as well as protection of one's right to be left alone. The right to privacy concerns one's peace of mind in that a person is allowed to be left alone without unwarranted publicity. Within a medical context, the law recognizes the patient's right against:

1. Appropriation or usage of the plaintiff's name or picture for defendant's sole advantage.
2. Intrusion by the defendant on the patient's seclusion or affairs.
3. Publication by the defendant of facts that place the patient in a false light.
4. Public disclosure of private facts about the patient by hospital staff or medical personnel.

Elements of invasion of privacy include:

1. An act that must intrude or pry into the seclusion of the patient.
2. Intrusion that is objectionable to the reasonable person.
3. An act or intrusion that intrudes or pries into private facts or publishes facts and pictures of a private nature.
4. Public disclosure of private information.

Information concerning the patient is confidential and may not be disclosed without authorization. Authorization may be either by patient waiver or pursuant to a valid reporting statute. Most hospitals and institutions have policies regarding who and under what circumstances information may be released. Liability could exist if nurses and hospital personnel fail to follow their published policies and procedures.

Nurses are to be cautioned about releasing information concerning current patients over the telephone. Even family members may not be privileged to patient information. The patient may elect not to disclose information concerning diagnosis and treatments to family members. Short of a valid reporting statute, the nurse may not violate this privacy right.

Frequently, relatives and friends call to inquire about the patient's status, diagnosis, or prognosis. Before releasing any information, the patient must authorize such release, and the nurse should verify who the inquirer is, since most patients allow release of information only to family and close friends. For callers who are not allowable recipients of patient knowledge, an appropriate response is to ask the caller to contact the family or relatives directly.

Patients have a right to their names as well as to their pictures. Pictures or photos may not be used, even for medical journals or technical publications, without proper authorization (*Vessiliades v. Garfinckel's, Brooks Brothers*, 1985). In that case, the court held that a plastic surgeon had violated the privacy of a patient when he allowed, without her consent or prior knowledge, "before" and "after" pictures to be used in promoting surgery procedures in a department store presentation and by a television station.

In limited circumstances, the newsworthiness of the event makes disclosure acceptable. The public's right to know can exceed the patient's right to privacy, as seen in the 1981 attempt on President Reagan's life or in the implantation of innovative life-support systems. Dr. Barney Clark (1982) would be an example of the latter, although his name might have been protected, as was done in the case of Baby K (1993).

Even though there may be a right to public knowledge, courts have not allowed the public disclosure to undermine a patient's dignity. Two landmark cases, *Barber v. Time, Inc.* (1942) and *Doe v. Roe* (1978), stand for the need to protect the patient's privacy rights. One cannot divulge so much information about the patient that the patient's identity becomes readily obvious.

Valid reporting statutes may allow disclosure of limited patient data. Nurses must protect the patient's privacy over and above what is required by disclosure statutes (*Prince v. St. Francis-St. George Hospital,* 1985). Chapter 7 discusses reporting statutes in more detail.

Defamation

Defamation, comprised of the torts of slander and libel, is the tort of wrongful injury to another's reputation (his or her good name, respect, and esteem). It involves written or oral communication to someone other than the person defamed of matters concerning a living person's reputation. A claim of defamation may arise from inaccurate or inappropriate release of medical information or from untruthful statements about other staff members.

Five elements are necessary to prove the quasi-intentional tort of defamation:

1. Defamatory language that would adversely affect one's reputation.
2. Defamatory language about or concerning a living person.
3. Publication to a third party or to several persons but not necessarily the world at large.
4. Damage to the person's reputation as seen by adverse, derogatory, or unpleasant opinion against the person defamed.
5. Fault on the part of the defendant in writing or telling another the defamatory language.

The tort may be harder to prove if the person affected is a public figure. The law recognizes that such public figures would have a greater possibility of publicly defending themselves than private persons, and could more easily explain or counteract the potentially defamatory statement. For example, politicians could call a press conference or request that the local newspaper write their version. A private housewife or everyday worker could not command such actions and thus has greater protection for this quasi-intentional tort at law.

Generally, no actual damages need to exist for slander (oral communications) but must exist for libel (written defamation). Exceptions include slan-

TABLE 6–3. QUASI-INTENTIONAL TORTS

Tort	Elements	Examples of Nursing Actions
Invasion of Privacy	Act must intrude or pry into person's seclusion. Intrusion must be objectionable to a reasonable person. Intrusion must concern private facts or publish facts and pictures of a private nature. It must be public disclosure of private information	Using patients' pictures without their consent or in a manner that was not authorized by them Releasing confidential information to others without patients' consent Giving status reports about patient to someone not authorized to receive such information
Defamation	Defamatory language about a living person adversely affects his/her reputation. Information is published to a third person. There is damage to reputation	Making false chart entries about a patient's life style or diagnoses Falsely accusing staff members in in front of visitors or other staff members

derous statements that concern contagious or venereal diseases, crimes involving moral turpitude, or comments that prejudice persons in their chosen profession, trade, or business. Two older but still applicable cases illustrate this point. *Schessler v. Keck* (1954) concerned a case wherein a nurse told a second person that a caterer was currently being treated for syphilis, and the false statement destroyed the catering business. *Farrell v. Kramer* (1963) concerned a similar defamatory statement.

The nurse is to be cautioned against defamatory statements in chart references to patients. For example, charting that a patient is a prostitute or acts "crazy" may raise potential liability issues. When a person exhibits unusual behavior, chart exactly the behavior as perceived rather than conclusory statements.

EXERCISE 6-2

Assume that you have to design a one-hour continuing education offering for nurses to learn more about intentional torts. What content should you include in the presentation? How should you present the information to the audience? How should you evaluate the effectiveness of your continuing education offering?

DEFENSES

In some instances, health care providers may commit an intentional tort and incur no legal liability. Called defenses, these specific instances and circumstances are the subject of the next chapter.

GUIDELINES: INTENTIONAL TORTS AND QUASI-INTENTIONAL TORTS

1. Recognize that the patient has several rights at law for freedom from intentional torts and quasi-intentional torts and that you must act to ensure these rights.

2. Know the elements of each of the intentional and quasi-intentional torts so that you will not violate the rights of your patients. Some torts are more common than others. You should know that the tort of battery is the most common one seen within the health care arena and possibly the easiest one to commit. Stop and think before making unwarranted contacts with patients.

3. Know that, in some limited circumstances, the absolute rights of the patient may be transgressed. Understand the full impact of the law in these limited areas, and seek legal guidance before transgressing the patient's rights.

4. Treat all patients with the same competent, courteous care that you would want for yourself and your loved ones.

5. Be particularly selective when answering questions about patients over the telephone. Recognize that patients have the right to refuse, unless there exists a state reporting statute to the contrary, to allow disclosure of details about their illness and prognosis to others, including close family members.

6. Be cautious of the patient who is also a public figure. Public figures, whether voluntarily placed before the public eye or not, are owed the same privacy and reputation rights as the private patient.

SUMMARY

Intentional torts, those willingly performed with knowledge and intent, occur in a variety of ways in health care settings. To avoid committing such torts, the nurse must first comprehend their importance at law, and then understand how easily (and frequently) they occur in clinical settings.

AFTER COMPLETING THIS CHAPTER, YOU SHOULD BE ABLE TO

- Define tort law.
- Define and differentiate between intentional and quasi-intentional torts.

- List the more commonly occurring intentional torts in health care settings and give an example of each.
- List the more commonly occurring quasi-intentional torts in health care settings and give an example of each.

APPLY YOUR LEGAL KNOWLEDGE

- How do intentional torts differ from negligence and malpractice?
- If a teaching session were to be given on intentional torts seen in clinical settings, which torts should be included? Would your answers differ if time were not limited and you could include additional materials?
- What can staff nurses do to protect patients against quasi-intentional torts?
- Does this differ from the nurse manager's role in preventing quasi-intentional torts?

REFERENCES

Anderson v. St. Francis-St. George Hospital, 614 N.E. 2d 841 (Ohio, 1992).

In the Matter of Baby K, 16 F.3d 590 (4th Cir.), cert. denied, 115 S.Ct. 91 (1994).

Baca v. Velez, 833 P.2d 1194 (App. New Mexico, 1992).

Barber v. Time, Inc., 348 Missouri 1199, 159 S.W. 2d 291 (1942).

Blackman v. Blackman for Rifkin, 759 P.2d 54 (Colo App., 1988), cert. denied (1988).

Doe v. Roe, 93 Misc. 2d 201, 400 N.Y.S. 2d. 958 (1978).

Farrell v. Kramer, 193 A. 2d 560 (Maine, 1963).

Foflygen v. R. Zemel, 615 A. 2d 1345 (Pennsylvania, 1992).

Keeton, W. P. (ed.) (1984). *Prosser and Keeton on the law of torts* (5th ed.). St. Paul, MN: West Publishing Company.

Loungbury v. Capel, 836 P.2d 188 (Utah, 1992).

Mohr v. Williams, 95 Minn 261, 104 N.W. 12 (1905).

Prince v. St. Francis-St. George Hospital, 484 N.E. 2d 265 (App. Ohio, 1985).

Schessler v. Keck, 271 P.2d 588 (California, 1954).

Schloendorff v. Society of New York Hospitals, 211 N.Y. 125, 105 N.E. 92 (1914).

Vessiliades v. Garfinkel's, Brooks Brothers, 492 A. 2d 580 (App. D.C., 1985).

Words and Phrases (1994). *Assault.* St. Paul, MN: West Publishing Company.

• seven

Nursing Liability: Defenses

PREVIEW

Health care providers are acutely aware of potential legal claims that may be filed against them. Much of this concern involves unknowns about the legal process and civil liability. But concern may also surface about possible defenses to lawsuits. This chapter explores possible legal defenses to nursing liability and how such defenses may lessen the individual practitioner's legal liability.

KEY CONCEPTS

defenses	abuse	assumption of the risk
consent	access	immunity
self-defense	qualified privilege	Good Samaritan laws
defense of others	release	statutes of limitations
necessity	exculpatory clause	products liability
truth	contribution (or comparative) negligence	collective liability
privilege		alternative liability
disclosure statutes	contributory negligence rule	

DEFENSES AGAINST LIABILITY

Several defenses are available to health care practitioners in the event that a legal claim or lawsuit is filed. *Defenses* are "arguments in support of or arguments used for justification" (Boyer et al., 1991, p. 198). Defenses may be based on statutory law, common law, or the doctrine of precedent. Defenses may also be classified according to the cause of action filed against them.

DEFENSES AGAINST INTENTIONAL TORTS

Some of the defenses against intentional torts include (1) consent, (2) self-defense, (3) defense of others, and (4) necessity.

TABLE 7–1. DEFENSES TO TORTS

Intentional Torts	Quasi-intentional Torts	Nonintentional Torts
Consent	Consent	Release
Self-defense	Truth	Contributory and comparative negligence
Defense of others	Privilege	Assumption of the risk
Necessity	Disclosure statutes	Immunity statutes
	Access laws	Statutes of limitations
	Duty to disclose laws	
	Qualified privilege	

Consent

Consent may be either oral, implied by law, or apparent. There can be no suit for a battery if the patient approved the touching. For example, Nurse Alicia is the medication nurse for a unit. She enters the patient's room with a syringe in one hand and an alcohol wipe in the other hand. As she enters the room she states, "Mr. Jones, I have your vitamin injection. In which arm would you prefer that I give it?" The patient extends his left arm and helps the nurse roll up his left sleeve with his right hand. *Apparent consent* has been given since the reasonable person would infer from the patient's conduct that he both understood what was said to him and that he consented to the injection.

Consent may also be *implied by law.* Many examples of implied consent occur in emergency settings. When the person is capable neither of giving nor of denying consent, the law adopts the granting of consent if the following four elements are met:

1. An immediate decision is made to prevent loss of life or limb.
2. The person is incapable of giving consent.
3. There is no reason to believe that consent would not be given if the patient was capable of such.
4. A reasonable person in the same or similar circumstances would give consent.

A more thorough discussion on consent may be found in Chapter 8.

Self-Defense and Defense of Others

Self-defense and *defense of others* may be justifiable to protect oneself and others in the area from harm. For example, a patient suddenly becomes combative, and there is imminent danger to the nursing staff as well as to other patients and visitors. The nurses are justified in forcibly restraining the patient, even though no order for restraints had been obtained. In such an example, the defense of others can be extended to include the defense of the patient as well. The caveat is that one can use only reasonable force, that which is necessary to prevent injury to oneself or to defend others in the situation.

In *Mattocks v. Bell* (1963), a landmark case in this area, a male medical student was allowed to strike a 23-month-old child on the cheek to free his finger from the child's mouth. In finding that no battery or assault occurred, the court concluded that no unnecessary force was used nor was the force applied inappropriately. The court did say, though, that it was not condoning the striking of the child. Information on the use of restraints is included in Chapter 13.

Necessity

Necessity, which is similar to self-defense, allows nurses to interfere with the patient's property rights to avoid threatened injury. For example, a suddenly combative patient approaches the staff with a knife or attempts to use a belt to strangle the nurse. This defense allows the nurse to take the knife or belt away from the patient. Thus, self-defense allows reasonable force against a person, while necessity allows the person's property to be confiscated. The caveat to remember is that a defense of necessity does not allow the nurse the right to search the patient's property. The defense of necessity mandates that the patient's property must be the threatening factor.

DEFENSES TO QUASI-INTENTIONAL TORTS

Consent

Consent may be a defense to the quasi-intentional torts of defamation and invasion of privacy as well as to the intentional torts. The nurse cannot be charged in a lawsuit with invasion of privacy if the patient allowed the nurse right of access to personal property. Consent does not need to be formal or well thought-out. Allowing a nurse to remove a nightgown from a piece of luggage would also constitute the patient's consent to notice a stash of drugs packed alongside the nightgown.

EXERCISE 7-1

A patient, who is suspected of being a drug substance abuser, asks the nurse to "Look in my shaving kit for my comb." While looking for the comb, the nurse sees a packet of a white, powdery substance. Thinking it might contain an illegal street drug, the nurse confiscates the packet. If the patient later brings suit for invasion of privacy for this occurrence, does the nurse have a valid defense? Would your answer change if, upon chemical analysis, no illegal drugs were found?

Truth

Truth is a valid defense against defamatory statements. Nurses should be aware that, in using this defense, the entire statement must be true and not merely parts of the statement. Someone who states that "Many patients have perished for want of her skill" must be able to show that the entire statement is truthful or face a possible defamation suit.

Truth may be a defense to defamatory statements, but may also lead to other torts such as invasion of privacy. Nurses, in proving the truth of a defamatory statement, may unwillingly make public facts that concern the nature of the patient's hospitalization or that the person was even a patient within a given setting. For example, for a nurse to prove that a specific patient was hospitalized for drug abuse, the nurse would need to divulge facts about the drug abuse that may invade the patient's privacy rights. As a practical matter this usually does not occur, since the injured party or patient forfeits this privacy right when filing the lawsuit.

Privilege

Privilege is another defense to defamation. *Privilege* is a disclosure that might ordinarily be defamatory under different circumstances, but that may be allowable to protect or further public or private interests recognized by law. Examples of privilege include the mandate to report persons with certain diagnoses or diseases or those suspected of abusing others.

Disclosure Statutes

Both federal and state laws compel disclosure of health-related information to proper agencies for the protection of the public. The reporting laws that exist require health care providers to be familiar not only with the types of information that must be disclosed, but also with the governmental agency requiring the information. The giving of required information is protected, and there may be liability for disclosing privileged information to the wrong governmental agency.

Disclosure statutes mandate the reporting of certain types of health-related information to protect the public at large. (Or a judge may mandate that certain information be disclosed by issuing a subpoena.) These statutes mandate that the health care providers or those standing in the place of health care providers voluntarily give the required information to the proper agency. The most common example of reporting statutes is vital statistics. All states require births and deaths to be reported, and a majority of states require an accounting of neonatal deaths and abortions.

Public health agencies may require a variety of disease states to be reported. Communicable and venereal diseases must be reported to protect the public. Additionally, some states require patients suffering from any type of seizure activity be reported to the state drivers' licensing agency. Cancer and other related diseases are to be reported in a handful of states.

If practitioners disclose only the limited information that they must disclose, there is no liability for the disclosure under either a defamation or invasion of privacy suit. These statutes therefore serve as a defense against both defamation and invasion of privacy.

Child abuse is reportable to child welfare offices and/or to other state designated offices. Such statutes usually require that suspected child abuse and suspected neglect be reported. *Abuse* incorporates physical, mental, and sexual assaults as well as physical, emotional, and medical neglect. Similar protection against abuse and neglect is currently being given adults in some states, particularly residents in nursing and convalescent homes.

Generally, nurses report any suspected cases through the administration of the institution. In most institutions, nurses report the suspected abuse to their immediate supervisors and treating physicians. All information concerning the notification is then documented in the patient's chart. Both civil and criminal liability may flow from the nonreport of such suspected cases, especially if further abuse or neglect occurs because of nondisclosure.

The landmark case of *Landeros v. Flood* (1976) held that a physician who fails to report suspected child abuse can be exposed for liability on the theory of medical malpractice. In that case, an 11-month-old was brought to the emergency center with a leg fracture. The fracture was the type for which a reasonable and careful physician would have started an investigation of possible abuse. Instead, the child was treated and released to her parents. Shortly afterwards, the child was admitted with severe and permanent injuries due to abuse. After being removed from her parents' care, this lawsuit was brought against the treating physician and health care institution.

In their findings, the court held that a hospital that, through its agents or employees, either knew or should have suspected that a child requiring care was a victim of abuse, and failed to report the case, could be held liable for the subsequent injuries done to the child by her abusers. The decision makes it clear that liability for failure to report suspected child abuse is a greater risk than reporting suspected child abuse that, upon investigation, proves to be erroneous.

Nurses could easily have been part of the *Landeros* case. Reporting laws grant immunity from prosecution to health care providers who do so in good faith and who report such violations to the correct governmental agency. This means that nurses who report a battered child to their supervisor and to the treating physician, following institution policy, have not violated the patient's or the parent's right of privacy. In fact, nurses are more open to liability if they fail to report the abuse. If the parents fail to assert the child's rights against the nurse for nondisclosure of abuse, the state child welfare agency could sue the nurse in a civil suit for the injuries inflicted on the child after the failure to disclose (*Kempster v. Child Protection Services of the Department of Social Services*, 1987).

Health care providers are protected when they report suspected child abuse, even if the subsequent investigation shows the report to be groundless. In *Heinrich v. Conemaugh Valley Memorial Hospital* (1994), a Pennsylvania Superior Court found that the hospital was immune for suit when a child abuse report, which later proved groundless, was filed. Pennsylvania's Child Protective Services Law mandates that suspected child abuse must be reported and that a plaintiff seeking to prove an injury resulting from a false report of abuse must show bad faith on the part of those reporting the suspected abuse. Courts presume good faith on the part of the health care providers unless that assumption is shown to be incorrect.

Remember, though, that violations of the statutes, even in good faith, may not protect the nurse from liability. In *Perez v. Bay Area Hospital* (1992), a child was examined in the emergency room for genital irritation. Medication was prescribed, the child instructed in proper hygiene, and a culture obtained. The child was discharged, and the culture came back negative for sexually transmitted diseases.

Two days later, the Oregon Children Services Division (CSD) received a phone call from an unnamed nurse at the defendant hospital, stating that the child had tested positive for gonorrhea. Later that day, a CSD employee and a local police officer went to the child's school, told the school secretary that there was reason to believe the child had been infected with a sexually transmitted disease, and the child was questioned. The child's mother was also questioned, in her home, by the CSD employee and the police officer. Later in the week, the mother was notified of the negative report by the defendant hospital.

The mother subsequently filed this cause of action, asserting that the CSD employee was "negligent in disclosing information and identifying misinformation." The court granted summary judgment for the defendants on the grounds that the CSD employee's disclosures were protected by the Oregon abuse reporting statutes.

On appeal, the mother argued that the CSD employee should have contacted the hospital independently to verify the report, and that failure to do so constitutes negligence. The defendants countered that the Oregon law requires that the CSD must immediately investigate reported abuse after receiving a report of suspected child abuse.

The trial court agreed with the plaintiffs and, had the case against the hospital been filed within the required statue of limitations, both the CSD employee and the defendant hospital would have been charged with negligence. Thus, very careful reporting of suspected abuse, according to the strict requirements of local and state law, is encouraged to prevent possible liability.

Access Laws

This group of statutory disclosure laws permits *access* to patient records and information without securing permission of the individual patient. The caveat is to know which individuals or agencies are allowed access to patient information. Workers' compensation statutes usually allow for access to medical records once a claim has been duly filed. If such a statute does not exist, the courts may rule that the filing of such a claim is a waiver under common law of the right of confidentiality in health-related information.

Access laws seldom involve staff and midmanagement nurses. Usually the medical records department and/or the administrative staff of the institution are apprised by the hospital attorney when charts may be accessed by law. Midmanagement nurses might become involved if access is sought to ongoing or current medical charts. This type of review of current records may be done in conjunction with the institution's Medicare and Medicaid reimbursement program. Before allowing access to medical records, nurses should take precautions. First, they should receive written confirmation of reviews from the hospital administration or the nursing service administration prior to the review. Then they should ascertain that the persons asking for access to the charts are the persons listed in the written confirmation, and ask for proof of identification as necessary. If any doubt persists concerning a chart review,

Guidelines: Disclosure Statutes

1. Know both federal and individual state laws concerning the duty to report versus privileges to access laws.

2. Report only the information that is required to the proper governmental agency, and ensure that others who have a duty to disclose health-related information do so promptly.

3. Reporting must be done in good faith (as with abuse statutes), and civil and criminal liability may be incurred for failure to report under a statutory duty to disclose.

4. With access laws, follow hospital policy carefully, and ensure that persons requesting access to medical records are allowed access by law. Ask for proper identification as needed.

5. If you work in home health care or community settings, you may be the only person with the first-hand information that is needed to file reports to the appropriate governmental agency.

6. Breach of confidentiality is usually considered unprofessional conduct and grounds for disciplinary action by the state board of nurse examiners. Report only the information required; no freedom from liability exists for information that was not required or for information that is given to other than the proper governmental agency.

nurses should contact their supervisors before allowing the charts to be seen. Finally, they should remain accessible to answer questions as needed. The reviewers may not clearly understand the system of charting, and nurses could be invaluable in interpreting the system to them.

Qualified Privilege

The defense of *qualified privilege* prevails when the person making the allegedly defamatory statements has a legal duty to do so, as in the instance where a nurse manager reports, in good faith, on the professional performance of a staff nurse. Qualified privilege legally negates any inference of malice because of the overriding public policy interest. When the quality of medical care is at issue, the reputation rights of health care professionals must concede to the greater social need.

Liability will not be imposed even if the communications are false as long as there is no malice and the communications are made in good faith to those persons with a need to know such facts. The court in *Wynn v. Cole* (1979) found no liability on the part of a director of a health department who provided a prospective employer with information concerning a specific nurse's abilities. Such privileged communications exist for assessments provided by former employers to prospective employers. The caveat to be watchful is threefold:

1. The communications must be made through appropriate channels to persons needing the information.
2. Liability may be granted for untruthful communications released with malice.
3. The communications should be worded in objective and observable behavioral terms rather than judgmental descriptions.

Defamation may be *mitigated* (lessened or reduced) by such factors as retraction (he or she did everything possible to rectify the previous statement) or by whether it was provoked or not. For example, the nurse may be provoked into a given statement by the anger and hostility aimed at the staff member by the patient or family. While not an excuse for the defamation, such mitigating factors may serve to lessen the damages awarded the plaintiff.

EXERCISE 7-2

Interview nurse managers in hospital and community settings about privileges and qualified privileges. How do the nurse managers use these doctrines in their respective clinical settings? Does one manager use one privilege more than another? Is there a trend in the use of privileges in the hospital versus community settings?

DEFENSES TO NONINTENTIONAL TORTS

Defenses to negligent actions include:

1. Release.
2. Contributory or comparative negligence.
3. Assumption of the risk.
4. Unavoidable accident.
5. Defense of the fact.
6. Immunity statutes.

Release

A *release* may be signed, during the settling of a claim, to prevent any and all future claims arising from the same incident. Once signed, the release bars (prohibits or prevents) future suits. In medical malpractice claims, a release is frequently a part of the out-of-court settlement. In effect the plaintiff states that the settlement is the only compensation for the negligent action.

Releases are distinguished from *exculpatory clauses* or *exculpatory contracts,* which are signed before care is given and seldom serve as a successful defense. Usually exculpatory contracts are signed to limit the amount of damages one receives in a suit or to prevent a future lawsuit based on the individual health care giver's actions. Such contracts usually fail on the grounds that they violate public policy. The court in *Cudnik v. William Beaumont Hospital* (1994) held that exculpatory agreements that completely release a hospital from liability for an employee's negligence, and that are signed by patients prior to receiving therapy, are against public policy and thus are invalid and unenforceable. The court further held that there are two exceptions to the rule invalidating exculpatory agreements for medical malpractice. One, experimental procedures are exempted as "they inherently require a deviation from generally accepted medical practices" (at 897). Two, agreements releasing medical care providers from liability after treatment, pursuant to a lawsuit settlement agreement, are valid and enforceable.

Contributory and Comparative Negligence

Contributory negligence and *comparative negligence* serve as defenses and in essence hold injured parties accountable for their fault in the injury. Fault by the plaintiff may occur for failure to follow prescribed treatments or for providing false information to the physician.

Many states once used an all-or-nothing *contributory negligence rule*: Patients who had any part in bringing about the adverse consequences were barred from receiving any compensation. Today most jurisdictions use comparative negligence and reduce the money award by the injured party's responsibility for the ultimate harm done. For example, in a $500,000 reward, if the plaintiff is found to be 30% responsible for the negligence, then the plaintiff is allowed a $350,000 award for damages. Some states further disallow compensation if the patient has 50% or greater responsibility in the ultimate harm done.

The court in *Parkins v. United States* (1993) held that the patient has a duty to conform reasonably to prescriptions and treatments and to follow reasonable and proper instructions given by health care providers. Failure to so conform will prevent recovery in a court of law.

Assumption of the Risk

A similar defense to contributory and comparative negligence is *assumption of the risk,* which states that plaintiffs are partially responsible for the consequences if they understood the risks involved when they proceeded with the action. Based on informed consent, this defense is further discussed in the next chapter.

Unavoidable Accident

This defense comes into play when nothing other than an accident could have caused the person's injury. For example, a staff member slips and falls in a patient's room. There is nothing on the floor that could have caused the accident and no one is at fault.

Defense of the Fact

This defense is used when there is no causation, direct or otherwise—no indication that the health care provider's actions were the cause of the patient's injury or untoward outcome. For example, the patient who receives an injection in the left arm and then experiences numbness and tingling in the right leg. The two events are not connected, and the defense to be plead is defense of the fact.

Immunity

Some states have enacted *immunity* statutes that serve to dismiss certain causes of action. The best example of a state immunity statute is the Good Samaritan statute. Because of the Good Samaritan laws, negligent actions against health care providers at scenes of accidents are rare.

Good Samaritan Laws

Legislation was at one time needed to encourage medical personnel to stop at the scene of an accident and to render appropriate medical care. In response to this need, all states have enacted **Good Samaritan laws,** which abrogate common law rescue doctrines in an effort to encourage health care providers to risk helping strangers in need of assistance, even when the health care providers have no duty to render such aid (*Jackson v. Mercy Health Center, Inc.,* 1993). While individual provisions of Good Samaritan laws vary greatly state to state, the laws have been instrumental in procuring necessary health care in emergency situations.

Good Samaritan laws are enacted to allow health care personnel and citizens trained in first aid to deliver needed medical care without unnecessary fear of incurring criminal and civil liability. The uniqueness of Good Samaritan laws is that they insulate health care practitioners from liability for rendering care at the scene of an accident.

Through such legislative acts, society, for its own good, has given health care providers immunity from negligent acts or omissions when acting as Good Samaritans at the scene of an emergency. State legislators have long recognized that persons who stop and render emergency care should be a protected class.

Dispute exists, however, over which persons should be protected and the extent to which the protection extends. Some states extend protection merely to licensed health care providers. Other states allow ordinary citizens to be covered under the legislation along with licensed health care providers. A newer trend is for states to mandate emergency assistance. Vermont was the first state to enact such a law requiring persons to assist others when exposed to grave physical harm as long as the assistance can be given without endangering themselves. Reasonable assistance should be given, and violation of the statute is punishable by fines (*Vermont Statutes Annotated,* 1968).

The need for Good Samaritan laws becomes apparent because there is generally no legal duty to render assistance to strangers in times of distress, unless so mandated by statute, or unless the individual just caused the stranger's distress. While one could argue that a moral or ethical duty should exist, no legal duty arises until the individual first initiates the giving of emergency care. Then the legal duty becomes one of reasonable or emergency care. Only when a person renders grossly negligent or wilful and wanton negligent care is the health care provider not protected by the Good Samaritan immunity. As a practical matter, malpractice suits against Good Samaritans are relatively rare.

Before proceeding under a Good Samaritan law, nurses must recognize that the acts vary greatly among states. Consequently, they must be aware of exactly what is covered by an individual state act. Nurses should look for the following information when reviewing an individual state act:

1. Who is covered as part of the protected class? Some states cover all persons who give emergency care, some cover only physicians and nurses, and a few state acts cover only in-state physicians and nurses.
2. Where does the coverage extend? All state acts allow for aid at the scene of the accident, emergency, or disaster, with some states mandating that such accidents, emergencies, or disasters be roadside occurrences. Other states allow for emergency care wherever the need is, be it in a hospital, doctor's office, or outside a medically equipped place. Still other states specifically limit coverage under Good Samaritan laws to areas outside the workplace. The nurse must know what qualifies as the scene of an emergency before rendering aid under the Good Samaritan laws.
3. What is covered? Some states protect the individual during transportation to a medical facility. Another group of states protect against failure to provide for further assistance.

Most states require that the care be given in good faith and that the care be gratuitous. Unfortunately, the acts may not define criteria to determine whether or not an emergency actually exists and what constitutes the scene of an emergency. Because of this, protection is uncertain in some states. To limit nurses' liability and allow them to participate in rendering needed care, they should adhere to the following guidelines (see chart page 105).

EXERCISE 7-3

Examine your state's Good Samaritan statutes. Are all health care providers included in the statutes? Are other qualified persons covered? How does the statute ensure that persons needing assistance will receive the needed help?

Guidelines: Good Samaritan Laws

1. Make your decision quickly as to whether or not you will stay and help. Remember that there is no common law duty to stop and render aid. Once you begin to provide care, you incur the legal duty to maintain a standard of reasonable emergency care.

2. Ask the injured person or family members for permission to help. Do not force your services if refused.

3. Care for the injured party where you can do so safely. This includes in the vehicle or at the exact site where the victim is found. Move the injured party only if you must do so without causing further harm and as needed to prevent further harm (eg, off a major highway).

4. Apply the rules of first aid: assess for and prevent bleeding, assess for the need to initiate cardiopulmonary resuscitation, cover the injured party with a blanket or coat, and so forth.

5. Continuously assess and reassess the person for additional injuries, and communicate findings of your assessment to the person or family members.

6. Have someone call or go for additional help while you stay with the injured party.

7. Stay with the person until equally or more qualified help arrives. Prevent unskilled persons from treating or moving the injured party.

8. Give as complete a description as possible of the care that you have rendered to the police and emergency medical personnel so that continuity of care exists. Give family members or police any personal items such as dentures, eyeglasses, and the like.

9. Do not accept any compensation (eg, money or gifts) offered by the injured party or family members. Acceptance of compensation may change your care into a fee-for-service situation and cause you to lose your Good Samaritan protection.

10. Should you choose not to stop and render aid, stop at the nearest phone and report the accident to proper authorities so that the injured party may be aided.

11. Review legislative actions periodically for any changes in your state's Good Samaritan laws. Know the Good Samaritan laws in other states before giving assistance.

STATUTE OF LIMITATIONS

Statutes of limitations specify time limits for initiating claims. Unless specific exceptions apply, a suit must be filed within the time limit or the cause of action is barred (prohibited by law). Typically individual states allow one to two years to file a malpractice suit: Injured parties must bring the suit within one to two years after they knew of the injury or had reason to believe that an injury was sustained. In the case of a minor, the statute of limitations may not begin to run (start) until the child reaches the age of majority, although a few states restrict this tolling (stoppage) of statutes of limitations until children reach their majority (Aiken and Catalano, 1994).

A case example involving statutes of limitations shows how it can be a valid defense in malpractice cases. In *Weathers v. Fulgenzi* (1994), an action was brought against a psychiatrist and a psychiatric clinic for professional malpractice. The patient was seen by Dr. Fulgenzi during the years 1981–1983. In 1989, she filed this malpractice action, and the trial court granted summary judgment to Dr. Fulgenzi and the psychiatric clinic because the two-year statute of limitations had expired in 1985 and no intervening events had occurred to toll the statute of limitation to a later date.

PRODUCTS LIABILITY

Products liability refers to the liability of a manufacturer, processor, or non-manufacturing seller for injury to a person or person's property by a given product. Under this type of action, the injured party may sue the maker of the product, the seller of the product, the intermediary distributors of the product, or all three entities. The landmark and leading case for imposing liability in this area of the law, irrespective of fault, is *Caprara v. Chrysler Corporation* (1981). In that case, the court declared that "the one in the best position to know of potential dangers and to have eliminated the same should respond to the injured party in damages" (at 124).

Theories of recovery for such products liability suits are based on either breach-of-warranty liability or strict liability. Under *breach-of-warranty liability,* the patient contends that the manufacturer or others in the chain of distribution breached either an expressed or implied warranty of fitness of the product. In a *strict liability action*, the plaintiff contends that the product is unreasonably dangerous due to a defect in its manufacture or design or due to inadequate labeling (*Corpus Juris Secundum*, 1984).

This area of law is really a mixture of tort and contract law. The expressed and implied warranties of fitness for a particular purpose and of merchantability are based in contract law. Tort law concerns the liability of a person in a civil action against the person or property of another and the violation of a duty owed the injured party. The warranties (from contract law) form the basis for finding liability without fault (from tort law) for injuries caused by the use of products.

The first hurdle for the plaintiff in products liability cases is to prove that a product has been sold rather than a service delivered. The distinction is crucial because a products liability action does not exist if there is no sale of a product. Some courts have held there was no responsibility since there was service, not the sale of a product (*North Miami General Hospital v. Goldberg*, 1993), while other courts have suggested that the hospital owes a higher duty of care to the patient since the patient has no voice in the equipment or products used (Fiesta, 1994).

A second issue for products liability cases concerns defining products as opposed to services. A product has been defined as a "thing produced by labor" or "something produced by nature or the natural process" (Boyer et al., 1991, p. 492). For years debate has centered around blood transfusions and whether they are the products or the services of a hospital. While some initial cases determined that blood transfusions were products for purposes of products liability cases, all jurisdictions, either by decisional law or by legislative statutes, have determined that blood transfusions by a hospital are a service incident to treatment and not a product sold by the hospital (Werthmann, 1984). More recent developments in this area concern whether a blood bank is a health care provider for purposes of statutes of limitations. In *Smith v. Paslode Corporation* (1993), the eighth circuit held that a blood bank was a health care provider in that the blood bank "provides health care services under the authority of a license or certification" (at 3). This minority opinion illustrates the difficulty courts have with determining the status of blood banks and blood products.

Along the same line, a series of court decisions determined that radiation treatments were services and not products, and that the dangers of the radiation treatment are not inherent in the radiation itself but result from (1) the professional medical decision to employ radiation therapy, (2) the manner in which it is administered, and (3) the amount given (*Dubin v. Michael Reese Hospital and Medical Center*, 1980).

A third issue concerns *unavoidably unsafe products*. To be considered unavoidably unsafe, a product must contain the following three criteria:

1. Its benefits must greatly outweigh its risks.
2. Its risks cannot be eliminated.
3. No safer product exists as an alternative.

If these three elements are proven, the manufacturer will be held liable only for injuries if there was failure to adequately warn of the risks. Prescription drugs usually are considered unavoidably unsafe, and case law concerns negligence for failure of inadequate warning rather than for product liability. One of the more interesting cases to date, *Detwiler v. Bristol-Meyers Squibb Company* (1995), has found liability against a physician who implanted a silicone breast implant. While the majority of the decision concerned statutes of limitations, the court held that silicone implants failed to meet the standard of unavoidably unsafe.

But contrast the preceding holding with the holding in *King v. Collagen Corporation* (1993). In that case, the plaintiff was denied damages for injuries caused by the antiwrinkle cream Zyderm because the corporation had submitted to and passed a rigorous premarket approval process required by the Federal Drug Authority. Thus the corporation was allowed a safe harbor from such claims as negligent design, failure to warn, and breach of warranty. This case may reopen this entire line of legal thought.

As a general rule, proper warning to the physician satisfies the drug manufacturer's duty to warn, since patients can obtain the drug only through the physician. Exceptions to this requirement, when the patient must be directly warned (such as through mass media newspaper communications) include situations in which (1) the drug may be given without an individual prescription (eg, with mass inoculation for polio), and (2) Federal Food and Drug Administration regulations require package inserts (*Lukaszewicz v. Ortho Pharmaceutical Corporation*, 1981). Newer state laws require that pharmacists have this same duty to warn when prescriptions are filled for individual patients.

Nurses' duty to warn patients of unavoidably unsafe prescription medications has not been delineated in the majority of jurisdictions, but it would seem reasonable to anticipate that their duty to warn will be incorporated into patient discharge education. Advanced nurse practitioners and nurses who, by legislative enactments, may prescribe medications are considered to have the same duty to warn as the physicians who prescribe medications.

COLLECTIVE AND ALTERNATIVE LIABILITY

Currently two theories are emerging to aid plaintiffs who previously could not prove which manufacturer was at fault. *Collective liability* stems from cooperation by several manufacturers in a wrongful activity that by its nature requires the participation of more than one wrongdoer (concert of action). All the wrongdoers' actions result in an inadequate industry-wide standard of safety as to the manufacture of a product (*enterprise liability*). *Alternative liability* applies when two or more manufacturers commit separate, wrongful or unreasonable acts, only one of which injures the plaintiff, but the plaintiff cannot identify the actual cause-in-fact defendant.

These theories rapidly emerged in light of the diethylstilbestrol (DES) lawsuits. Women who were injured by the drug directly and through their offspring attempted to sue manufacturers for failing to adequately test and label the drug and thus to warn of its risks. But it was virtually impossible to identify the manufacturer of the particular DES they took. This occurred because of (1) inadequate long-term record keeping by pharmacies, (2) the widespread practice of prescribing generic drugs, and (3) the failure of the DES tablets to identify the manufacturer. Under the newer liability theories, injured women and their daughters gained compensation for the industry's failure to adequately test the drug on fetuses and to warn of its risks. (See generally *Abel v. Eli Lilly and Company*, 1984, and *Collins v. Eli Lilly and Company*, 1984).

CAVEATS IN PRODUCT LIABILITY LAWSUITS

Before deciding that a products liability action exists, several points need to be comprehended and remembered:

1. States often follow strict liability in medical or health-related causes of actions. Not to allow a strict liability cause of action would place an unfair burden on the plaintiff. Indeed, even with such a cause of action, compensation has been denied persons injured in the health care settings.
2. For a products liability cause of action to exist in most jurisdictions, the defendant must be a commercial supplier or be determined to be a commercial supplier.
3. The cause of action must be based on a sold product and not a service, or no action will exist under products liability.
4. There may also be a negligence cause of action. If the defendant passes all the hurdles and successfully defends against a products liability cause of action, the plaintiff may still be able to prove negligence.

EXERCISE 7-4

Think of all the equipment and products that you use daily in the care of clients. Think of all the pharmaceutical agents that you give to patients during the course of an average day or shift. What precautions do you take to further ensure the safe, competent care of clients?

SUMMARY

Defenses are available to health care providers to justify or partially explain their actions. Defenses explored in this chapter include those against intentional, quasi-intentional, and negligent torts, statutes of limitations, and product liability. Used correctly, these defenses can lessen the individual practitioner's potential liability.

AFTER COMPLETING THIS CHAPTER, YOU SHOULD BE ABLE TO

- Define the term "defenses," and give examples of defenses that may be used against intentional torts, quasi-intentional torts, and negligent torts.
- Explain the concept of statute of limitations, including the importance of this statute in the health care field.
- Define and explain products liability defenses.

APPLY YOUR LEGAL KNOWLEDGE

- Which of the available defenses are commonly used by professional nurses? Why?
- How do statutes of limitations protect professional nurse defendants? Do they also protect the injured parties?
- Can product liability defenses prevent injured parties from showing negligence and liability against professional nurse practitioners?

REFERENCES

Abel v. Eli Lilly Company, 343 N.W. 2d 164 (Michigan, 1984).

Aiken, T. D. and Catalano, J. T. (1994). *Legal, ethical, and political issues in nursing.* Philadelphia: F. A. Davis Company.

Boyer, M., Ellis, K., Harris, D. R., and Soukhanov, A. H. (Eds.). (1991). *The American heritage dictionary* (2nd ed.). Boston: Houghton Mifflin Company.

Caprara v. Chrysler Corporation, 52 N.Y. 2d 114 (New York, 1981).

Collins v. Eli Lilly Company, 342 N.W. 2d 37 (Wisconsin, 1984).

Corpus Juris Secundum (1984). 72 Products Liability.

Cudnick v. William Beaumont Hospital, 525 N.W. 2d 891 (Mich. Ct. App., 1994).

Detwiler v. Bristol-Meyers Squibb Company, 884 F. Supp. 117 (DSNY, 1995).

Dorney v. Harris, 482 F. Supp. 323 (D. Colo., 1980).

Dubin v. Michael Reese Hospital and Medical Center, 393 N.E. 2d 588 (Ill. App., 1979), rev'd. 415 N.E. 2d 350 (Illinois, 1980).

Fiesta, J. (1994). *20 legal pitfalls for nurses.* Albany, NY: Delmar Publishers.

Flower's Case, Cro. Car. 211, 79 Eng. Rept. 785 (1632).

Goetzman v. Wichern, 327 N.W. 2d 742 (Iowa, 1982).

Heinrich v. Conemaugh Valley Memorial Hospital, 648 A. 2d 53 (Pennsylvania, 1994).

Jackson v. Mercy Health Center, Inc., 884 P. 2d 839 (Oklahoma, 1993).

Kempster v. Child Protective Services of the Department of Social Services, 515 N.Y.S. 2d 807 (New York, 1987).

King v. Collagen Corporation, No. 92-1278, 1993 US App., LEXIS 432 (1st Cir., January 15, 1993).

Landeros v. Flood, 551 P.2d 389, 17 Cal.3d 399 (California, 1976).

Lukaszewicz v. Ortho Pharmaceutical Corporation, 510 F. Supp. 961 (E.D. Wisc., 1981).

Mattocks v. Bell, 194 P.2d 307 (D.C. App., 1963).

McKee v. Moore, 648 P.2d 21 (Oklahoma, 1982).

North Miami General Hospital v. Goldberg, No. 87-337 (Fla. App. Ct., February 23, 1993).

Parkins v. United States, 834 F. Supp. 569 (D. Conn., 1993).

Perez v. Bay Area Hospital, 829 P.2d 700 (Or. App., 1992).

Probst v. Albert Einstein Medical Center, 440 N.Y.S. 2d 2 (App. Div., 1981).

Providence Hospital v. Truly, 611 S.W. 2d 127 (Tex. App., 1980).

Racer v. Utterman, 629 S.W. 2d 387 (Mo. App., 1981).

Richard v. Southwest Louisiana Hospital Association, 383 So. 2d 83 (La. App., 1980).

72 Corpus Juris Secundum Supp. (1975). Products Liability, p. 10.

Smith v. Paslode Corporation, WL 392245 (8th Cir., 1993).

Tatham v. Hoke, 469 F. Supp. 914 (W.D. N.C., 1979).

Thomas v. St. Joseph Hospital, 618 S.W. 2d 791 (Tex. App., 1981).

Vermont Statutes Annotated, Title 12, Sec. 519 (1968).

Weathers v. Fulgenzi, 884 P.2d 538 (Oklahoma, 1994).

Werthmann, B. (1984). *Medical malpractice law: How medicine is changing the law.* Lexington, MA: Lexington Books.

Wynn v. Cole, 284 N.W. 2d 144 (Mich. App., 1979).

· eight

Informed Consent and Patient Self-Determination

PREVIEW

In the past, informed consent was a matter concerning the patient and the physician, a concept capable of being delegated to the nurse as the physician thought best. Too often the consent was automatic and uninformed. Patients and their loved ones allowed the paternalistic health care system to do as it saw fit and asked far too few questions. Fortunately this trend has changed, and nurses must understand the concept of informed consent to ensure that patient consent is truly valid and informed. Extensions of the concept of informed consent are patients' rights in research and patient self-determination. This chapter explores the essential characteristics of consent, the power to consent, requirements for patients' consent in research, and patient self-determination through living wills and durable power of attorney for health care.

KEY CONCEPTS

consent	waiver	living will
informed consent	competency at law	natural death act
informed refusal	legal guardian or representative	durable power of attorney for health care (DPAHC)
expressed consent		
implied consent	minor	medical durable power of attorney (MDPA)
standards of disclosure	in loco parentis	
reasonable or prudent patient standard	court order	medical or physician directive
	right of refusal	do not resuscitate directives
medical disclosure laws	patient self-determination	hospice center
therapeutic privilege	substituted judgment	assisted suicide

ROLE OF CONSENT

Generally the health care provider's right to treat a patient, barring true emergency conditions or unanticipated happenings, is based on a contractual relationship that arises through the mutual consent of parties to the relationship. *Consent* is the voluntary authorization by a patient or the patient's legal representative to do something to the patient. Consent is based on the mutual consent of all parties involved, and the key to true and valid consent is patient comprehension.

Consent becomes an important issue from a legal perspective in that patients may sue for a battery (unconsented touching) if they do not consent to the procedure or treatment and the health care provider goes ahead with the procedure or treatment. This means that patients may bring a lawsuit and be awarded damages even if they were helped by the procedure or treatment. The more current trend, though, is to argue consent under a negligence or malpractice cause of action.

Consent is an issue in its own realm. Consent does not always become a factor in a malpractice suit, although it may be a concurrent issue in a malpractice suit. Consent concerns the health care provider's right to treat an individual, not the manner in which the treatment was delivered. Thus one can deliver safe, competent care and still be sued for lack of consent.

The right to consent and the right to refuse consent are based on a long recognized, common law right of persons to be free from harmful or offensive touching of their bodies. In a landmark case during the early part of this century, the court declared the reason for consent, and that case is still quoted today when referring to the consent doctrine. "Every human being of adult years has a right to determine what shall be done with his own body, and a surgeon who performs an operation without his patient's consent commits an assault for which he is liable in damages" (*Schloendorff v. Society of New York Hospitals,* 1914, p. 93).

Thus two concepts are involved: (1) the prevention of a battery and (2) the person's right to control what is done to his or her body. Because of these rights, the health care provider has a duty to obtain consent prior to treating a patient. Consent therefore is not contingent on a request for information or clarification by the patient but must be actively sought by the health care practitioner.

CONSENT VERSUS INFORMED CONSENT

Consent, technically, is an easy yes or no. "Yes, I will allow the surgery" or "No, I want to try medications first, then maybe I will allow the surgery." Patients may not understand or may understand only vaguely what they are allowing.

The law concerning consent in health care situations is based on *informed consent,* which mandates to the physician or independent health care practitioner the separate legal duty to disclose needed material facts in terms that patients can reasonably understand so that they can make informed choices. There should also be a description of the available alternatives to the proposed treatment, along with the risks and dangers involved in each alternative. Failure to disclose the needed facts in understandable terms does not negate the consent, but it does place potential liability on the practitioner for negligence. In other words, without any consent given, the practitioner may be sued for a battery (an intentional tort). Without informed consent, practitioners open themselves to potential lawsuits for negligence.

The doctrine of informed consent has developed from negligence law as the courts began to realize that, while consent may have been given, not enough information was imparted to form the foundation of an informed decision. The right to informed consent did not become a judicial issue until 1957. In a landmark decision, the California courts found a doctor negligent for failing to explain the potential risks of a vascular procedure to a patient who was subsequently paralyzed by the procedure (*Salgo v. Leland Stanford, Jr., University Board of Trustees,* 1957).

Some courts have extended the right to informed consent to what might be called *informed refusal.* The practitioner may be liable for failure to inform the patient of the risks of not consenting to a therapy or diagnostic screening test. *Truman v. Thomas* (1980) was one of the first cases to recognize this important corollary to informed consent. In that case, the court awarded damages against a physician for failure to inform the patient of the potential risks of not consenting to a recommended Papanicolaou (Pap) smear.

INCLUSIONS IN INFORMED CONSENT

To be informed, patients must receive, in terms they can understand and comprehend, the following information:

1. A brief, but complete explanation of the treatment or procedure to be performed.
2. The name and qualifications of the person to perform the procedure and, if others will assist, the names and qualifications of those assistants.
3. An explanation of any serious harm that may occur during the procedure, including death if that is a realistic outcome. Pain and discomforting side effects that may occur during the procedure and following the procedure should also be discussed.
4. An explanation of alternative therapies to the procedure of treatment, including the risk of doing nothing at all.
5. An explanation that patients can refuse the therapy or procedure without having alternative care or support discontinued.
6. The fact that patients can still refuse, even after the procedure or therapy has begun. For example, all of the radiation treatments need not be completed.

TYPES OF INFORMED CONSENT

Consent may be obtained in a variety of ways. Consent may be expressed or implied, written or oral, complete or partial.

Perhaps the easiest means of obtaining informed consent is when the consent is expressed. *Expressed consent* is consent given by direct words, written or oral. For example, after the nurse informs the patient that he or she is going to start an intravenous infusion, the patient says, "Okay, but could you put the needle in my left hand, since I am right-handed?" As a rule, expressed consent is the type most often sought and received by health care providers.

Implied consent is consent that may be inferred by the patient's conduct or that which may legally be presumed in emergency situations. Implied consent has its foundation in the classic case of *O'Brien v. Cunard Steamship Company* (1899). In that case, a ship's female passenger joined a line of people receiving vaccinations. She neither questioned nor refused the injection. In fact, she willingly held out her arm for the vaccination. Later she unsuccessfully brought suit for battery.

In the preceding example, rather than saying that he or she would allow an intravenous infusion to be started, suppose the patient merely extended a left arm and said nothing. The reasonable practitioner would infer from the conduct that the patient both understood the therapy and consented by action. Implied consent is frequently obtained by health care practitioners for minor procedures and routine care.

Implied consent may be presumed to exist in true emergency situations. For such consent, patients must not be able to make their wishes known, and a delay in providing care would result in the loss of life or limb. An important element in allowing emergency consent is that health care providers have no reason to know or believe that consent would not be given were the patient able to deny consent. For example, the health care provider may not wait until the patient loses consciousness to order treatment that the patient had previously refused, such as a blood transfusion for a known Jehovah's Witness patient.

Consent may be *implied by law,* as in the instance where the patient is a minor and the parent or state, standing in the place of a parent, consents to treatment. The law implies the minor's consent for the treatment.

Consent may be given *orally* or may be reduced to *writing.* Unless state law mandates written consent, the law views oral and written consent as equally valid. As a precaution, health care providers should recognize that oral consent is much more difficult to prove should consent or lack of consent become a legal issue. As a convenience and to prevent such court issues, most health care institutions require written consent.

Consent may be *partial or complete.* Patients may authorize the entire treatment or procedure or only part of the proposed therapy. For instance, if the patient authorizes a breast biopsy but refuses to sign the consent form for a mastectomy based on the biopsy results, only a biopsy may be performed. The health care practitioner would then need to have a separate consent form signed before performing the mastectomy, should such surgery prove necessary.

STANDARDS OF INFORMED CONSENT

The various jurisdictions apply **standards of disclosure** for informed consent in one of three manners. These tests or standards of disclosure have evolved to assure that patients are informed in their decisions and to allow a means of determining the adequacy of the disclosure.

The majority of states use a *medical community* standard, sometimes referred to as the reasonable medical practitioner standard. This standard evolved from the landmark *Karp v. Cooley* (1974) decision and is based on a model of medical paternalism. The standard requires that the medical or independent practitioner "disclose facts which a reasonable medical practitioner in a similar community and of the same school of medical thought would have disclosed regarding the proposed treatment" (*Karp v. Cooley,* 1974, p. 411). This standard is fluid and changing, based on the prevailing medical thought and community, and is established at court through expert medical witness testimony. Generally, the patient must be told about inherent risks, but not necessarily unexpected risks that could occur after the treatment or procedure is initiated. Disclosure must include serious injuries that could occur, and courts favor more rather than less facts for full disclosure.

The last two tests involve the **reasonable** (or **prudent**) **patient standard.** One test, an *objective patient standard,* is based on disclosure of risks and benefits as determined by the needs of what a prudent person in the given patient's position would deem material. Thus this standard is also known as the *pru-*

dent patient standard or *material risk standard*. Material facts are factors that may make a significant difference to the reasonable and prudent patient. It is imperative that the person has enough information on which to make a decision, including material risks (*Joswick v. Lenox Hill Hospital*, 1986; *Arato v. Avedon*, 1993). The court in *Korman v. Mallin* (1993) stated that the "determination of materiality is a two-step process: (1) defining that existence and nature of the risk and the likelihood of occurrence; and (2) whether the probability of that type of harm is a risk which a reasonable patient would consider" (at 1149).

The second reasonable patient standard is based on a *subjective patient standard*, or the individual patient standard, which requires full disclosure that a particular patient, rather than a reasonable person, would have wanted to know. The fact finder must determine what risks were or were not material to the patient's decision with respect to the treatment accepted or refused. No expert testimony is required on the scope of disclosure, although such expert testimony may be required to establish risks and alternatives to therapy. Only a handful of states have adopted this standard.

Some states have attempted to bypass the three tests of disclosure by statutorily defining what must be disclosed to a patient prior to therapy or surgery. These **medical disclosure laws** mandate that certain risks and consequences be printed on the face of the consent form in language that the patient can be reasonably expected to understand.

Some states have adopted no one standard for disclosure, but rely on individual case-by-case analysis, while others restrict informed consent to certain types of procedures such as operative or surgical procedures (*Jones v. Philadelphia College of Osteopathic Medicine*, 1993). A newer collaborative model for informed consent has been proposed by Piper (1994). This new standard proposes that the patient and physician define jointly what informed consent means to them. Such a standard would assign at least four responsibilities to patients: (1) to communicate their values and expectations of treatment to the physician; (2) to ask questions and seek clarification in patient–physician discussions; (3) to evaluate symptoms and report subjective impressions of how well treatment is satisfying their individual goals and values; and (4) to make reasonably good faith efforts to participate appropriately in treatment (Piper, 1994, p. 310).

Arguments for standards of full disclosure center on four key points:

1. Patients actually assume all the risks since their bodies and lives are ultimately affected.
2. Informed consent mandates increased communications between the patient and the health care provider. With increased communications, one is less apt to violate the informed consent standards, and one is more likely to fully answer patients' questions.
3. Informed consent creates better health awareness by the consumer and ultimately encourages better health care practices.

4. Informed consent increases the quality of medical care because the health care provider is forced to explain all risks and benefits of the proposed procedure and to outline alternatives for the patient, thus selecting the best type and quality of care needed.

To bring a successful malpractice suit based on informed consent, the plaintiff must be able to prove, by a preponderance of the evidence, all of the following:

1. There was a duty on the part of the physician to know of a risk or alternative treatment.
2. There was a duty on the part of the physician to disclose the risk or alternative treatment.
3. There was a breach of the duty to disclose.
4. If the case is in a reasonable patient standard jurisdiction, a reasonable person in the plaintiff's position would not have consented to the treatment if he or she had known of the outstanding risk.
5. The undisclosed risk caused the harm or the harm would not have occurred if an alternative treatment plan was selected.
6. The plaintiff suffered damages.

EXERCISE 8-1

Explore your own state requirements for standards of informed consent. How did you go about discovering these standards? Do elective procedures and emergency situations use the same standard of informed consent?

EXCEPTIONS TO INFORMED CONSENT

The courts recognize four exceptions to the need for informed consent in circumstances in which consent is still required. These include:

1. Emergency situations.
2. Therapeutic privilege.
3. Patient waiver.
4. Prior patient knowledge.

From a practitioner standpoint, consent is still needed to prevent charges of a battery, but the informed consent requirements are eased.

Emergencies give rise to implied consent. Some courts have recognized that if there is time to give information, a limited disclosure may be valid. If no time exists or if the patient is incapable of understanding by virtue of the physical disability, then no information need be given.

Therapeutic privilege, which has its origins in the common law defense of necessity, allows primary health care providers to withhold information and any disclosures that they feel would be detrimental to the patient's health. The detrimental nature of the information must be more than fear that the information would lead to the patient's refusal. It must be a recognized and documented increased anxiety in the patient. Physicians, in using this exception, must be able to show that full disclosure of material facts would be likely to (1) hinder or complicate necessary treatment, (2) cause severe psychological harm, or (3) be so upsetting as to render a rational decision by the patient impossible (Rozovsky, 1990).

Therapeutic privilege is not favored by the courts and comes into play only when the patient is severely and emotionally disturbed and the current medical status presents an imminent danger to the patient's life. Some courts have held that a relative must concur with the patient decision to consent and that the relative must be given full disclosure, while other courts have held no relative need give concurrent consent. Once the risk to the patient has abated, the physician or independent practitioner must fully disclose the previously withheld information to the patient.

The patient may also agree to a *waiver* of the right to full disclosure and still consent to the procedure. The caveat to be avoided in this instance is that the health care provider cannot suggest such waiver. The waiver, to be valid, must be initiated by the patient.

Prior patient knowledge involves patients to whom the risks and benefits were fully explained the first time they consented to the procedure. Liability does not exist for nondisclosure of risks that are public or common knowledge or that patients had previously experienced.

ACCOUNTABILITY FOR OBTAINING INFORMED CONSENT

The physician or independent practitioner has the responsibility for obtaining informed consent (*Petriello v. Kalman et al.,* 1990). Individual hospitals have no responsibility for obtaining informed consent unless (1) the physician or independent practitioner is an employee or agent of the hospital, or (2) the hospital knew or should have known of the lack of informed consent and took no action. Court cases and individual state statutes have repeatedly upheld this last principle.

The institution or hospital becomes responsible for informed consent only if those primarily responsible for ensuring that informed consent is obtained are employed by the hospital or institution or only if the hospital fails to take appropriate actions when informed consent is not obtained and the hospital is aware of that omission (*Lincoln v. Gupta,* 1985, and Cushing, 1991). In *Lincoln,* the court concluded that the patient should discuss risks of procedures with the physician, who "is the best person to inform the patient about the procedure and where to obtain proper services and facilities" (at 315).

Attorneys argue both sides of the accountability issue as it relates to the hospital or institution. However, most providers in the medical profession feel that allowing liability, and thus allowing the hospital to monitor consult procedures and the actual disclosure of material facts on which to base informed consent, would destroy the professional relationship with the patient.

Nurses' Roles in Obtaining Consent

Nurses who are not independent practitioners may become involved in obtaining informed consent in one of several ways. Given that consent must be obtained for all procedures and treatments, not just for medical procedures, one realizes the vast impact of this doctrine. This does not mean that nurses obtain written consent each time they give an injection or turn a patient. Most nursing interventions rely on oral expressed consent or implied consent that may be readily inferred through the patient's actions.

What the doctrine of informed consent means is that nurses must continually communicate with patients, explaining procedures and obtaining their permission. What it also means is that patients' refusal to allow a certain procedure must be respected. Know the state laws on allowing patients to refuse life-sustaining treatment. Even if they validly refuse life-sustaining treatment, nurses could face charges for honoring or failing to honor this request. Each state has its own laws and applications of the laws. If patients are unable to communicate, permission may be derived from their admission to the hospital or obtained from their legal representatives.

A very real concern for nurses is in obtaining consent for the nursing aspects of medical procedures in which the primary procedure is performed by another practitioner. An example of such a concern is with postoperative care. Should the patient be taught about postoperative care before surgery, or should the nurse wait until after the surgery has been performed? Who is responsible for teaching postoperative care—the primary practitioner or the nursing staff? The answers from a legal perspective are far from clear. Possibly the best way to handle this dilemma is for the nurse to wait until after the patient has consented to the surgical procedure to give postoperative care information. This approach prevents interference with the physician–patient relationship and avoids potential conflicting explanations. Another approach is to have postoperative teaching materials and films developed to orient the patient to the entire procedure. This approach may be augmented by having a nurse available for questions or clarifications as needed. Many hospitals have implemented this approach with major procedures and operations such as heart catheterizations, vascular arteriography, and open heart surgery.

A third area of concern for nurses is in obtaining informed consent for medical procedures provided completely by another practitioner. This obvious area of concern was perhaps the first one identified by most nurses. For years, nurses have been the health care providers obtaining the patient's consent for surgical or medical therapies performed by physicians. Some hospitals continue to permit nurses to obtain the patient's signature on the consent form. Other hospitals, to avoid this potential liability, prohibit nurses from obtaining signatures on consent forms.

Nurses must understand that physicians may legally delegate the responsibility of obtaining the patient's informed consent to the nurse. Physicians delegate this task at their own peril, for most medical practice acts hold that the physician is the responsible party for obtaining informed consent. Thus any deficiencies in the informed consent as obtained by the nurse may be imputed back to the responsible physician. Nurses so delegated act in the role of the physician or independent practitioner, and they must ensure that all material information is given to patients in language that they can understand. Therefore nurses may incur potential liability along with the delegating physician for the patient's informed consent (*Hoffson v. Orentreisch*, 1989). Any additional information that the patient requests should be supplied by the physician, and the nurse is well advised to contact the physician immediately rather than attempt to talk a reluctant patient into the proposed procedure.

Some hospitals have begun to prohibit the medical practitioner from delegating the accountability for obtaining informed consent to nurses. Once nurses become an integral part of the informed consent process, then the hospital also assumes liability under the doctrine of respondent superior.

Nurses also have an important role if patients subsequently wish to revoke their consent or if it becomes obvious that their already signed, informed consent form does not meet the standards of informed consent. Most nurses have been faced with the problem of what to do when it becomes all too clear that patients do not understand the procedure to be performed or when they believe that there are no major risks or adverse consequences inherent to the procedure. Remember, nurses and the hospital may incur liability if there is reason to know that the standards of informed consent have not been met. In such a case, nurses should contact their immediate supervisors and the responsible physicians. Both persons need to be informed of patients' changes of mind or lack of comprehension.

EXERCISE 8-2

A patient is admitted to your surgical center for a breast biopsy under local anesthesia. The surgeon has previously informed the patient of the procedure, risks, alternatives, desired outcomes, and possible complications. You give the surgery permit form to the patient for her signature. She readily states that she is aware of the procedure and risks, has no additional questions, and she signs the form without hesitation. Her husband, who is visiting with her, tells you that he is afraid something may be said during the procedure that will alarm her. What do you do at this point? Do you alert the surgeon that informed consent has not been obtained? Do you request that the surgeon revisit the patient and reinstruct her about the surgery? Is there anything more that you should do?

CONSENT FORMS

Essentially two types of consent forms are presently in use. The *blanket consent form* that is required prior to admission is sufficient for routine and customary care. Routine and customary care may also be implied from the patient's voluntary admission into the hospital, so that this initial blanket consent form is needed only for insurance coverage and assignment of benefits.

Specific consent forms provide information, such as the name and description of the procedure to be performed, to be specifically named. Usually the form also includes a section stating that (1) the person who signed the form was told about the medical condition, risks, alternatives, and benefits of the proposed procedure, and (2) any and all questions have been answered. With this type of form, the physician and hospital could show that no battery occurred because consent was given. However, the plaintiff may still be able to convince a court that informed consent was not given.

A second type of specific consent form attempts to prevent this second possibility. This second specific type of form is a detailed consent form that lists the procedure, consequences, risks, and alternatives. Many states are now mandating this type of form through statutory medical disclosure panels.

Most of the latter forms have the following elements:

1. Signature of the competent patient or a legal representative.
2. Name and full description of the proposed procedure.
3. Description of risks and alternatives of the proposed procedure, including nontreatment.
4. Description of probable consequences of the proposed procedure.
5. Signatures of one or two witnesses according to state law.

With such detailed forms, nurses should remember three things. First, witnesses are not required to make the consent valid. Witnesses merely attest to the competency of the patient signing the form and to the genuineness of the signature, not that the patient had all the information needed to make an informed choice (Switzer, 1995). Although nurses need not be witnesses for the consent form to make it valid, if they observe the signature and chart that such information was given at the time of the signing of the consent form, they would make excellent witnesses in a medical malpractice case. Second, consent may be withdrawn at any time. There is nothing in the written form that precludes patients' right to withdraw their consent at will. Third, consent forms, although strong evidence of informed consent, are not conclusive in and of themselves. Several challenges have surfaced, including (1) technical language that precluded reasonable patients from understanding what they actually signed, (2) a signature that was not voluntary but was coerced or forced, and (3) incompetency of the signer due to impairment by medications previously received.

Consent forms are considered to be valid until withdrawn by the patient or until the patient's condition or authorized treatments change significantly. Some hospitals use a 30-day guideline, but most hospitals prefer to have no set guidelines. Such guidelines could become cumbersome for patients with chronic, disabling diagnoses or for patients who gave valid consent and then became incompetent to renew or resign new consent forms.

WHO MUST CONSENT?

Equally important to giving patients all material facts needed to make an informed choice is that the correct person(s) consent to the procedure or therapy. Informed consent becomes a moot point if the wrong signature is obtained.

Competent Adult

The basic rule is that if the patient is an adult according to state law, only that adult can give or refuse consent. Most states recognize 18 as the age at which one becomes an adult, although some actions might serve to classify the person as an adult prior to the legal age, such as in the case of marriage. The adult giving or refusing consent must be competent to either sign or refuse to sign the necessary consent forms. *Competency at law* means that (1) the court has not declared the person to be incompetent, and (2) the person is generally able to understand the consequences of his or her actions. There is a strong legal presumption of continuing competency.

The actual determination of legal competency is not necessarily the function of the psychiatric medical staff. It is usually made based on the assessment of the person by a physician or other member of the health care profession. Often this assessment is performed at the time informed consent is requested. Consultation with other health professionals is always a possibility and should be performed if there is (1) underlying mental retardation, (2) an obvious mental disorder, or (3) a disease that affects the patient's mental functioning. Courts generally have held that there is a strong presumption of continued competency. Such cases involved persons either whose minds sometimes wandered or who were disoriented at times, and, in one case, an individual who was confined to a mental institution. In each case, the court sought evidence to show that the person was capable of understanding the alternatives to the procedure as proposed and could fully appreciate the consequences of refusing consent to the procedure (*In Re Milton*, 1987).

There are two exceptions to the legal adult's right to give or to refuse informed consent. The hospital must seek and abide by the decision of (1) a court-appointed guardian and (2) a person with a valid, written power of attorney. Such persons will present themselves to the hospital administration if they have previously been appointed and if the adult patient is incapable of giving or refusing consent.

Incompetent Adult

The *legal guardian or representative* is the person who is legally responsible for giving or refusing consent for the incompetent adult. Because the law is allowing someone other than the adult to make decisions for the adult, guardians and representatives have a narrower range of permissible choices than they would if deciding for themselves. Some states also insist that the known choices of the patient be considered first. Any expressed wishes concerning therapy or refusal of therapy made while the patient was still fully competent should be evaluated and followed if at all possible.

To be appointed as a legal representative or guardian, the court must first declare the adult incompetent. The court will then appoint either a temporary or a permanent guardian. If the court has reason to believe the adult is only temporarily incapacitated, then it will appoint a guardian until the adult is able to once again manage his or her affairs.

Guardians are usually selected from family members because the law feels that such persons will have the patient's best interests at heart and are in a position to best know the patient's desires. If the spouse of the incompetent adult is also elderly and ill, an adult child may be the appointed guardian.

Some persons are never adjudicated as incompetent by a court of law, and in selected states the family is asked to make decisions for the incompetent patient. For example, an automobile accident may render the patient incapable of making decisions and giving consent, and the physician will frequently ask the family about medical matters for the unconscious patient. The order of selection is usually:

1. Spouse.
2. Adult children or grandchildren.
3. Parents.
4. Grandparents, adult brothers, and sisters.
5. Adult nieces and nephews.

The practitioner is cautioned to validate state laws and judicial decisions because *family consent* may not be valid consent in a handful of states. Lack of valid consent may become a court battle, especially if the practitioner acts on family consent and there was disagreement among family members as to the course of action to take.

Minors

Most states recognize a child under 18 as a *minor.* Parental or guardian consent is necessary for medical therapies unless (1) the emergency doctrine applies, (2) the child is an emancipated or mature minor, (3) there is a court order to proceed with the therapy, or (4) the law recognizes the minor as having the ability to consent to the therapy. Some states also allow *in loco parentis* or the ability of a person or the state to stand in the place of the parents. Look to statutory law to see who may consent in the absence of a parent. If there is a family consent doctrine, it will be a grandparent, adult brother or sister, or adult aunt or uncle. A newer trend is allowing minor parents to consent for their children's medical and dental treatments.

As with adults, the law applies the doctrine of implied consent with medical emergencies, unless there is reason to believe that the parents would refuse such therapy. An example could be the child of Jehovah's Witness parents. Medical personnel would have reason to believe that the parents might not consent to the giving of blood. The best course for the medical staff to follow if there is doubt about whether consent would be forthcoming is to seek a court order for the therapy unless there is a true emergency or life-threatening condition.

If the child's parents are married to each other or have joint custody, usually either parent can sign the consent form or make treatment decisions. If divorce results in a sole custody arrangement or in total abrogation of parental rights, then generally the parent with custody is considered the party to give or deny consent.

Such issues are state-specific, and there are important exceptions to general rules. For example, a Georgia court has ruled that a do-not-resuscitate order could not be enforced without the signatures of both parents (Rutherford, 1994).

Emancipated minors are persons under the legal age who are no longer under their parent's control and regulation and who are managing their own financial affairs. Some states require the parent to completely surrender the right of care and custody of the child to prevent runaways from coming under this classification. Such emancipated minors may validly consent for their own medical therapies. Examples of emancipated minors are married persons, underage parents, or those in the armed service of their country. Some states allow college students, living away from their parents, to fall in this category.

Mature minors may also consent to some medical care. This is a relatively new concept that is gaining legal recognition. Its origin is in family law and involves the right of the child to make a choice as to which parent will have custody of the child following a divorce. The concept of a mature minor was recognized as early as 1957 (*Masden v. Harrison*, 1957). The mature minor is someone, between the ages of 14 to 17, who is able to understand the nature and consequences of the proposed therapy, and who is making his or her own decisions on a daily basis, and who is independent.

The medical practitioner is encouraged to seek parental consent along with the consent of the mature minor in most circumstances. Such a practice aids in limiting potential liability and encourages family involvement.

Obtaining valid informed consent when minors declare themselves to be emancipated or sufficiently mature to consent in their own stead can be problematic. When there is a question of valid consent, the best course of action is to temporarily postpone any elective procedure or treatment until it is determined if the minor can consent within state law. If a true emergency presents, then the practitioner may proceed under an emergency consent doctrine. The practitioner should carefully document in the medical record the existence of valid informed consent or the need for emergency care.

The law also recognizes the right of minors to consent for some selected therapies without informing their parents of the treatment. The reason for these exceptions is to encourage minors to seek needed treatment. Informing the parents of the treatment might prevent the minors from receiving the necessary therapy. Instances for which minors may give valid consent include:

1. The diagnosis and treatment of infectious, contagious, or communicable diseases.
2. The diagnosis and treatment of drug dependency, drug addiction, or any condition directly related to drug usage.
3. Obtaining birth control devices.
4. Treatment during a pregnancy as long as the care concerns the pregnancy.

Court orders may be obtained for the care of minors if the parents refuse to consent to needed procedures or treatment, although there is a trend toward nonintervention unless treatment is needed to save a life. For example, hospitals have often obtained court orders for blood transfusions when the parents have refused consent for the transfusion. In *In re Hamilton* (1983), the court ordered chemotherapy for a 12-year-old girl when the parents refused consent based on religious grounds. That court overruled the parents to improve the quality of the child's life during her dying.

EXERCISE 8-3

John Smith, a 20-year-old college student, is admitted to your institution for additional chemotherapy. John was diagnosed with leukemia five years earlier and has had several courses of chemotherapy. He is currently in an acute active phase of the disease, although he enjoyed a 14-month remission phase prior to this admission. His parents, who accompany him to the hospital, are divided as to the benefits of additional chemotherapy. His mother is adamant that she will sign the informed consent form for this course of therapy, and his father is equally adamant that he will refuse to sign, since "John has suffered enough." You are his primary nurse and must assist in somehow resolving this impasse. What do you do about the informed consent form? Who signs it? Why?

GUIDELINES: INFORMED CONSENT

Two criteria must be satisfied:

1. The consent is given by one who has the legal capacity for giving such consent, such as a(n):
   a. Competent adult.
   b. Legal guardian or representative for the incompetent adult.
   c. Emancipated, married minor.
   d. Mature minor.
   e. Parent, the state, or a legal guardian of a child.
   f. Minor for the diagnosis and treatment of specific disease states or conditions.
   g. Court order.
2. The person(s) giving consent must fully comprehend:
   a. The procedure to be performed.
   b. The risks involved.
   c. The expected or desired outcomes.
   d. Any complications or untoward side effects.
   e. Alternative therapies, including no therapy at all.

RIGHT TO REFUSE CONSENT

The right of consent involves the *right of refusal.* If persons have the right to consent, then they also have the right to refuse to give consent. The right of refusal continues even after primary consent is given. Patients or guardians need only to notify the health care giver that they no longer wish to continue with the therapy. In some limited circumstances the danger of stopping therapy poses too great a harm for the patient, and the law allows its continuance. For example, in the immediate postoperative period the patient cannot refuse procedures that assure a safe transition from anesthesia. Likewise, the patient may not refuse immediate care for life-threatening arrhythmias following a myocardial infarction if that refusal would worsen the patient's condition. After the arrhythmias have abated, the patient may refuse further therapy.

The right for such refusal may be based on the common law right of freedom from bodily invasion or the constitutional rights of privacy and religious freedom. The right of refusal is not without potential consequences. The patient or guardian must be informed that the right of refusal may mean—and most often does mean—that the patient's physical condition continues to deteriorate and may hasten death. The right of refusal may also mean that third-party reimbursement may be denied, since most insurance policies have a clause that denies or limits reimbursement for refusing procedures that would aid in the diagnosis or reduction of the injury or illness.

Limitations on Refusal of Therapy

The state may deny a patient's right of refusal in several instances. These state rights exist to prevent committing crimes and to protect the welfare of society as a whole. Limitations on refusal include:

1. Preservation of life if the patient does not have an incurable or terminal disease.
2. Protection of minor dependents.
3. Prevention of irrational self-destruction.
4. Maintenance of the ethical integrity of health professionals by allowing the hospital to treat the patient.
5. Protection of the public's health.

In cases filed to enforce the right to refuse care, the courts balance individual rights against societal rights (*Jefferson v. Griffith Spalding County Hospital Authority*, 1981; *Norwood Hospital v. Munoz*, 1991; *Thor v. Superior Court*, 1993; *Leach v. Akron General Medical Center*, 1984). In *Leach*, the court found that a patient has the right to refuse therapy based on a privacy right. In this case, the patient was incompetent and the issue was whether to allow the patient to forego life-sustaining treatment.

LAW ENFORCEMENT

Often medical personnel are requested by the police and other law enforcement personnel to draw blood, remove stomach contents, remove bullets, and the like for the purpose of gathering evidence to be used against a suspect. The suspect will often refuse to give consent to the proposed treatments and procedures. As a health care provider, can you legally do as requested? Or will you open yourself to a potential lawsuit for battery?

The Supreme Court of the United States attempted for several years to answer these questions for the health care provider. In *Rochin v. California* (1950), the court ruled that the "removal of stomach contents shocks the conscience" and refused to permit the test results on the stomach contents from being introduced into evidence (at 757). Six years later the court ruled that blood drawn from an unconscious person could be introduced into evidence, showing that the driver was legally intoxicated (*Breithaupt v. Adams*, 1957).

Finally, with the landmark case of *Schmerber v. California* in 1966, the court gave the health care provider some criteria for cooperating with law enforcement officials while staying relatively liability free. Five conditions must be present and documented:

1. The suspect must be under formal arrest.
2. There must be a likelihood that the blood drawn will produce evidence for criminal prosecution.
3. A delay in drawing the blood would lead to the destruction of the evidence.
4. The test is reasonable and not medically contraindicated.
5. The test is performed in a reasonable manner (at 763).

Remember, though, that state law may supersede the law enforcer's request, that is, in most states hospital or health care providers have no legal duty to perform the test as requested by the law enforcement official. State law may dictate who and under what circumstances blood may be involuntarily drawn.

INFORMED CONSENT IN HUMAN EXPERIMENTATION

Using vulnerable groups of people for research poses many potential problems because of the ease with which the subjects can be coerced. This is especially true of the mentally disabled, children, and prisoners. The major issue, other than coercion, seems to be that of informed consent.

Whenever research is involved, be it a drug study or a new procedure, the investigator(s) must disclose the research to the subject or the subject's representative and obtain informed consent. Federal guidelines have been developed that specify the procedures used to review research and the disclosures that must be made to ensure that valid, informed consent is obtained.

Since 1974, the Department of Health and Human Services (HHS) has required that an institutional review board (IRB) examine and approve the research study prior to any funding from HHS. This institutional review board determines whether subjects will be placed at risk and, if so, if the following criteria are met:

1. Risks to subjects are outweighed by the benefit to the subject and by the importance of the knowledge to be gained by doing the research.
2. The rights and welfare of the subject will be protected.
3. Legally effective consent will be secured prior to starting any data collection.

Specific requirements that the institutional review board must assure before approving the research study are that:

1. Risks to the subjects are minimized.
2. Risks to the subjects are reasonable in relation to anticipated benefits, if any, to the subjects and to the importance of the knowledge that may reasonably be expected to result.

3. Selection of subjects is equitable.
4. Informed consent will be sought from each prospective subject or the subject's legally authorized representative.
5. Informed consent will be appropriately documented.
6. Where appropriate, the research plan makes adequate provision for monitoring the data collected to ensure the safety of the subjects.
7. Where appropriate, there are adequate provisions to protect the privacy of subjects and to maintain the confidentiality of data.
8. Where some or all of the subjects are likely to be vulnerable to coercion or undue influence, such as persons with acute or severe physical or mental illness or persons who are economically or educationally disadvantaged, appropriate additional safeguards have been included in the study to protect the rights and welfare of these subjects (45 CFR, Section 46.111).

The federal government has also mandated the basic elements of information that must be included to meet the standards of informed consent. These basic elements include:

1. A statement that the study involves research, an explanation of the purposes of the research, and the expected duration of the subject's participation, a description of the procedures to be followed, and identification of any procedures that are experimental.
2. A description of any reasonably foreseeable risks or discomforts to the subject.
3. A description of any benefits to the subjects or others that may reasonably be expected from the research.
4. A disclosure of appropriate alternative procedures or courses of treatment, if any, that may be advantageous to the subject.
5. A statement describing the extent, if any, to which confidentiality of records identifying the subject will be maintained.
6. For research involving more than minimal research, an explanation as to whether any compensation and an explanation as to whether any medical treatments are available if injury occurs and, if so, what they consist of or where further information may be obtained.
7. An explanation of whom to contact for answers to pertinent questions about the research and research subjects' rights and whom to contact in the event of a research-related injury to the subject.
8. A statement that participation is voluntary, refusal to participate will involve no penalty or loss of benefits to which the subject is otherwise entitled, and the subject may discontinue participation at any time without penalty or loss of benefits to which the subject is otherwise entitled (45 CFR, Section 46.116).

The information given must be in language that is understandable by the subject or the subject's legal representative. No exculpatory wording may be included, for example, a statement that the researcher incurs no liability for the outcome to the subject. Subjects should also be advised of (1) any additional costs that they might incur because of the research, (2) potential for any foreseeable risks, (3) rights to withdraw at will, with no questions asked or additional incentives given, (4) consequences, if any, of withdrawal before the study is completed, (5) a statement that any significant new findings will be disclosed, and (6) the number of proposed subjects for the study.

Excluded from these strict requirements are studies that use existing data, documents, records, or pathological and diagnostic specimens, if these sources are publicly available or the information is recorded so that the subjects cannot be identified [45 CFR, Section 46.101 (b), 1981]. Other studies that involve only minimal risks to subjects, such as moderate exercise by healthy adults, may be expedited through the review process (45 CFR, Section 46.110, 1981).

Before proceeding under these specific guidelines, state and local laws must be reviewed for laws regulating research on human subjects. Proposals involving new investigational drugs or devices must meet Federal Drug Administration regulations (21 CFR, parts 50, 56, 312, 314, & 812).

PATIENT SELF-DETERMINATION

Patient self-determination involves the right of individuals to decide what will, or will not, happen to their bodies. Usually the right of self-determination is addressed in issues surrounding death and dying, but self-determination concerns all aspects of consent and its refusal.

THE ISSUE OF CONSENT

Before one can discuss the patient's right to die or to forego life-sustaining procedures, one must address the issue of informed consent. Competent adults have long been recognized as having the right to refuse medical treatment, unless the state can show that its interests outweigh that right. Examples of such overriding state interests include:

1. Protecting third parties, especially minor children.
2. Preserving life, especially that of minors and incompetents.
3. Protecting society from the spread of disease.

Competent adults may decide which treatments they will receive and which they will refuse. Usually any decision to forgo medical treatment will need to survive a period in which the health care receiver is incompetent. Many states have attempted to help this classification of patient by statutory enactments.

Often patients express their desires in oral form. In some states these oral wishes have been upheld by the judiciary. The courts examined documentation of these wishes and usually determine if the persons knew of their terminal condition when expressing their wishes or whether they were talking, in general terms, about future care when they became terminally ill. The courts have

GUIDELINES: RIGHTS OF PATIENTS IN RESEARCH

1. Informed consent is the first hurdle to valid human experimentation. Nurses must ascertain that the patient or legal representative understands that a research study will be involved and that the patient or legal representative has a basic understanding of the research to be performed (nature of the study, expected results of the study, and the like).

2. The patient or legal representative must be given the choice to participate or not. This entails the giving of information in understandable terms and in sufficient quantity so that the patient or legal representative can make an informed choice of participation.

3. Patients or legal representatives must know that they can choose to terminate participation at any point in the research study. This may be done without penalty, forfeiture of quality care and treatment, or loss of dignity.

4. Patients or legal representatives should be aware of who is conducting the research study and how to contact this person(s) at any given time. All questions should be answered for them, as needed, by the principal investigator.

5. Patients should be free from any arbitrary hurt or intrinsic risk of injury. Any physical or mental risks that they may be exposing themselves to should be explained as fully as possible when the initial informed consent is obtained. Likewise, medical care or treatment for such incurred risks should be made available to patients by the researcher, and patients or legal representatives should be aware of these considerations at the time of the initial informed consent.

6. Patients always retain their right to privacy and confidentiality. If at all possible, they should never be capable of being identified through the research study, but a coding system should be devised and followed. If not possible, patients should be known to as few persons as can be allowed by the research design.

7. The quality of research in which human subjects are involved is important. Institutional review boards should exist for all institutions in which human subjects are used for ongoing research studies. Institutional review boards should look first to the expected outcomes of the study and to that which is being studied in deciding if human persons may be used as subjects.

8. While the rights of the minor and of the mentally or developmentally disabled person are no greater than those of the competent adult subject in a research study, the need to protect these rights is greater. These persons are more likely not to understand the nature of the research or the fact that they can terminate their participation at will; they are also more easily coerced into becoming subjects for the proposed research study. Nurses must guard against such happenings and ascertain that valid legal representation exists for such underaged or disadvantaged persons.

been reluctant to enforce generalities, and vague talk about potential happenings in the future usually have been held to have little weight by the court.

For years, legal experts have concluded that competent adults have the right to refuse medical treatment, even if the refusal is certain to cause death, a view that is consistent with the majority of states to decriminalize suicide. But it was not until 1984 that an appellate court directly confronted an issue where a clearly competent patient refused necessary life-sustaining treatment. In *Bartling v. Superior Court* (1984), the California Court of Appeal's decision was eased because the patient died before the case was resolved. That tentativeness of the court was overcome by the next case to present itself, *Bouvia v. Superior Court* (1986).

The issue addressed in *Bartling* concerned the right of a competent adult patient, with a serious illness that was probably incurable but not necessarily terminal, over the objections of his physicians and the hospital, to have life-support equipment disconnected despite the fact that the withdrawal of such devices would hasten his death. Mr. Bartling, a severe emphysemic patient, entered the hospital for depression. While hospitalized, a tumor was noted on x-ray, and during the subsequent biopsy his lung collapsed. Despite aggressive therapy, Mr. Bartling was trached and ventilator-dependent at the time this cause of action was heard. Though Mr. Bartling died during the course of the appeal, the appellate court held that the "right of a competent adult to refuse medical treatment is a constitutionally guaranteed right which must not be abridged" (*Bartling v. Superior Court*, 1984, at 192).

In *Bouvia v. Superior Court* (1986), the court addressed many of the same issues. Bouvia, a 28-year-old patient with severe cerebral palsy, sought removal of a nasogastric tube, inserted and maintained against her will for the purpose of involuntary forced feedings. Here the court wrestled not only with the right of a competent adult to refuse medical therapy, but also with the facility's obligation to serve the autonomous interests of patients, as defined by those patients. In *Bouvia*, those autonomous decisions included medical support to prevent further pain and suffering during the dying process.

The legal history of the right of competent patients to forego life-sustaining treatment is provided in a clear and accurate way through these two California opinions. The very strong unanimous court in *Bouvia* also demonstrates the consensus absent in 1984 that was beginning to solidify by 1986.

Incompetent patients present a totally different picture. The first court case to challenge the judiciary in this respect was the *Quinlan* case (*In re Quinlan*, 1976). In a lengthy decision, the New Jersey Supreme Court held that, although patients generally have the right to refuse therapy, guardians for the incompetent usually do not. "The only practical way to prevent destruction of the [privacy] right is to permit the guardian and family of Karen to render their very best judgment . . . as to whether she would exercise it in these circumstances" (at 664).

That court allowed the father of Karen Quinlan to authorize the withdrawal of life support systems for Karen. The decision was a difficult one to reach because Karen did not meet the Harvard criteria for brain death. While she was respirator-dependent at the time of the court case, she had some brain activity on the EEG and some reflex movements. The decision was also difficult because it conflicted significantly with a precedent-setting New Jersey case that held that one should always save a life, even if the patient's objection to life-saving procedures was based on religious beliefs (*John F. Kennedy Memorial Hospital v. Heston*, 1971).

The decision reached by the court in *Quinlan* was to allow Karen's father the right to remove Karen from life support systems. It should be clear, however, that the father made the final decision. The court system gave him the right to make the ultimate decision, but did not influence that decision.

The next significant decision in this area of the law was *Superintendent of Belchertown State School v. Saikewicz* (1977). Here the Massachusetts Supreme Court deviated from the Quinlan case in two significant ways:

1. This court used the doctrine of **substituted judgment** (subjective determination of how persons, were they capable of making their opinions and wishes known, would choose to exercise their right to refuse therapy) to decide what Joseph Saikewicz would have wanted to be done with his right to refuse therapy.

2. No ethics committee was suggested by the court. Unlike Quinlan, the Saikewicz opinion met with general disfavor because the court totally rejected the notion that these types of decisions should be made by families and physicians with the aid of ethics committees. Indeed, the Saikewicz court held that the decision to discontinue therapy "must reside with the judicial process and the judicial process alone" (at 475).

Eichner v. Dillon (1980), the third case to define allowing patients the right to forego life-sustaining procedures, restricted the termination of extraordinary life support treatments to the patient who was terminally ill or in a "vegetative coma characterized as permanent or irreversible with an extremely remote possibility of recovery" (at 468). *Eichner* also combined the substituted judgment doctrine as followed in *Saikewicz* with the *best interest* test (personal preferences made while the now incompetent patient was rational and capable of stating what he or she would want in the event of a catastrophic happening), as derived from *Quinlan*. While not a perfect solution, the decision seemed to soften the negative impact of *Saikewicz*.

The final decision concerning the incompetent patient's right to die seems to have been settled in 1990. In *Cruzan v. Director, Missouri Department of Health* (1990), the court made explicit that the right to die issues will be decided on a state-to-state basis and that there will be little, if any, United States constitutional limits on what states may do. Following the *Cruzan* decision, cases have allowed more latitude to family members and courts have struggled to find instances where patients had made some expression, however fleeting, about their desires for sustaining life with artificial or life support measures.

Two recent cases exemplify those points. In *In re Fiori* (1995), a Pennsylvania court held that a hospital amy terminate life support treatment for a patient in a persistent vegetative state without a court order if the hospital obtained the consent of close family members and the consent of two physicians. The court limited this holding to patients in a persistent vegetative state with no cognitive powers, with no chance of recovery, and with no clearly expressed preference for termination. In a previous case, *Grace Plaza of Great Neck, Inc., v. Elbaum* (1993), the court held that, where doubt exists as to an incompetent's desired course of treatment, a judicial determination is necessary before life support can be terminated. The court further stated that proof of a patient's desires, such as through a living will or prior statement, serves to limit a provider's autonomy in denying termination of treatment.

LIVING WILLS

Living wills, started in the 1960s, gained popularity following these three cases. A *living will* is a directive from competent individuals to medical personnel and family members regarding the treatment they wish to receive when they can no longer make the decision for themselves (Figure 8-1). The living will is not necessary if patients are competent and capable of making their wishes known. It becomes important when previously competent persons become seriously ill and incompetent.

Usually the language of a living will is broad and vague. It gives little direction to the health care provider concerning the circumstances and actual time the declarant wishes the living will to be honored. There is typically no legal enforcement of the living will, and medical practitioners may choose to abide by the patient's wishes or to ignore them as they see fit. There is also no protection for the practitioner against criminal or civil liability, and many physicians have been afraid to proceed under a living will's direction for fear that family members or the state will file charges of wrongful death.

NATURAL DEATH ACTS

To protect the practitioner from potential civil and criminal lawsuits and to ensure that patients' wishes are followed when they are no longer able to make their wishes known, a special type of living will, known as the *natural death act*, was enacted into law. These natural death acts are legally recognized living wills in that they serve the same function as living wills but with statutory enforcement, and virtually all states have enacted some form of natural death legislation. Recognizing that physicians may be unwilling to follow the directive, several of these laws require a reasonable effort on the part of physicians to transfer patients to a physician who will abide by these wishes.

Statutory provisions for natural death acts vary from state to state. Generally, persons over 18 years may sign a natural death act. Such persons must be of sound mind and capable of understanding the purpose of the document that they sign. The natural death act document is usually a declaration that

LIVING WILL DECLARATION

To My Family, Doctors, and All Those Concerned with My Care

I, _____, being of sound mind, make this statement as a directive to be followed if for any reason I become unable to participate in decisions regarding my medical care.

I direct that life-sustaining procedures should be withheld or withdrawn if I have an illness, disease or injury, or experience extreme mental deterioration, such that there is no reasonable expectation of recovering or regaining a meaningful quality of life.

These life-sustaining procedures that may be withheld or withdrawn include, but are not limited to:

**SURGERY   ANTIBIOTICS   CARDIAC RESUSCITATION
RESPIRATORY SUPPORT   ARTIFICIALLY ADMINISTERED FEEDING AND FLUIDS**

I further direct that treatment be limited to comfort measures only, even if they shorten my life.

You may delete any provision above by drawing a line through it and adding your initials.

Other personal instructions:

These directions express my legal right to refuse treatment. Therefore, I expect my family, doctors, and all those concerned with my care to regard themselves as legally and morally bound to act in accord with my wishes, and in so doing to be free from any liability for having followed my directions.

Signed _____ Date _____
Witness _____ Witness _____

PROXY DESIGNATION CLAUSE

If you wish, you may use this section to designate someone to make treatment decisions if you are unable to do so. Your Living Will Declaration will be in effect even if you have not designated a proxy.

I authorize the following person to implement my Living Will Declaration by accepting, refusing and/or making decisions about treatment and hospitalization:

Name _____
Address _____

If the person I have named above is unable to act on my behalf, I authorize the following person to do so:

Name _____
Address _____

I have discussed my wishes with these persons and trust their judgment on my behalf.

Signed _____ Date _____
Witness _____ Witness _____

FIGURE 8-1. EXAMPLE OF A LIVING WILL. *(COURTESY OF SOCIETY FOR THE RIGHT TO DIE, NEW YORK, NY.)*

withholds or withdraws life-sustaining treatment from patients should they ever be in a terminal state. The natural death act must be in written form, signed by the patient, and witnessed by two persons, each of whom is 18 years or older.

Some states also specify that the witnesses to the natural death act not be:

1. Related to the patient by blood or marriage.
2. Entitled to any portion of the estate of the patient by will or intestacy.
3. Directly financially responsible for the patient's medical care.
4. The attending physician, his or her employee, or an employee of the facility in which the declarant is a patient.
5. The person who, at the request of the patient, signed the declaration because the patient was unable to sign.

Other states incorporate some of these restrictions.

The form of the natural death act also varies from state to state. Some states provide no suggestion as to the contents of the document, while other states have a mandatory form that must be filled in by the declarant. Still other states suggest a form but provide that additional directions may be added if they are not inconsistent with the statutory requirements. For states that have no set form, private organizations have suggested formats for these special living wills.

Once signed and witnessed, most natural death acts are effective until revoked, although some states require that they must be reexecuted every five years. In some states the patient who is pregnant may not benefit from the provisions of the natural death act during the course of the pregnancy. It may be advisable for the declarant to review, redate, and resign the natural death act every year or so. This assures family members and health care providers that the directions contained in the natural death act reflect the current wishes of the patient.

The natural death act may be revoked by physical destruction or defacement, by a written revocation, or by an oral statement indicating that it is the person's wish to revoke the previously executed natural death act. Some states have fewer restrictions on revocation; for example, the revocation may take place without regard to the mental condition of the patient, and the revocation is ineffective until the attending physician is notified of it.

Once a valid natural death act exists, it is effective only when the person becomes qualified, that is, the person is diagnosed to have a terminal condition and the removal or withholding of life support systems would merely prolong the patient's process of dying. Most states require that two physicians certify in writing that any procedures and treatments will not prevent the ultimate death of the patient but will serve only to postpone death in a patient with no chance of recovery. Medications and procedures used merely to prevent the patient's suffering and to provide comfort are excluded from this definition.

Today, many states also allow an oral invocation of a natural death act and/or another person to invoke a natural death act for the patient. States were exploring a variety of options to ensure that natural death acts met the needs of patients when the durable power of attorney for health care became more prominent.

DURABLE POWER OF ATTORNEY FOR HEALTH CARE

The *durable power of attorney for health care (DPAHC)* or the *medical durable power of attorney (MDPA)* allows competent patients to appoint a surrogate or proxy to make health care decisions for them in the event that they are incompetent to do so. These legislative enactments were the next logical step following limitations with living wills and natural death acts. No longer did the family or health care provider need to guess if this was the time that the patient would have wanted the living will to be followed, because there was a person, given the authority of the patient to either accept or refuse care, to speak for the patient.

Power of attorney is a common law concept that allowed one person (an agent) to speak for another (the principal), and that is a concept of the agency relationship. At common law, the power of attorney terminated upon the death or incapacity of the principal. To prevent this occurrence, when the patient most wanted the power of attorney to be effective, legislatures adopted the Uniform Durable Power of Attorney Act. This act sanctions the right of an individual to grant a durable power of attorney—one that would be valid even if the principal was incapacitated and legally incompetent.

Under most of the Durable Power of Attorney for Health Care Statutes, individuals may designate agents to make medical decisions for them when they are unable to make such decisions. The power includes the right to ask questions, select and remove physicians from the patient's care, assess risks and complications, and the right to select treatments and procedures from a variety of therapeutic options. The power also includes the right to refuse care and/or life-sustaining procedures. Health care providers are protected from liability if they abide, in good faith, on the agent's decisions.

Agents further have the authority to enforce the patient's treatment plans by filing lawsuits or legal actions against health care providers or family members. Agents have the right to forego treatment, change treatment plans, or consent to additional treatment. In short, they have the full authority to act as the principal would have acted. Thus the durable power of attorney for health care is the best form of substituted judgment available for an otherwise incompetent patient.

Most patients are cautioned to appoint persons as agents who understand what the patient would want and who are capable of making those hard decisions. Friends, relatives, or spouses may be appointed as agents. And most states allow patients or potential patients to appoint subsequent agents. In the event the first named person cannot serve or is unwilling to serve in this capacity, then a second or third person has the principal's authority. Without this latter provision, patients' wishes might still not be honored.

MEDICAL OR PHYSICIAN DIRECTIVES

Some states allow for a directive that lists a variety of treatments and lets patients decide what they would want, depending on the patient's condition at the time. For example, the patient can select life-sustaining therapy if the condition is not terminal to disallowing life-sustaining therapy if the condition is terminal and irreversible. Generally known as a *medical* or *physician's directive,* this document has legal worth comparable to that of the living will.

UNIFORM RIGHTS OF THE TERMINALLY ILL ACT

The Act, adopted in 1989, is narrow in scope and limited to treatment that is merely life-prolonging and to patients whose terminal condition is incurable and irreversible, whose death will occur soon, and who are unable to participate in treatment decisions. The Act's sole purpose is to provide alternative ways in which terminally ill patients' desires regarding the use of life-sustaining procedures can be legally implemented.

This Act was passed because no two states have identical living will or natural death act provisions. And perhaps the Act was passed because the political nature of the right to die had driven the legislature to enact virtually meaningless statutes to avoid political fallout.

Many of the provisions of the Act look identical to some state natural death act provisions. For example, the qualified patient must be diagnosed as terminal, and life-sustaining procedures would only prolong the dying of the patient. Physicians who are unwilling to comply with patients' requests not to begin or continue life support procedures should take all necessary steps to transfer the patient to a physician who will comply. And patients diagnosed as being in a persistent vegetative state are not qualified patients.

PATIENT SELF-DETERMINATION ACT OF 1990

In November 1991, the Patient Self-Determination Act of 1990 was enacted into law as part of the Omnibus Budget Reconciliation Act of 1990. This Act, in direct response to the Nancy Cruzan case in Missouri, mandates that patients must be queried about the existence of advanced directives and that such advanced directives must be made available to them, if they so wish.

In 1983, Nancy Cruzan was involved in a one-car automobile accident. She was discovered lying facedown in a ditch without cardiac or respiratory functioning, and life support was started. She eventually was diagnosed as being in a persistent vegetative coma and her parents requested the removal of artificial hydration and nutritional support. The trial court allowed such removal because Cruzan "expressed thoughts at age 25 in a somewhat serious conversation with a friend that if sick or injured she would not wish to continue her life unless she could live at least halfway normal" (*Cruzan v. Director, Missouri Department of Public Health*, 1990, at 2843). The Supreme Court of Missouri reversed that decision, stating that such statements were unreliable for the purpose of determining her intent and further held that the family was not entitled to direct the termination of her treatment in the absence of a living will or "clear and convincing, inherently reliable evidence absent here" (at 2844).

The United States Supreme Court held that states had the authority to impose legal requirements on decisions to discontinue therapy for incompetent patients. The case was then remanded back to trial level in Missouri and, on retrial, the court concluded that the friend's statement of Nancy Cruzan's desires was sufficient to allow the removal of the feeding tube. Ms. Cruzan died on December 16, 1990.

Justice Scalia, in his separate concurrence, praised states for beginning to grapple with the issue of terminating medical treatment through legislation. Almost every state recognizes some form of advanced directive, from living wills to durable powers of attorney for health care. The problem, though, is that few people prepare advance directives. Thus the Patient Self-Determination Act was passed to ensure that persons knew about such advanced directives and that they would be assisted in making such directives, if they so desired.

The Act merely lets people know about existing rights, and does not create any new rights for patients. Nor does it change state law. Perhaps the Act has served as incentive for more states to pass durable powers of attorney for health care statutes, but it does not mandate such passage. The Act does not require that patients execute advanced directives. It merely provides for patient education about such directives and provides assistance for patients wishing to execute these directives. The legislation specifically states that providers may not discriminate against a patient in any way based on the absence or presence of an advanced directive.

Nor does the Act legislate communication or conversation. Yet one of its purposes is to encourage communication and conversation about existing directives, at a time when the patient is competent to understand and to execute advanced directives.

DO-NOT-RESUSCITATE DIRECTIVES

Some health care organizations have initiated *do-not-resuscitate directives* that patients may execute upon admission to health care institutions. Per the patient's request, the physician will then follow hospital policy in attaching the orders to the patient's record. Most institutions require documentation that the patient's decision was made after consultation with the physician regarding the patient's diagnoses and prognosis. The order should then be reevaluated according to institution policy.

New York State has enacted a do-not-resuscitate statute that establishes the hierarchy of surrogates who may request a do-not-resuscitate status for incompetent patients and has also mandated that all health care facilities inquire of patients as they are admitted their desires concerning resuscitation. The act was promulgated by worry over the overuse of cardiopulmonary resuscitation. Frequently, the issue concerning do-not-resuscitate turns on whether the patient was fully informed when a physician ordered a no-code for the patient. *Payne v. Marion General Hospital* (1990) represents the first case in this area of the law.

Find out what your hospital does about advanced directives. How are the patients made aware of these options and who assists them in completing these directives? If patients come to your institution with advanced directives, how are staff alerted to their existence? Is there provision for ensuring the validity of advanced directives prior to a patient's death? Give your suggestions for a more effective use of such documents.

HOSPICE CARE

Some terminally ill patients sidestep the need for natural death acts and living wills by entering hospice centers. A *hospice center* allows patients to receive the nursing and medical care that is required and to be kept comfortable, without the fear that they will be resuscitated or placed on life support systems when death occurs. Some states are also beginning home hospice care to allow patients to receive the benefits of hospice centers in their own homes.

Congress recognized the need for such terminal care apart from the hospital setting and authorized Medicare reimbursement for hospice care (P.L. 97-248, 1982). Medicare reimbursement is limited to six months, and this does not indicate that Congress meant that patients with a longer life expectancy should seek or accept more aggressive care.

The problem encountered with hospice centers is that usually the patients seeking such care are competent, the very same patients who could refuse heroic care if they were in a formal hospital setting. Problems encountered with allowing patients to die are usually confined to the incompetent, hospitalized patient.

ASSISTED SUICIDE

Although suicide as a crime has been abrogated in all states, most states still prohibit *assisted suicide.* Some states treat assisted suicide harshly, while other states prohibit only causing suicide, not assisting it. Washington, Oregon, and

GUIDELINES: ADVANCED DIRECTIVES

1. Nurses should review the state statutes and provisions for durable powers or attorney for health care, natural death acts, and living wills. Realize that the requirements may vary greatly state to state, and have the in-hospital attorney hold classes for nurses so that the staff is fully aware of any statutory requirements and the means by which these advanced directives are enforced.

2. Review the hospital policy and procedure manual for any hospital guidelines in this area. If no policies exist, suggest to the committee or persons responsible for policies the need for guidance in this area.

3. Should a patient or family tell you that he or she has a signed advanced directive, make that known to the physician and the hospital administration immediately. Document the existence of the declaration in the patient's medical record, and ask for a copy of the declaration for the medical record.

4. Should the patient revoke the declaration or tell the nurse that he or she desires to revoke the declaration, the nurse is obligated to document the revocation in the record and to immediately notify the attending physician and hospital administration. This is true even if the competency of the patient is questionable since some statutes allow for revocation even if the declarant is not of sound mind.

5. It is advisable that nurses not be witnesses to the living will or natural death act, since many natural death acts forbid a witness from being employed by the attending physician or facility in which the patient is hospitalized. Usually a friend or someone unrelated to the patient serves as witness.

6. Should there be a copy of the living will or natural death act in the patient's medical record, read it carefully to ascertain the scope of its provisions. Clarify the declaration while the patient is still competent. Document in the medical record any clarification that the patient gives to you, and ensure that the attending physician also understands the scope of the declaration.

7. In most states, nurses or other persons may write and sign advanced directives as proxies of competent patients. Here nurses must be sure that patients are of sound mind, since competency is an important issue in the execution of the directive. Document in the record what occurred and the circumstances that made it necessary for a second person to sign for the patient (such as partial paralysis).

8. Assist the family members in this time of crisis by being available and by answering as many of their questions as possible. Tell the family members of any existing ethics committee or other persons available to talk with them. Remember that they need time to internalize what is happening, especially if they are called on to concur with the patient's directive or to insist on the implementation of the patient's directive.

California have tried, through legislation, to pass assisted suicide statutes. While these measures have either failed or are being challenged through the court system, it seems likely that they will pass at some future date. And many predict that the Supreme Court will be the judiciary body to finally attempt to come to terms with this issue.

The Oregon Death with Dignity Act, passed by the voters in November 1994 and now under judicial review, will allow physicians to write a lethal drug prescription for a competent, terminally ill adult who is a resident of the state. Other provisions that must be met before the prescription is written include:

1. Both the attending physician and a consulting physician must certify that the patient has no more than six months to live.
2. The patient must make both an oral and written request for the prescription, followed by a second oral request 15 days or more after the first request.
3. The attending physician must refer the patient for counseling if a psychological illness or depression is suspected.
4. The doctor must wait at least 48 hours after the third request before prescribing the medication.

Michigan is the state that has dealt with this issue in great degree. Because of Dr. Jack Kevorkian's "death machine," assisted suicide has taken on new meaning. Michigan originally filed murder charges against Kevorkian, but they were dismissed. Michigan then passed a statute "prohibiting one who has knowledge that a person intends to commit suicide from intentionally providing the physical means or participating in the physical act by which the person attempts or commits suicide," but the prohibition does not apply to "withholding or withdrawing by a licensed health care professional" (Kamisar, 1993, p. 37). The Michigan law is currently being challenged.

The nurse's role in this area is still developing. The American Nurses Association opposes the movement and opposes nurses' participation in either assisted or active euthanasia because it violates the ethical traditions embodied in the *Code for Nurses* (American Nurses Association, 1994). In Michigan, the Michigan Nurses Association has come out in support of the legalization of assisted suicide for "competent persons whose suffering cannot be relieved or satisfactorily reduced with alternative strategies" (Michigan Nurses Association, 1994).

If nurses are asked directly by the patient to assist with a suicide, they must refuse—but look beyond the request to what the patient may be saying. The patient may be expressing a need for greater pain control or for someone to talk with about the fears of a terrible death. At this time, nurses must be clear that they cannot assist the patient in this aspect, but may be able to assist with procuring medications for more effective pain control or by supplying needed forms to assist the patient with advanced directives. Another avenue may be to ensure that patients speak with a chaplain, with representatives of their faith, or with a social worker. Ensure that patients know that someone cares and assist them in every legal, ethical way.

SUMMARY

This chapter has detailed informed consent from a variety of aspects: from the competent person's consent for minor surgery to the incompetent person's right to die without life-sustaining procedures and devices. The American public places great value and respect in people's right to determine what will happen to them. Nurses must understand and use the legal measures that ensure one's right to control his/her own destiny.

AFTER COMPLETING THIS CHAPTER, YOU SHOULD BE ABLE TO

- Define informed consent, comparing and contrasting it with consent.
- Describe means of obtaining informed consent, including expressed, implied, oral, written, complete, and partial.
- Compare and contrast three standards of informed consent.
- Describe four exceptions to informed consent.
- Describe who has responsibility for obtaining informed consent.
- Describe the types of consent forms in use in health care settings.
- Analyze whose signature must be obtained to ensure informed consent.
- Describe one's right to refuse consent for medical care.
- Describe the patient's right either to give or to deny consent for research.
- Describe advanced directives including living wills, natural death acts, and durable power of attorney for health care and do-not-resuscitate directives.

APPLY YOUR LEGAL KNOWLEDGE

- How does the distinction between consent and informed consent have implications for professional health care providers?
- What should the nurse do when told by patients that they have an advanced directive?
- How does the nurse decide if a patient's consent is truly voluntary and informed?
- Should nurses have a role in securing informed consent?

REFERENCES

American Nurses' Association. (1994). *Position statement on assisted suicide*. Washington, DC: Author.

American Nurses' Association. (1994). *Position statement on active euthanasia*. Washington, DC: Author.

Arato v. Avedon, 858 P. 2d 598 (California, 1993).

Bartling v. Superior Court, 163 Cal. App. 3d 186, 209 Cal. Rept. 220 (Cal. App. Ct., 2d Dis., 1984).

Blazevic, D. J. & Keenan, K. P. (1993). Informed consent. *The Brief* (2), 20–25, 42–43.

Breithaupt v. Adams, 352 U.S. 432 (1957).

Bouvia v. Superior Court, 179 Cal. App. 3d 1127, 225 Cal. Rept. 297 (Cal. App. Ct., 2d Dis., 1986).

Cruzan v. Director, Missouri Department of Health, 110 S.Ct. 2841, 102 L.E.D. 224 (1990).

Cushing, M. M. (1991). Demystifying informed consent. *American Journal of Nursing, 91*(11), 17–19.

Eichner v. Dillon, 73 App. Div. 2d 431, 426 N.Y.S. 2d 517 (2d Dept., 1980).

Hoffson v. Orentreish, 543 N.Y. 2d 242 (New York, 1989).

Grace Plaza of Great Neck, Inc., v. Elbaum, 82 N.Y. 2d 10 (New York, 1993).

In re Fiori, 652 A. 2d 1350 (Pennsylvania, 1995).

In re Hamilton, 657 S.W. 2d 425 (Tenn. App., 1983).

In re Milton, 29 Ohio App. 3d 20, 505 N.E. 2d 255 (Ohio, 1987).

In re Quinlan, 70 N.J.10, 335 A. 2d 647 (1976).

Jones v. Philadelphia College of Osteopathic Medicine, 813 F. Supp. 1125 (Pennsylvania, 1993).

Kamisar, Y. (1993). Active versus passive euthanasia: Why keep the distinction? *Trial, 29*(3), 32–37.

Jefferson v. Griffin Spalding County Hospital Authority, 247 Ga. 86, 274 S.E. 2d 457 (1981).

John F. Kennedy Memorial Hospital v. Heston, 58 N.J. 576 (1971).

Joswick v. Lenox Hill Hospital, 510 N.Y.S. 2d 803 (New York, 1986).

Karp v. Cooley, 493 F. 2d 408 (5th Cir., 1974).

Korman v. Mallin, 858 P. 2d 1145 (Alaska, 1993).

Leach v. Akron General Medical Center, 13 Ohio App. 3d 393, 469 N.E. 2d 1047 (Ohio, 1984).

Lincoln v. Gupta, 370 N.W. 2d 312 (Michigan, 1985).

Madison v. Harrison, #68651 (Massachusetts, 1957).

Michigan Nurses' Association. (1994). *MNA Human Rights/Ethics Committee position statement on assisted voluntary self-termination.* Okemos, MI: Author.

Norwood Hospital v. Munoz, 564 N.E. 2d 1017 (Massachusetts, 1991).

O'Brien v. Cunard Steamship Company, 154 Mass. 272, 28 N.E. 226 (1899).

Patreillo v. Kalman et al., 576 A. 2d 474 (Connecticut, 1990).

Payne v. Marion General Hospital, 549 N.E. 2d 1043 (Ind. App. 2d Dis., 1990).

Piper, A., Jr. (1994). Truce on the battlefield: A proposal for a different approach to medical informed consent. *The Journal of Law, Medicine, and Ethics.* 22(4), 301–313.

Public Law, 97–248 (1982).

Rochin v. California, 342 U.S. 165 (1950).

Rozovsky, F. A. (1990). *Consent to treatment: A practical guide* (2nd ed.). Boston: Little, Brown and Company.

Rutherford, M. (1994). Small patients, big legal risks. *RN,* 57(9), 51–57.

Salgo v. Leland Stanford, Jr., University Board of Trustees, 317 P.2d 170 (Cal. Dis. Ct. App., 1957).

Schmerber v. California, 384 U.S. 757 (1966).

Schloendorff v. Society of New York Hospitals, 211 N.Y. 125, 105 N.E. 92 (1914).

Superintendent of Belchertown State School v. Saikewicz, 373 Mass. 728, 370 N.E. 2d 417 (1977).

Switzer, K. H. (1995). Informed consent for inserting a CVC. *American Journal of Nursing,* 95(6), 66–67.

The Patient Self-Determination Act, Sections 4206 and 4751 of the *Omnibus Reconciliation Act of 1990,* Public Law 101-508, November 1990.

Thor v. Superior Court, 855 P.2d 375, 21 Cal. Rept. 2d 357 (California, 1993).

Truman v. Thomas, 27 Cal. 3d 285, 611 P.2d 902 (1980).

45 CFR, sec. 46.111, 46.101(b), 46.110, and 46.116.

21 CFR, parts 50, 56, 312, 314, and 812.

· nine

Documentation and Confidentiality

PREVIEW

A major responsibility of all health care providers is that they keep accurate and complete medical records. Much of what is collected and recorded is very sensitive information. Understanding the need for clear and concise records, as well as knowing which portions of the record may be discovered and introduced during trials, should enable nurses to be proficient recorders of patient care. This chapter presents guides for documentation, including both the patient record as well as incident reports, and for issues of confidentiality.

medical records	retention of records	patient's right to privacy
standards for record keeping	omnia praesumuntur contra spoliatorem	confidentiality of medical records
effective documentation	patient access to medical records	common law duty to disclose
computerized charting		
charting by exception	incident, variance, situation, or unusual occurrence report forms	
alteration of records		

MEDICAL RECORDS

Medical records and a medical records library are mandated by federal governmental and nongovernmental agencies. Additionally, agencies, such as the Joint Commission for the Accreditation of Healthcare Organizations (JCAHO), and state and local rules and regulations further define this complex area.

From a nursing perspective, the most important purpose of documentation is communication. The *purposes of medical records,* as identified by JCAHO, are as follows:

1. Assist in planning patient care and in continuing the evaluation of the patient's condition and ongoing treatment.
2. Document the course of the patient's medical evaluation, treatment, and change in condition.
3. Document communication between the practitioner responsible for the patient and any other health professional who contributes to the patient's care.
4. Assist in protecting the legal interest of the patient, the hospital, and the practitioner responsible for the patient.
5. Provide data for use in continuing education and in research (1995).

Thus such documents not only record what has transpired but also serve as a vital communication link among members of the health care team and further educational and research programs.

To accomplish the primary purposes of record keeping, the JCAHO *Accreditation Manual for Hospitals* also specifies **standards for record keeping.** These standards attempt to ensure:

1. Patient identification.
2. Medical support for the selected diagnoses.
3. Justification of the medical therapies used.
4. Accurate documentation of that which has transpired.
5. Preservation of the record for a reasonable time period.

Although the *Accreditation Manual for Hospitals* previously specified only in-patient care, the latest edition dictates that the same high standards apply to emergency care patients, patients seen through the hospital's ambulatory clinics (outpatients), and patients seen in conjunction with a hospital-based home health care program (JCAHO, 1995).

CONTENTS OF THE RECORD

The basic information that should be recorded for any patient includes:

1. Personal data such as name, date of birth, gender, marital status, occupation, and person(s) to be contacted for emergencies.
2. Financial data such as the health insurance carrier with assignment of rights, patient employer, and person responsible for payment of the final bill.
3. Medical data.

These last data entries form the bulk of the record and include, but are not limited to, a history of signs and symptoms, diagnoses, treatments, medical tests, laboratory results, consultation reports, anesthesia and operating room records, signed informed consent forms, progress notes, respiratory therapy records, and nurses' notes. In some states and in some instances, marital status may not be recorded. For example, some states prohibit the inclusion of the parents' marital status on birth certificates to prevent the stigma of illegitimacy.

The accreditation standards also specify that the documentation of nursing care reflect the individual patient's status. Thus nurses' notes should address patient needs, problems, limitations, and responses to nursing interventions. Individualized, goal-directed nursing care is provided to patients through the use of the nursing process. Each patient's nursing needs are assessed by a registered nurse at the time of admission or within the period established by the nursing department/service policy. Patient education and patient/family knowledge of self-care are given specific consideration in the nursing plan. The plan of care is documented and reflects current standards of nursing practice (JCAHO, 1995).

The observations charted should lead to nursing diagnoses. Pertinent patient quotes about symptoms and feelings should be included in the medical record. It is advisable to use some form of nursing process in charting so that no pertinent information is overlooked or forgotten.

Documentation must show continuity of care, interventions that were used, and patient responses to the therapies implemented. Nurses' notes are to be concise, clear, timely, and complete. Even if the patient condition does not change, the absence of change should be recorded at least once per shift. The complete patient assessment performed by the nurse caring for a selected patient should be reflected, in its entirety, in the patient's medical record.

EFFECTIVE DOCUMENTATION

The American legal system has helped nurses recognize what must be included in charting and, through case law, has given tips on how to chart entries correctly. These tips for *effective documentation* are enumerated in the following paragraphs.

Make an Entry for Every Observation

If no mention has been made of a change in a patient's condition, the jury can infer that no observation of the patient was conducted. In *Javis v. St. Charles Medical Center* (1986), the physician had ordered hourly assessments of the patient's fractured leg to assess for the development of compartment syndrome, and required immediate notification if changes occurred in the patient's condition. While initial assessments were made and recorded, there was evidence in the chart of sporadic assessments. At 4:00 AM on the day that the patient's condition changed, there was a notation of normal circulation, movement, and pulsation in the patient's extremity. When the physician saw the patient at 8:30 AM on the same day, the foot was pulseless, white, and painful. No intervening notations could be found on the record. One could argue that such assessments were most likely performed and not charted, but at some time there had been a significant change in the patient's condition. The jury in this case concluded that, since there were no records, there were likewise no observations and decided against the nursing staff and the hospital. The lesson from this case is that even routine checks of patients must be recorded because failure to record such data leads to the inference that the patient had not been checked.

Follow Up as Needed

Merely charting changes in patient status may not be adequate. The landmark decision of *Darling v. Charleston Community Memorial Hospital* (1965) showed that follow-up measures must be taken. James Darling, an 18-year-old high school football player, had broken his leg during a Saturday afternoon game and had the leg casted at the local hospital. Following the casting, he was admitted for observation. The nursing staff continued to assess Darling's casted leg, noting repeatedly in the patient record his deteriorating condition, the foul odor being emitted from the casted extremity, and the patient's ever-increasing pain. The nurses shared their observations with the primary physician, but took no further action when the primary physician failed to take corrective action.

The court concluded that the follow-up and evaluation of the patient's responses were equally important to the initial assessment, that the nurses had a further duty to the patient, and that merely assessing and charting Darling's condition were insufficient. The court also inferred that proper documentation, no matter how accurate and timely it is, can never be a substitute for quality nursing care. Rather, the nursing staff should have reported their observations and lack of subsequent medical interventions to the nursing supervisor. The supervisor should have consulted the medical chief for the service.

Complete records, though, may help to protect the staff from legal liability. In a classic Kentucky case, periodic observations plus accurate charting, coupled with timely physician contact and medical management, allowed a jury to conclude that there was no liability against either the nursing staff or the physician (*Engle v. Clarke*, 1961). This principle has since been upheld in a number of cases (Miller, 1990).

Read the Notes before Giving Care

Few nurses have been encouraged to read the nurses' notes prior to giving care and/or charting. By taking the time to read the entry prior to the current one, nurses may note if there has been a change in the patient's condition. Even physicians have a duty to read nurses' notes, concluded the court in a 1988 case. There a patient's leg incision failed to heal properly following heart bypass surgery. After the patient continued to mention her discomfort and a discharge from the leg incision persisted, the nurse made an entry in the record. The patient continued to experience problems with her leg and a year after the initial surgery, x-rays revealed that hemoclips had been left in her leg.

The defendants prevailed because no medical expert witness was called to testify. If there had been expert testimony, both the physician and the hospital would have had difficulty explaining why no one, particularly the surgeon, paid attention to the patient's complaint or the nurses' notes. The court concluded that the nurses' notes literally and figuratively stand out "like a red flag" (*Regan Report on Nursing Law*, 1988, p. 1).

Always Make an Entry, Even If It Is Late

Record entries must be timely, charted as close to the happening as possible. Time dulls even the best memories, and nurses may have to strain to recall what actually transpired. Too often valuable information is then omitted for the lack of recall. If one must chart after the fact, it is more important that all pertinent data are included rather than preserving the chronological order of the chart. To show timeliness, remember to include the complete date and time of charting in the entry. The use of military or 24-hour time has aided in the accuracy of timed entries.

There is no rule against charting out of time sequence, and a late entry is far superior to no entry at all. However, the longer the time interval between the actual patient care and the charting of the care, the more the court may become suspicious that the additional entry was made merely to prevent liability. If a late entry is made, the nurse may want to add a note stating why the entry is late or to explain why the charting had not been done earlier. Such a note could be as simple as "First day back from three scheduled days off" or "Patient chart unavailable at 03:00."

Make the Chart Entry after the Event

Never chart in advance of an event, treatment, or medication. The patient may not tolerate the procedure as had been intended or may not take the medication, or the nurse may have been unable to complete the intended treatment. For example, another patient on the unit arrests or needs assistance immediately, and the already charted procedure is never completed. Or the patient may be in a full code and the vital signs as recorded show an acceptable heart rate, respiratory rate, and blood pressure. While it seems a small issue, if it can be shown that the nurse charted in advance, an attorney may be able to lessen the nurse's credibility in the eyes of a jury.

Use Clear Language

For years, nurses have been taught to use somewhat vague terminology in charting rather than drawing conclusions. Entries were used as "appears to be asleep," "seems to be resting comfortably," or, even more vague, "had a good night." These types of entries were thought to protect the nurse against drawing conclusions or being accused of making medical diagnoses. In looking at such vague verbiage, today's attorney is inclined to ask questions that cast doubt on the nurses' observational powers or that serve to imply that what the nurse actually saw was quite different from what was charted. Thus, nurses should use objective, definite terms so that there is no doubt about the certainty of the entry.

Be Realistic and Factual

Nurses should also chart a realistic picture of patients, particularly those who refuse to comply with therapeutic regimes or who are difficult to care for because of abusive and threatening language. These patients may well have a less than satisfactory outcome, especially if they were noncompliant. Charting what patients say, instances of noncompliance, and threats against nursing personnel helps to prevent such cases from coming to court. Prospective attorneys will be hesitant to represent clients who caused or contributed to their unsatisfactory outcomes.

Noted observations should be factual and should describe objectively the patient's symptoms, appearance, and behaviors. Avoid any language of blame or negligence in charting. If needed, use quotation marks to include actual patient statements. Never use conclusory statements without giving supportive objective data, such as "Patient states he was tying to climb over the bedrail and that is why he fell."

Chart Only Your Own Observations

It is advisable that nurses refrain from charting for other nurses, unless absolutely necessary. For example, the physician insists on giving an injection and the nurse notes that medication received by the patient, as well as the person who administered it. Because patient records may be used in a variety of courts, nurses doing the charting will be unable to remember particulars about the patient, diagnoses, and nursing care. Yet they will be called to testify since their names appear on the chart. For the same reason, chart only what is observed or assessed.

Some institutions still require that professional nurses chart or "cosign" charts for unlicensed personnel. Charting for others or cosigning notes makes the charting nurse potentially liable for care, observations, or omissions as charted. Always read and investigate what has been charted before cosigning. Nurses should further investigate ways of changing such policies.

Correct Charting Errors

The legal system has also given guidance on how to rectify charting errors. There is adequate case law to support the contention that, if errors appear in part of the record, the jury could find that errors might just as easily exist elsewhere as well, and thus the entire record could be found to be erroneous. Recognizing that anyone could make an error or misspell a word, the error in question should have a single line drawn through it with the correct entry placed above or next to the error. Also include the time and date of the correction, and initial or sign the correction to show by whom, when, and why a new notation was made. The nurse may also explain the correction with an entry such as "Entry made on wrong chart" or "Spelling error." To avoid charting on another patient's chart, each page of the patient's medical record should be stamped with the patient's name, medical record number, and other institution identifiers.

If the reason for striking a portion of the chart is self-evident, no additional note need be made and the nurse should just initial the cross-out. For example, a misspelled word is crossed out, and the correctly spelled word appear next to the entry. Frequently this is seen when the word "right" is crossed out and "left" inserted, or vice versa. Obviously, the wrong extremity was first charted, and then the correct extremity was identified.

Many institutions discourage the use of "error" (such as "spelling error" or "error in charting") when correcting a chart entry. There is some concern that using the word "error" may be interpreted as though the entire entry is in error, and nurses are urged to avoid using the word on the chart.

Nurses should never, under any circumstance, totally obliterate the entry, tape a new entry over the erroneous entry, or use a more imaginative way to prevent the reading of the error in their charting. Correction fluid was not invented to obliterate a medical record entry and should not be used for this purpose. Such obliterations or erasures serve only to raise suspicion and questions. Innocent though the entry may be, it is hard to defend a lawsuit with altered records. In *Ahrens v. Katz* (1984), white-outs of part of the nursing notes in the original chart were discovered and the records x-rayed so that the injured party's counsel could determine what the nurse had originally written.

For the same reason, charts should never be destroyed or recopied, for the question is always asked "What was the nurse trying to hide?" Additionally, records should not be altered if nurses know that a lawsuit is pending. The attorney for the patient already has a copy of the record and additions or changes will not be on that copy. Thus, the patient's attorney will introduce that a new version of the chart has been made.

Physicians do not have the right to demand that nurses alter records, nor may physicians alter nurses' notes. In *Henry v. St. John's Hospital* (1987), a patient in active labor was administered 6 cc of Marcaine IM in each hip by the resident, and the nurse recorded the drug, dosage, and person administering the medication in the nursing notes. After the neonate was born with fetal distress, the resident went back and amended the dosage to a lesser amount. The court found against the resident and defendant hospital.

Attorneys for injured patients examine charts for evidence that materials have been included later or that a part of the record has been totally replaced. Examples of such alterations include:

1. Writing crowded around existing entries.
2. Changes in slant, pressure, uniformity, or other differences in handwriting.
3. Use of different pens or typewriters to write a single entry.
4. Additions of different dates written in the same ink, while original entries were written in a separate, but consistent ink.
5. Differences between pages as to folds, stains, offsets, holes, tears, and type of paper used.
6. Use of forms not in use at the purported time of entry.
7. Use of later years (1996 for 1995), especially if corrected (Nygaard and Deubner, 1988).

A different color of ink was the clue that the record had been altered in *Rotan v. Greenbaum* (1959). The plaintiff died from an allergic reaction to penicillin, which had been ordered during treatment for mumps. The record indicated that the penicillin was given "for mumps and pharyngitis." However, the words "and pharyngitis" were written in a different color ink, clearly because penicillin would be an appropriate treatment for pharyngitis, while not an appropriate therapy for mumps.

Above all, the record must be readable and charted in ink. One of the primary purposes of charting is to communicate with other health care workers about the patient's condition, response to therapies, and progress. If nurses cannot write clearly and their writing cannot be read, then they should print the entry. There is no communication if the primary entry maker is unable to make the entry clear.

Writing should be legible and only standard, institution-approved abbreviations used. If nurses have difficulty remembering an abbreviation or frequently confuse the abbreviation among several meanings, they should not use it. It is far better to spell out an entry than to be unable to explain the abbreviation to the jury. And counsel for the injured party frequently reviews the records with the author during deposition, insisting that each illegible word and comment be explained.

Nurses' notes should be organized and written as neatly as possible. Writing sloppy notes may have no bearing on the quality of care delivered. However, opposing attorneys will make the observation that, if nurses are disorganized and sloppy in charting, then they are most likely disorganized and sloppy in the delivery of nursing care. Many jurors will accept that as true.

Since documentation is done to communicate to other health care deliverers the status of the patient, never invent new abbreviations that have meaning only to one or two persons or to one nursing unit in the hospital. Such self-coined abbreviations hinder rather than assist the communication process. A second and equally valid reason not to coin new abbreviations is that nurses are likely not to remember what they meant when asked by opposing counsel. It is difficult to show quality, competent care when the primary nurse is unable to ascertain what happened to the patient.

Perhaps the best reason not to use self-coined abbreviations is because of how they appear to the patient or what they signify. In a 1990 case, the family had been concerned about the quality of health care delivery during the elderly patient's hospital stay. The family brought suit, especially after they discovered the "PBBB" notation in the physician's progress note stood for "pine box by bedside." The case settled before going to court. (Mariqels, 1990).

Identify Yourself after Every Entry

At the conclusion of all entries, nurses identify themselves by their full names and titles, whether or not they have been previously identified. Some institutions allow nurses to use initials at the conclusion of a page entry if they have signed the bottom portion of the page, where all personnel charting are identified by name and status.

Use Standardized Checklists or Flow Sheets

To prevent routine care from being omitted from the chart and to ensure that frequent observations are both performed and charted, many hospitals have adopted graphic sheets or flow sheets. Even checking that patients have received take-home instruction sheets are significant in preventing subsequent liability (*Roberts v. Sisters of St. Francis*, 1990). These simple checklist approaches to charting are legally valid and prevent the need for long chart entries. This method also seems to prevent some of the short-hand charting that left large gaps in the chart.

GUIDELINES: WHAT THE CHART SHOULD CONTAIN

1. All the information that is necessary to communicate the patient's progress:
   a. Initial assessment data.
   b. Description of actual and/or potential problems.
   c. Record of all procedures, treatments, medications, and care.
   d. Record of health teaching.
   e. Description of patient reactions to treatments, procedures, medications, and teaching.
   f. Record of actions taken and persons contacted.
2. Information presented in a form that communicates the patient's progress, that is, notes that:
   a. Are made at the time of or immediately following the event recorded, with correct times and dates.
   b. Are written and properly signed by the person doing or observing the event being recorded.
   c. Are made in chronological order.
   d. Are free of omissions, personal opinions, generalizations, and ambiguous abbreviations.
   e. Are concise, precise, spelled correctly, accurate, and unambiguous.
   f. Are legible and neat.
   g. Have no unused spaces or blank lines.
3. Information that is recorded from a legal perspective:
   a. Record of the obvious: Record what you actually saw, did, or communicated to another.
   b. Do not allow inaccuracies to be charted: Record what actually happened, even if you wish you had done something differently.
   c. Do not obliterate an entry: Draw a single line through an error, mark it as a mistaken entry, and sign it using your first initial, last name, and correct title.
   d. Do not destroy parts of the record: Follow the same advice as for obliteration of an entry.
   e. Describe events and behaviors: Do not use labels or medical terms you are unsure of in charting.
   f. Document all communications to others and any intermediary steps taken; if you question an order, document that you recontacted the physician and clarified the order.
   g. Record all routine assessments and nursing care; help develop a flow sheet for more accurate records, if needed.

Leave No Room for Liability

One last point to remember is that the nurse should chart on all lines in sequence and ensure that additional entries cannot be squeezed in later. Blank spaces allow others to enter information over the previous nurse's signature, in which case the previous nurse may then be legally liable for the entry.

EXERCISE 9-1

For the last two of your patients (or any two patients), compare the nursing notes against the guidelines presented in this chapter. Can they be written more completely to adhere to the guidelines? If the answer is yes, do so. Has this exercise changed your opinion of the importance of nursing documentation? Explain your answer.

COMPUTERIZED CHARTING

Many institutions have adopted, either in part or in whole, *computerized charting.* The use of computers makes the recording of facts more accurate and does it more promptly than in manual charting, particularly when bedside computers are used. Nursing information systems (NIS) also allow for accuracy at all stages of the nursing process, from assessment to evaluation. In fact, some systems prompt nurses if a portion of the nursing process is omitted. Perhaps one of the more important reasons for computers in hospitals is the improved patient care that results with computers. Necessary test and laboratory results are instantly available, medication errors are reduced, and problems with charting, such as illegible writing, misspellings, unapproved abbreviations, and the time needed for writing entries, are eliminated.

Issues of concern with using computers for hospital records usually focus on patients' rights to privacy and confidentiality. Actually, a properly designed and implemented computer program offers more security than do more traditional charting procedures. Security is enhanced because:

1. There are fewer points of access into the system.
2. Each person's access can be restricted to a limited scope of information.
3. The information sought through individual access codes can be monitored, making misuse easier to detect.

CHARTING BY EXCEPTION

This abbreviated system of charting radically differs from the more traditional methods of charting. *Charting by exception* requires only documentation of significant or abnormal findings, and previously entered standardized or expected results are not entered into the chart. The charting by exception format uses preprinted guidelines, such as nursing diagnosis-based standardized care plans and protocols, flow sheets, and graphic records to show the progress, or lack of progress, of the patient. Bedside charting is increased, so that health care workers have immediate access to patient data. Charting by exception streamlines documentation by combining three essential elements:

1. Standards of nursing care.
2. Flow sheets.
3. Bedside access to chart forms.

Institutions can personalize charting by exception to fit their own needs. For example, they can either use only the preprinted guidelines or individualize patient care within the preprinted guidelines. In the latter case, however, the institution must establish standards that are uniformly used by all health care personnel and establish normal findings and expected outcomes, so that all significant data are considered when assessing patient outcomes.

Charting by exception is not without some legal perils. Charting by exception may fail to provide enough information to alert practitioners to potential problems. For example, in *Lama v. Borras* (1994), the patient underwent surgery for a herniated disc. Two days later, there was an entry noting that the surgical dressing was "very bloody," and pain at the site of the incision was noted on the following day. By the fourth day postoperatively, the surgical dressing was again "soiled," and severe incisional pain was noted on the fifth day postoperatively. On the sixth day after surgery, the physician diagnosed diskitis and began antibiotic therapy.

Review of the patient's chart failed to show what happened during the time that the patient's dressing became bloody and he experienced increasing pain. Vital signs and medications are charted, but important details, such as the status of the incision or the duration and intensity of pain, were not charted. Lacking, too, are possible nursing and medical interventions that should have accompanied the changing surgical drainage and pain or any communications that occurred between the nursing and medical staff.

The jury in this case concluded that more complete charting could have answered questions that charting by exception failed to answer. The jury also concluded that the infection might have been diagnosed sooner if more traditional charting methods had been followed. "Intermittent charting failed to provide the sort of continuous danger signals that would be the most likely to spur early intervention by a physician" was the final holding of the court (at 278). The court further found that this type of charting failed to meet the regulations of the Puerto Rico Department of Health, which requires qualitative nurses' notes to be recorded for each patient by each nursing shift.

Charting by exception may make it impossible to show the attentiveness of the nursing staff to patients, particularly patients in whom complications develop. Charting by exception may not assist nurses in being able to defend themselves, because even they cannot re-create what was done and not done for an individual patient. Remember that it may be two years before nurses know that a lawsuit is filed.

ALTERATION OF RECORDS

Essentially two types of *alterations of records* may be necessary to ensure a truthful, accurate record. The first concerns *minor errors,* such as those that occur in spelling, notations of laboratory data, incorrect phraseology, and the like. These types of errors are usually corrected by the person making the entry at the time of the entry or shortly after the entry was made. The error should be marked through with a single line, and then the correct information should be entered, timed, dated, and signed. Never erase or obliterate incorrect entries, since such actions raise suspicion in jurors' minds.

The second type of alteration concerns *substantive errors,* such as incorrect test data, omitted progress notes, incorrect orders, and the like. Only administrative staff or the primary physician should correct such substantive errors, and all persons misled by the error should be contacted and advised of the correct information. Correction for these types of errors include the addition of new materials with the explanation of why they were necessitated, who made the addition, the date, and the time.

An addendum to the record by a physician or other health care provider should not be seen as proof of an error. Occasionally, an addendum may be written based on new information that was just received. However, since a patient's record should reflect as closely as possible concurrent treatment and observation, adding information at a later date is unusual. The further away in time the charting occurs, the more suspicious a reviewer can be about the provider's purpose.

Patients may wish to correct or modify an entry in the medical record. Usually the patient is permitted to add to the original chart a letter of explanation regarding the modification or addition. Staff agreeing with the letter of modification or addition may also add their own letters of support. This approach preserves the original document while clarifying the source and nature of the change.

RETENTION OF RECORDS

Health care facilities have a responsibility to maintain and protect patient records (*Fox v. Cohen,* 1980). This obligation, **retention of records,** is codified in state statutes that impose a clear duty on facilities not to lose or destroy records within certain time frames. The time frame usually coincides with state statutes of limitations for medical negligent causes of action.

Record retention varies according to state law, with the majority of states preserving records for the period of time in which suits may be filed (state statutes of limitations) or for five years, whichever time interval is longer. As a practical matter, most institutions save records for longer periods.

The impact of lost medical records can be devastating to meeting the burden of proof. If records are lost, are incomplete, or have disappeared, the court tends to presume negligence and juries have no difficulty finding for the injured party. Known as *omnia praesumuntur contra spoliatorem* ("all things are presumed against a despoiler"), courts have allowed such disappearances and lack of records to suggest a presumption of guilt. In *May v. Moore* (1982), the Alabama Supreme Court held that even testimony about a physician's lost records (and this physician had a record of losing charts when the outcome was bad) was admissible and was sufficient to create an inference of negligent treatment.

The destruction of medical records may be performed to protect confidentiality, and destruction should be complete. Should patients request the destruction of their medical records prior to the retention interval lapsing, many courts favor sealing the record over total destruction. Sealing preserves the record while preventing its discovery.

OWNERSHIP OF THE RECORD

Because the chart is the business record of the institution, the hospital is the rightful owner of the entire record. Correspondingly, individual physicians own the chart records of patients seen in their offices. Courts have recognized this right of hospital ownership by declaring that, since hospital records are essential to proper administration, the records become the property of the hospital.

This ownership right of hospitals to their business records does not preclude the patients' property rights in the same records. The patient generally has the right to all the information contained within the record and to a copy of the original record. (The hospital may charge the patient a reasonable fee for the copy.) Some exceptions are made for certain psychiatric records, and state law may forbid patients access to some psychiatric records.

ACCESS TO MEDICAL RECORDS

Besides a legal right to the record, there are some practical reasons for allowing the *patient access to medical records.* Allowing patients access to their medical records helps to dispel feelings that the physician was lying about the severity of their illnesses or that the physician was unsympathetic to their illnesses. Allowing access also helps reassure patients that their care was based on actual medical findings.

Most states require that the record be completed prior to the patient's right of access, and statutes have been enacted to establish procedures for patient access. For example, the policy may provide that access be between the hours of 9 AM to 5 PM Monday through Friday and only when a hospital representative is present to answer questions. It is also generally recognized that competent patients can authorize this right of access to others. These others include insurance carriers, legal representation, and outside professionals acting on behalf of the patient.

One of the problems concerning patients' access to medical records arises when patients are incompetent, minors, or die prior to exercising their rights. In such instances, others may be able to authorize access to a patient record. As a general rule, guardians of incompetent patients stand in the place of the patients and can authorize access. If there is no court-appointed guardian, hospitals may rely on the authorization of the next of kin or the person responsible for authorization and payment of the medical treatment.

Access may be refused if family confidences or information about anyone other than the patient would be needlessly disclosed through access to a mentally incompetent patient's medical record. *McDonald v. Clinger* (1982) denied access of a patient record to a spouse with a showing that such disclosure would cause a danger to the patient, spouse, or other person.

Access to the charts of minors also presents a recurring problem, especially in the event of treatment for sexually transmitted diseases, pregnancy, or substance abuse. As a rule, if minors are authorized under state law to consent to their own care, then parents will not have a right of access to the record. Additionally, the payment for care may help to decide access questions. If minors, even mature minors, rely on their parents for payment of care, then the parents may have the right of access to the record or of disclosure from the primary health care provider.

In the event of a patient's death, the next of kin or the executor of the estate may authorize access to the record. If the spouse has predeceased the patient, it would be advisable to obtain the authorization of all adult children rather than rely on the authorization of only one of them.

Access may be gained to a patient record by law. Examples of *access by law* include subpoenas of records if the party's mental or physical condition is relevant to the lawsuit, billing fraud by the health care provider is suspected, and if there is a statutory duty of disclosure.

In *Florida Department of Health and Rehabilitative Services v. V.M.R., Inc.* (1991), a warrant was issued allowing the Florida Department of Health and Rehabilitative Services to enter a women's medical center and inspect the clinic's premises and records. The clinic and two patients moved to quash the warrant, claiming that the medical records could not be released without written authorization from patients. The court agreed and noted that, although there may be an exception to the privacy provisions in limited circumstances, no such exception had been accorded this agency. Additionally, the court found that the agency's right to examine records did not extend to such personal information as a patient's name, address, and medical history. The impact of such decisions respects the state's authority to regulate, but the power does not allow a governmental agency to make private medical records public.

A second concern with access is the patient's right to privacy and confidentiality. Such privacy rights encourage candor by the patient and optimize proper medical treatment and diagnosis. Privacy rights also allow nurses to be truthful and open in their assessments and recording of patient care. For example, in *Head v. Colloton* (1983), the Iowa Supreme Court held that the records of a potential donor for a bone marrow transplant were hospital records and, as such, were exempt from release as public records under the state's freedom of information law.

In general, health care providers involved in the direct care of the patient have access to the record, and records should be housed where they will be the most accessible for patient care providers. This encourages prompt recording as well as quality patient care. Administrators and hospital staff members have access for the purposes of auditing, billing, quality assurance, and defending potential claims.

Researchers may also have access to medical records. Staff members and qualified students generally may review charts for research purposes without prior patient consent. If the institution receives federal funding, an internal or external review panel to protect the rights of human subjects is required prior to allowing researchers access to medical records.

INCIDENT REPORTS

Incident, variance, situation, or unusual occurrence report forms were originally designed to be part of the overall risk management or quality assurance effort of any health-oriented institution. JCAHO standards dictate the establishment of an incident reporting system (1995), with the main functions of incident reports being the review and evaluation of patient care. If one uses the definition of an *incident* to be an unfavorable deviation of expectations involving patient care, which may be the result of medical management, it is easy to see that incident reports were devised to augment and improve the quality of patient care. Other obvious uses of such forms are to enhance the hospital's in-service educational offerings, to alert hospital administrative staff to potential problem areas, to minimize injuries from the incident, and to decrease the likelihood of similar incidents in the future.

Incident reports may serve to aid the hospital attorney in planning defense strategy and in deciding whether a case should be litigated or settled out of court. The hospital's liability carrier frequently asks for such reports when investigating claims. Because of the confidential status of these reports in most states, nurses traditionally have been instructed to be candid in their remarks on incident reports so that the quality of care can be upgraded.

The confidentiality of incident reports is rooted in the doctrine of *hospital or business record privileged communication*. While not a common law right, hospitals have long declined to divulge such reports, arguing that disclosure would make the incident report virtually useless.

In today's legal atmosphere, more and more justices are ruling that plaintiff's, through their attorneys, have a right to discover incident reports. Declaring that plaintiffs must still show the need for their right to incident reports, several cases have allowed discovery.

Guidelines: Incident Reports

1. The incident report should be initiated by someone who directly observes the incident or by the first person to arrive at the site of the incident.

2. Incorporate patients' accounts of the happening into incident reports, and state their comments as direct quotes. If patients are unable to give an account, describe exactly what you witnessed or discovered. For example, "The patient fell out of bed" is appropriate if you actually saw the fall. Statements such as, "Patient found on floor at foot of bed," or "Patient states, 'I was trying to get up and lost my balance'" are more appropriate if you were the first person to discover the patient on the floor.

3. Write only the facts. Do not infer assumptions or draw conclusions. Do not add what you would like to have done after the fact. Above all, never imply liability. A question such as, "How could this incident have been prevented?" should be left unanswered or answered in the negative.

4. Have other witnesses assist you in preparing the report and have them cosign the final report.

5. If appropriate, have the patient or injured party seen by a physician and document any actions taken and treatment given.

6. Avoid writing in the medical record that an incident report was completed, or else it will become incorporated by reference into the patient's chart. Document what happened and the actions taken if the incident report involved a hospitalized patient.

7. Forward the report to nursing service, the hospital attorney, the quality assurance committee, and anyone else so designated by hospital policy.

8. Ensure that only one copy of the report exists. If other departments or committees would like to see the report, the original may be forwarded to them in succession.

9. Should your hospital require multiple copies of incident reports, initiate action to reduce the number of copies to one.

Nurses must exercise caution in completing these reports and should always fill out the forms as though they are discoverable. No language that admits liability should be included, and there should be no mention of the incident report form having been completed in the patient's chart. Indicating that there is an incident report, *incorporates by reference* the incident report into the chart and makes it as discoverable as the original patient chart. The ideal incident report is a checkoff list, with a limited area for a brief, written description of the occurrence.

It is also advisable to abandon multiple copies of the form because such copies tend to deny a privileged communication. For an incident report to be considered privileged under the attorney-client privilege, it is ideally completed and forwarded directly to the hospital attorney or the in-house representative.

EXERCISE 9-2

Acquire a copy of your facility's incident or variance report form. Does the form adhere to the guidelines suggested in this chapter? Explain how it does or does not. Design a form that could be substituted for the current form.

FAXING OF MEDICAL RECORDS

Using fax machines to send health information is another way to ensure that material is received promptly and accurately. However, difficulty arises in assuring the *patient's right to privacy.* JCAHO requires that facilities have safeguards in place that protect the security and confidentiality of computerized and paper-based records (1995). Thus, medical information should only be faxed if urgently needed, and it must be accompanied by a signed release form. Accompanying all medical faxes should be a cover sheet indicating (1) the confidentiality of the material and (2) the party to whom it is to be given. Additionally, fax machines should be located in an area with restricted access.

CONFIDENTIALITY OF MEDICAL RECORDS

The primary reason for the *confidentiality of medical records* is to promote candor by patients and health care providers to optimize medical and nursing treatment. The second reason for confidentiality is that violation of the right opens health care providers to potential lawsuit. Confidentiality respects patient privacy issues. In *Morris v. Consolidated Coal Company* (1994), a physician disclosed information about a patient to his employer, and the court held that the patient had a cause of action against the physician for breach of the duty of confidentiality.

REPORTING AND ACCESS LAWS

The law compels disclosure of medical information in contexts other than discovery or testimony. Reporting laws require that information be given to governmental agencies, both federal and state. Examples include vital statistics, child abuse, elder abuse, public health, and wounds.

Some statutes do not mandate reporting, but allow access to medical records without the patient's permission. Examples of such access laws include workers' compensation, state public records laws, and federal freedom of information act.

COMMON LAW DUTY TO DISCLOSE

The *common law duty to disclose* recognizes a duty to disclose medical information in limited circumstances. Persons who could have avoided injury if information were disclosed have filed successful lawsuits against those with a duty to disclose.

Contagious Diseases

When dealing with contagious diseases, health care providers have a duty to warn others at risk for exposure unless forbidden by statute. This includes family members and health care providers, among others. In most states there is no duty to warn all members of the public individually, but states vary on this requirement. For example, the State Supreme Court in Georgia has held that a hospital could be held liable for the death of a patient from meningitis. The child's friend had been diagnosed and treated for meningitis at Oconee Memorial Hospital, and the hospital failed to notify persons who had had contact with the child during the contagious period (*Phillips v. Oconee Memorial Hospital*, 1986).

Threats to an Identified Person

Some courts have ruled of the duty to warn identified persons when a patient has made a credible threat against them. The first decision to impact this duty was *Tarasoff v. Board of Regents of the University of California* (1976). In that case, a nonhospitalized psychiatric patient told his psychiatrist that he would kill his former girlfriend. The threat to kill was made more than once, and there was no doubt in the psychiatrist's mind that the patient could make good his threat. After Tarasoff was killed, her parents brought this lawsuit for wrongful death, and the court concluded that the psychiatrist or his employer had a duty either to warn the potential victim or to warn others who could have advised the victim of her potential danger. In a later decision, *Thompson v. County of Alameda* (1980), the same court clarified the scope of this duty to warn by ruling that only threats to readily identifiable persons created a duty to warn, and there is no corresponding duty to the public at large.

Courts have since split on this duty to warn. *Hamman v. County of Maricopa* (1989) ruled that foreseeable victims had to be warned even without specific threats, and *Peterman v. State* (1983) held that the duty to warn extended to unidentifiable victims. Courts have extended this duty to warn to include property damage, imposing a liability on a counseling service when a patient of theirs burned his parents' barn (*Peck v. Counseling Service*, 1985), while other courts have held that there is no duty to warn even readily identifiable victims (*Shaw v. Glickman*, 1980). Perhaps the safest course of action to follow in states that have yet to rule in this area is to follow the California rule and warn identified individuals of credible threats when the patient is not detained.

A trend is beginning to extend this duty to warn to the general public. For example, in *Kathleen K. v. Robert B.* (1984), the court allowed a woman to sue her sexual partner for deliberate and/or negligent failure to warn her that he had genital herpes. A more recent case, *Reisner v. Regents of the University of California* (1995), held that a man who discovered in 1990 that he had contracted the AIDS virus from his girlfriend may sue a physician for failing to inform her she had received contaminated blood in 1985.

LIMITATIONS TO DISCLOSURE

Several statutory and common law limitations on disclosure have evolved that assist in preserving confidentiality and impose sanctions for some violations of confidentiality.

Substance Abuse Confidentiality

Special federal rules deal with confidentiality of information concerning patients treated or referred for treatment for substance abuse. These rules apply to any facility receiving federal funding, including Medicare and Medicaid reimbursement. These rules prevent disclosure, and even acknowledgment of the patients' presence in the facility.

Information may be released with the patient's consent, if the consent is written and contains all of the following elements:

1. The name of the person or program to make the disclosure.
2. The name or title of the person or organization to receive the disclosure.
3. The name of the patient.
4. The purpose of the disclosure.
5. How much and what kind of information is to be disclosed.
6. The patient's signature.
7. The date of the signature.
8. A statement that the consent may be revoked.
9. The date when the consent will automatically expire.

A court order, including a subpoena, does not permit the release of information unless these nine elements are all met (42 CRF, 1988).

Child abuse reports may be made under state law without patient consent or court order, but release of records to child abuse agencies must have consent or an order. Staff members must be oriented to these rules. In *Heng v. Fos-*

ter (1978), a nurse successfully challenged her dismissal for failure to report a fellow staff member's theft of patient files by establishing the reasonableness of her belief that the federal regulations prohibited the report.

HIV/AIDS Confidentiality

Special characteristics of HIV, AIDS, and the AIDS epidemic present new and unique challenges to health care providers trying to maintain patient confidentiality, while meeting their obligations to disclose medical information. First, widespread fear of AIDS and ignorance about its transmission have made concerns of privacy and confidentiality even more important and urgent. If information about a person's AIDS infection or HIV positivity reaches employers, insurers, schools, or friends, it may have disastrous effects. And confidentiality is at the heart of HIV and AIDS testing, for most individuals will not submit to HIV testing and counseling unless there is assurance of confidentiality.

Second, the fact that the transmission of AIDS and HIV is not through close proximity or casual contact limits the need for disclosure of information about infection. This argument can be expounded both as a need not to warn, since the rate of infection is somewhere around .0001 per exposure, to an affirmative duty to warn, particularly in the transmission to unborn children.

Third, the fact that AIDS at present is incurable (though medications now exist to retard the full-blown event) makes prevention all the more essential. One can use this statement to argue either for strict confidentiality to allow persons to be tested and counseled, or for limited confidentiality to protect persons who may be exposed.

States have adopted a variety of legislative and administrative approaches to confidentiality and disclosure of information regarding AIDS and HIV. All states now require physicians to report AIDS cases to state health departments, and a number of states also require the reporting of HIV infection. The majority of states have adopted statutes maintaining the strict confidentiality of AIDS-related information, including California, Florida, and Massachusetts. Other states have passed statutes permitting the disclosure of AIDS testing to certain persons or under certain circumstances, such as Texas (disclosure to spouse permitted), Georgia (disclosure to spouse, sexual partner, or child permitted under limited circumstances), and New York (disclosure permitted if the infected person refuses to do so after counseling and a warning that the physician will disclose the information if the infected person does not do so).

A number of states permit the state health department to engage in contact tracing or partner notification. Some states notify all sexual and needle-sharing contacts, while others have chosen a more limited means of notifying contacts, such as the contact of all individuals who have received infected blood products. Health care providers are urged to investigate their state statutes in this regard.

EXERCISE 9-3

You have been appointed to a panel to establish a national standard for nursing documentation. The purpose of this panel is to assist in preventing future litigation centering around documentation. What types of uniform charting forms should be developed? Why? Can one form or one set of forms be developed for national usage? List the pros and cons of a national standard for documentation.

SUMMARY

Medical records ensure that communications concerning individual patients—including patients' diagnoses, treatments, procedures, interventions, and response to those treatments, procedures, and interventions—will be available to health care providers. Communications also exist for research, quality assurance, third-party payors, and legal defense. This chapter has outlined the reasons for written communication, explained how to document effectively, and stated general rules when patient data may be disclosed to others.

AFTER COMPLETING THIS CHAPTER, YOU SHOULD BE ABLE TO

- List and explain the five purposes of medical records.
- Define and describe basic information to be included in the medical record.
- List and give examples of ten guidelines for accurate documentation.
- Analyze the concepts of:
    Alteration of records.
    Retention of records.
    Ownership of medical records.
    Access to medical records.
    Computerized charting.
- Describe four important aspects of incident reports.
- Compare and contrast charting by exception to traditional charting.
- Define confidentiality and relate that concept to:
    Substance abuse conferences.
    AIDS/HIV conferences.
    Access laws.
    Child/elder abuse conferences.

APPLY YOUR LEGAL KNOWLEDGE

- How can a staff member ensure confidentiality in clinical settings?
- What makes charting effective? How can professional nurses ensure that their charting is effective?
- After learning the purposes and guidelines for documentation, how might one design a better chart?

REFERENCES

Ahrens v. Katz, 595 F. Supp. 1108 (N.D. Georgia, 1984).

California Health and Safety Code, Section 199.21.

Darling v. Charleston Community Memorial Hospital, 33 Ill. 2d 326, 211 N.E. 2d 253 (1965), cert. den'd. 383 U.S. 946 (1965).

Engle v. Clarke, 346 S.W. 2d 13 (Kentucky, 1961).

Florida Department of Health and Rehabilitative Services v. V.M.R., Inc., No. 90-2779, 1991 Fla. App. Lexis 6122 (July 2, 1991).

Florida Statutes Annotated, Section 14A, Section 381609 (2)(f).

Fox v. Cohen, 406 N.E. 2d 178 (Ill. App. Ct., 1980).

42 CFR 1988.

Hamman v. County of Maricopa, 775 P. 2d 1122 (Arizona, 1981).

Head v. Colloton, 331 N.W. 2d 870 (Iowa, 1983).

Heng v. Foster, 63 Ill. App. 3d 30, 379 N.E. 2d 688, 19 Ill. Dec. 816 (1st Dis., 1978).

Henry v. St. John's Hospital, 512 N.E. 2d 1044 (Illinois, 1987).

Hiatt v. Groce, 215 Kan. 14, 523 P. 2d 320 (1974).

Javis v. St. Charles Medical Center, 713 P. 2d 620 (Oregon, 1986).

Joint Commission for the Accreditation of Healthcare Organizations. (1995). *Accreditation manual for hospitals.* Oakbrook Terrace, IL: Author.

Kathleen K. v. Robert B., 198 Cal. Rept. 273 (Cal. App., 1984).

Lama v. Borras, 16 F.3d 473 (1st Cir. [PR] 1994).

McDonald v. Clinger, 84 A.D. 2d 482, 446 N.Y.S. 2d 801 (4th Dept., 1982).

McKinley's-*New York Public Health Law*, Section 2782(4)(a) and (b).

Massachusetts General Legislative Chapter 111, Section 70f.

Mangels, L. (1990). Chart notes from a malpractice insurer's hell. *Medical Economics*, November 12.

May v. Moore, 424 So. 2d 596 (Alabama, 1982).

Miller, R. D. (1990). Problems in hospital law. In R. D. Miller (6th ed.), *Patient information* (pp. 287–315). Rockville, MD: Aspen Publishers, Inc.

Morris v. Consolidated Coal Company, 446 S.E. 2d 648 (West Virginia, 1994).

Nygaard, D. A. and Deubner, S. J. (1988). Altered or lost medical records. *Trial 24* (6), 6–55.

Peck v. Counseling Service, 146 Vt. 61, 499 A. 2d 422 (1985).

Peterman v. State, 100 Wash 2d 421, 671 P. 2d 230 (Washington, 1983).

Phillips v. Oconee Memorial Hospital, 290 S.C. 192, 348 S.E. 2d 836 (South Carolina, 1986).

Regan Report on Nursing Law (1988). *29*(6), 1.

Reisner v. Regents of the University of California, 37 Cal. Rept. 2d 518 (Ct. App. 1995).

Roberts v. Sisters of St. Francis, 566 N.E. 2d 662 (Illinois, 1990).

Rotan v. Greenbaum, 273 F. 2d 830 (D. C. Cir. 1959).

Shaw v. Glickman, 45 Md. App. 718, 415 A. 2d 625 (1980).

St. Francis Regional Medical Center v. Hale, 752 P. 2d 129 (Kansas, 1988).

Tarasoff v. Board of Regents of the University of California, 17 Cal. 3d 425, 551 P. 2d 334 (1976).

Thompson v. County of Alameda, 27 Cal. 3d 741, 614 P. 2d 728 (1980).

Vernon's *Annotated Texas Revised Civil Statutes*, Article 4419b-1, Section 9.03.

· ten

Professional Liability Insurance

PREVIEW

With the advent of the malpractice crisis of the 1970s, health care providers rapidly became acutely aware of the vast scope of potential lawsuits that could be filed against them, either individually or collectively. This malpractice scare served to alert health care providers of their unique vulnerability. Lawsuits could be filed by any health care consumer at almost any time. Physicians quickly acquired and increased their liability coverage. Nurses, like their physician counterparts, should not be without professional liability insurance. This chapter explores issues that nurses should consider and investigate when choosing a policy that will give them the best protection should a lawsuit be filed against them.

INSURANCE POLICIES

An *insurance policy,* sometimes called an *insuring agreement,* is a formal contract between the insurance carrier and an individual or corporation. For a stated premium (a fee per year), the insurance policy provides the insured party or *policy holder* with a specific dollar amount of protection when certain injuries are caused by the person(s) insured by the policy. The conditions of the coverage and the extent of coverage are detailed in the policy itself.

Regardless of the policy chosen, all *professional liability* policies share some common elements. The policies provide payment for a lawyer to represent the insured nurse in the event of a claim or lawsuit. Most insurance carriers insist that the nurse use a lawyer whom the insurance company has on retainer because this ensures both the nurse and the insurance carrier that the selected lawyer will be versed in medical malpractice issues. All policies specify the limits of legal liability. Insurance carriers pay settlements or jury awards but do not cover the cost of any moral obligations that nurses might feel they owe the injured party.

TYPES OF POLICIES

Insurance policies are classified in essentially two ways. The first way is as either occurrence-based or claims-made insurance coverage. *Occurrence-based policies* cover the nurse for any injuries arising out of incidents that occurred during the time that the policy was in effect, known as the *policy period.* This holds true even if the subsequent lawsuit is filed after the policy has expired and the policy was not renewed by the policy holder. *Claims-made policies* provide coverage only if an injury occurs and the claim is reported to the insurance company during the active policy period or during an uninterrupted extension of that policy period. The uninterrupted extension, or *tail,* allows the claims-made policy to be enforced for a specific period of time following the policy period.

The occurrence-based policy is preferable for most nurses since lawsuits may not be filed immediately, particularly in cases involving children and neonates. Claims-made coverage is adequate if the policy is continuously renewed and kept active or if a tail is purchased for extended coverage. If you have any doubt regarding the coverage needed, consult the insurance agent.

A second way of classifying insurance policies is as individual, group, or employer-sponsored coverage. *Individual coverage* is the broadest type of coverage and is specific to the individual policy holder. This type of policy covers the *named policy holder* on a 24-hour basis, as long as actions fall within the scope of professional nursing practice, including both paid services and voluntary services. This type of policy is tailored to meet the needs of the individual nurse. *Group coverage* involves insuring a group of similarly licensed professionals and may be advantageous in some private clinics or businesses. Group coverage is frequently obtained by professional practitioners where all the insured individuals practice during office hours and have essentially the same job descriptions. *Employer-sponsored coverage,* which is obtained by institutions, is perhaps the narrowest of coverage for individual nurses since they must first show that they are practicing within the scope of their employment as well as within the scope of professional nursing practice. Those covered are called the *insureds,* or they may be referred to as *former insureds for acts committed while insured.* Employer-sponsored coverage is favored by the institution since the coverage is written specifically for the business and its major concerns.

EXERCISE 10-1

Using your own professional clinical area, list arguments for purchasing either occurrence-based or claims-made insurance policies. Which coverage would be best for you as an individual policy holder?

DECLARATIONS

The first part of the policy is known as the **declarations.** Included under this section are the policy holder's name, address, covered professional occupation (such as general staff nurse, advanced family nurse practitioner, or emergency center staff nurse), and the covered time period. This section also lists the company's limits of liability coverage and state requirements for information that may modify the policy.

LIMITS AND DEDUCTIBLES

The insurance policy should have a section marked *limits of liability.* This section usually has language about two separate dollar figures. For example, it could read $500,000 each claim, $1,000,000 aggregate, or $1,000,000 each claim, $3,000,000 aggregate. These dollar figures indicate what the insurance company will pay during a given policy period. The company will pay up to the lower limits for any one claim or lawsuit and up to the upper limits of the policy during the entire policy period.

All claims arising from the same incident or occurrence are considered a *single claim* for purposes of the insurance coverage. For example, if a professional nurse inadvertently gave patient A the medications that were ordered for patient B, both patients could file suit for injuries caused by this single medication error. Most insurance companies would consider these two separate lawsuits as a single claim (arising from the same incident) and would pay up to the lower limits of the policy. The upper limit figure or aggregate figure is the total amount that the insurance carrier will pay for all claims made in a calendar year or policy period.

Deductibles include any amounts that the insurance carrier deducts from the total amount available to pay for plaintiff damages. Some policies deduct the amount paid for the nurse's legal defense from the total limits of liability.

ADDITIONAL CLAUSES IN INSURANCE POLICIES

Exclusions are items not covered in the insurance policy. In professional liability policies, exclusions frequently describe circumstances or activities that prevent coverage of the insured party. Exclusions also include the absence of appropriate licensure or certification. These exclusions may be covered in the policy under the general title *reservation of rights,* so-called because the company reserves the right to deny coverage once the facts are known. When and if it is determined that a restricted activity has been involved, then the insured nurse must reimburse the insurance company for expenses incurred for the legal defense. Other insurance companies insist that insured nurses pay all expenses out of pocket until it is shown that an excluded activity has not been involved.

Some of the more common examples of excluded activities involving inappropriate behavior include:

1. Criminal actions.
2. Incidents occurring while the insured was under the influence of either drugs or alcohol.
3. Physical assault, sexual abuse, molestation, habitual neglect, licentious and immoral behavior toward patients whether intentional, negligent, inadvertent, or committed with the belief that the other party was consenting.
4. Actions that result in punitive damages to the plaintiff.

More recent additions to this list include exclusion for the transmission of AIDS/HIV from the health care provider to a patient and exclusions for expanded roles in nursing. Sometimes this last exclusion is worded as "exclusions for liability incurred in the position of proprietor, superintendent, or executive officer of a clinic, laboratory, or business enterprise."

Exclusions also include any claims or suits resulting from the practice of a profession that does not appear on the certificate's declarations. Nurses should alert their insurance company when there is a change in professional status to ensure that they are fully covered during the policy period.

Terms in the *coverage* section indicate when the insured is actually covered and for what activities. Policies that have fairly broad coverage sections include language similar to the following: "... professional services by the individual insured, or by any persons for whose acts or omissions such insured is legally responsible ..." will be covered in this policy. Such verbiage indicates that the insureds are covered both for their own actions and for actions performed by nurses under their direct and indirect supervision. This coverage is vital for nurses who hold supervisory positions, such as nursing supervisors, charge nurses, and nursing faculty.

Defense costs are included in most policies. These include all reasonable and necessary costs occurred in the investigation, defense, and negotiation of any covered claim or suit. Most companies pay these in addition to the limits of liability. Additionally, if the nurse is required to appear before the state board of nursing or a governmental regulatory agency, the company pays attorney fees and other costs resulting from investigation or defense of the proceeding, up to $1,000 per policy period. This latter amount is in addition to the coverage limits.

Covered injuries outlines the types of injuries and provisions that the insurance company will honor. Usually insurance companies include personal (bodily) injury, mental anguish, property damage, personal injury to a patient such as invasion of privacy, libel, and slander, and economic damages such as covered injuries. The lawsuit must specifically note that the suit is for monetary damages. In other words, the insurance company covers the cost of litigation and awards if money damages are involved. The insurance company does not cover the cost of litigation if the action sought is a specific performance, as in the instance of a lawsuit brought to prevent a nurse practitioner for performing medical acts. *Sermchief v. Gonzales* (1983) is a good example of such a specific performance lawsuit.

The *supplementary payments* section includes provisions for additional payments to the insured party. Some policies may supplement lost earnings or reasonable expenses incurred by the insured as well as the cost of appeal bonds and costs of litigation charged against the insured. These latter provisions may also be termed *defense costs.*

Conditions or *coverage conditions* outline the insured nurse's duties to the insurance carrier in the event a claim or lawsuit is filed, provisions for cancellation of the policy, prohibition of assignment of the policy, and subrogation of rights. Many insurance policies cover policyholders only if they give written

Guidelines: Professional Liability Insurance Policies

1. Read the policy carefully before purchasing it and ask for explanations as needed. Make sure that the policy augments an employer-sponsored policy or adequately protects your interests if you are independently employed.

2. Make sure that the per-claim and aggregate coverage limits are adequate for your specific nursing needs. As a double check, scan your geographic area for the tendency of nurses to be named in lawsuits and for the average dollar damages being awarded plaintiffs.

3. Check on any information that relates to malpractice claims in your area. Resources to be explored include the local law library, insurance carriers, health claims arbitration boards, and hospital attorneys.

4. Look to see that the policy gives you optimal coverage. It should be occurrence-based coverage and include protection for both your direct professional actions as well as the professional actions of those you supervise. If your area allows only the purchase of claims-made coverage, investigate the availability and cost of a tail for the policy. Investigate other options that are covered by the policy. Does this policy cover appeal bonds or supplementary benefits? Can you select your own counsel or request a settlement out of court?

5. Understand the exclusions of the policy. Are you still covered if you accept a job as an independent practitioner? If the exclusions also exclude your job description, as in the instance of advanced practice nurses, investigate additional insurance policies.

6. Be aware that there are areas of nursing practice in which the risk of lawsuits is higher. These areas include, but are not restricted to, critical care areas, home health care, emergency centers, the operating room, and maternal and child health areas. Thus the need for individual coverage is most acute.

7. Above all remember that you are a member of a profession with the potential to have lawsuits constantly filed against it. Do not consider practicing professional nursing without the valuable protection provided by liability insurance.

notice to the insurance carrier immediately upon the filing of a claim or lawsuit and forward to the insurance carrier every demand, notice, summons, or other process received.

Also in this section are the nurse's right to select counsel and the right to request a settlement. Most policies allow the insurance carrier to settle without the policyholder's consent and deny the policyholder the right to retain counsel apart from the insurance company. As explained under general provisions, most insurance companies prefer to retain attorneys known to have expertise in medical matters, rather than allow the insured the right to obtain attorneys unknown to them.

EXERCISE 10-2

Using the sample policy found in Appendix B, find the various provisions that were just discussed, including:

1. Limits of liability.
2. Declarations.
3. Deductibles.
4. Exclusions.
5. Reservation of rights.
6. Covered injuries.
7. Defense costs.
8. Coverage conditions and supplementary payments.

Did you have difficulty finding some sections? Would this policy be worth purchasing for your own liability coverage? Why or why not?

INDIVIDUAL VERSUS EMPLOYER LIABILITY COVERAGE

Should nurses have individual professional liability coverage, or should they rely on the employer's insurance policy in the event of a malpractice action? Many nurses have been assured by hospital administrative staff and by competent lawyers that they can depend on the hospital's insurance policy to cover them in the event of a subsequent legal action. However, the truth is that nurses who relied on hospital policies most often were not adequately protected monetarily, nor were they adequately represented by legal counsel in the lawsuit.

There are several reasons for this situation. First, many institutional liability insurance policies have limited coverage and cover employees only while they are performing work as hospital employees. Thus private duty nurses and off-duty employees are automatically excluded from coverage. Likewise, nurses who volunteer their professional services are not covered. School nurses and community or home health care nurses may not be covered at all in most medical insurance policies, though the trend is to protect these nurses in the performance of their employment.

Second, the hospital's policy is designed to meet the needs of the large institution, and hospital attorneys may not be able to protect the individual nurse's best interests. For example, the hospital may elect to settle out of court rather than pursue a particular case, even though the nurse's best interests can be served only through a court hearing. Also, should the hospital wish to bring an indemnity claim against the nurse for the incident that triggered the lawsuit, the hospital policy neither covers the nurse nor pays for his or her representation. *Indemnity* claims are those brought by the employer for monetary contributions from the nurse or nurses whose actions or failure to act caused the original patient injury.

Finally, most hospital insurance policies do not have supplementary payments for the nurse-defendant. This means if nurses incur additional expenses in investigating the claim or lose days of work defending the claim, then they must cover the expenses out of pocket.

Employer-based coverage, though, is a good starting point for prudent nurses. They should either ask to see and read the hospital policy or ask about specific provisions in the employer-sponsored coverage and then acquire their own individual coverage to augment the employer's policy. Nurses should also take into consideration the following factors:

1. The type of nursing that they normally do (staff versus charge versus supervision).
2. The dollar amount of the average awards in their geographic area.
3. The unit or type of nursing in which they normally work (critical care versus general medical-surgical nursing).
4. The propensity for lawsuits against nurses in that geographic area.

The hospital attorney can provide nurses with information regarding trends in malpractice in their locality. Then nurses should find a policy that provides the necessary coverage. They can extend coverage as their job status changes or as they expand their practice roles.

EXERCISE 10-3

Consult with your risk manager or institution's legal counsel. What types of provisions are made in the institution's policy for individual nurses? What type of coverage should nurses working in the institution purchase?

REASONS TO PURCHASE INDIVIDUAL LIABILITY INSURANCE

Nurses need liability insurance for several reasons:

1. Perhaps the most convincing reason is that defending against a lawsuit, no matter what the merit of the case, is costly. There are attorney fees, court costs, costs of discovery, not to mention the actual award (or settlement) if the defendant is found negligent. Few nurses can sustain such financial strain without insurance coverage.

2. Professional liability insurance is relatively inexpensive. Many nurses can purchase adequate coverage for between $50 and $150 a year.

3. A popular reason for insurance coverage is the assurance of adequate protection against a lawsuit. Malpractice is not synonymous with incompetence or guilt; even the most conscientious nurses could be sued for performing their actions below the acceptable standard of care if an untoward happening occurs and they are in the direct line of causation. For example, the physician orders a new medication for a patient. The nurse could correctly administer the medication and still be sued if the patient has a violent reaction to the medication. One's mental health is well worth the cost of the insurance policy.

4. Having one's own professional liability insurance does not automatically trigger an employee indemnity lawsuit. But should the institution choose to sue the nurse, he or she is protected.

5. The fact that professionals assume accountability for their own actions or omissions is an additional reason for acquiring liability coverage. Inherent in accountability is responsibility (and the ability to pay) should the plaintiff be negligently injured by the professional's actions or omissions.

6. Malpractice insurance premiums are currently a tax-deductible business expense.

ARGUMENTS FOR PROFESSIONAL LIABILITY INSURANCE

There is no good reason for nurses to be caught in a lawsuit without professional liability insurance. A favorite argument of many in-hospital attorneys is to remind nurses that they are more lawsuit-prone if they have an individual insurance policy. However, in today's society nurses are, in essence, the conduit either to the hospital's potential liability or to the physician's potential liability through the doctrine of respondeat superior or through a dual servant role. In fact, in some state tort reform acts, the amount of economic liability against individual defendants may be limited. Thus, nurses may find themselves named in more, not fewer, lawsuits as attorneys seek means to find additional sources of revenue for injured clients. It is immaterial to the patient bringing the lawsuit whether or not the nurse has insurance. In fact, when injured parties originally file the lawsuit, they have no idea of whether the nurse is insured. But it should matter greatly to nurses, since the cost of defense could very well financially destroy them. In most states the judgment remains open until satisfied or dropped. That means that nurses may be paying on a prior judgment for several years after the judgment, or in states that allow garnishment of wages for adjudicated debts, their wages may be garnished for several years after the initial judgment.

EXERCISE 10-4

Poll nurses with whom you work about the advantages of professional liability insurance. Do they have individual policies? List their reasons for either having or not having their own policies. What are the top one to three reasons in either case? Were the reasons valid or rationalizations? List the arguments that you would use to educate nurses about the value and necessity of having individual professional liability insurance coverage.

SUMMARY

Individual malpractice insurance may not prevent potential liability, but it does assist the nurses if a lawsuit is filed or they are named parties in a lawsuit. Policies, though difficult to understand at first glance, are really not that difficult once the reader understands the various terms and phrases.

AFTER COMPLETING THIS CHAPTER, YOU SHOULD BE ABLE TO

- List elements common to all professional liability insurance policies.
- Differentiate the types of professional liability insurance policies available commercially to professional nurses.
- Identify issues to be considered when deciding between individual coverage, group coverage, and employer-sponsored coverage.
- List and refute reasons given against having individual coverage.

APPLY YOUR LEGAL KNOWLEDGE

- What do the terms and language in insurance policies mean to the policyholder?
- Are some insurance policies more desirable for nurses who work in different clinical areas of the hospital?
- Are there times when it would be advisable to have no individual professional liability coverage?

REFERENCES

How to read and understand your professional liability insurance policy. (1995). *The American Nurse,* *27*(8), 22–23.

Lippmann, H. (1993). Malpractice protection: How much is enough? *RN, 56*(5), 61.

Sermchief v. Gonzales, 600 S.W. 2d 683 (Missouri, en banc 1983).

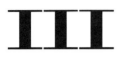

III

IMPACT OF THE LAW ON THE PROFESSIONAL PRACTICE OF NURSING

• eleven

Nurse Practice Acts, Licensure, and the Scope of Practice

PREVIEW

Throughout the years an elaborate system of licensure and credentials for health care providers has evolved to ensure that only qualified persons deliver health care. Both licenses and credentials have as their primary purpose the protection of the public at large. Through proper issuance of licenses and credentials, qualified health care providers are distinguished from unqualified persons. The first group is given a license to practice, while the latter group is prohibited from harming society in a health care role. This chapter outlines the relationship between state nurse practice acts, entry into professional practice, and the scope of practice issues.

KEY CONCEPTS

credentials	endorsement	standing orders
professional licensure	licensure by examination	joint statements
mandatory licensure	licensure by waiver	scope of practice
permissive licensure	temporary license	continuing education
institutional licensure	disciplinary action	National Practitioner Data Bank (NPDB)
nurse practice acts	diversion programs	certification
grandfather clause	articulation with medical practice acts	
reciprocity		

CREDENTIALS

Credentials are proof of qualifications, usually in written form, stating that an individual or organization has met specific standards. Two types of credentials are used in health care: licensure and certification.

PROFESSIONAL LICENSURE

Professional licensure is the legal process by which an authorized authority grants permission to a qualified individual or entity to perform designated skills and services in a jurisdiction where practice would be illegal without a license. Licenses are issued by governmental agencies and are enforced by the police power of the state. For nurses, the authorized authority is the *state board of nursing* or the *state board of nursing examiners*. The qualified individual is the candidate for licensure, and this candidate is either a graduate nurse who has successfully completed all requirements for licensure or a nurse with licensure in another state. The designated skills and services are professional nursing actions.

Licensure is enacted through state legislative action. Licensure statutes measure minimum competency of the person licensed and are intended to protect health care consumers. Licensure laws, an example of a state's exercise of its police power, protect the public against unqualified practitioners.

Individual state legislative bodies enact into law their specific licensing procedures, stating which professions must be licensed to practice within the state. In most states physicians and dentists were the first professionals to be licensed, with nurses generally the next licensed professional. Part of the statutory law in all jurisdictions of the United States is the state nurse practice act. Each state, the District of Columbia, and territories of the United States have individual nurse practice acts.

State Boards of Nursing

Individual legislators do not directly enforce statutory law. Nurse practice acts are enforced through the state board of nursing or the state board of nurse examiners. This board is created by language in the selected nurse practice act and is ultimately accountable to the legislators for professional nursing within a jurisdiction. A board of nursing has no greater authority than that which the statute, enacted by the legislature, grants to it. Therefore, the board of nursing is limited by the language of the nurse practice act.

State boards of nursing are mandated in the state nurse practice acts. The specific act sets the number of members of the board, qualifications for membership, and the term of appointment. States vary in the numbers of persons on the board, and currently there are 7 to 17 members on the state boards of nursing. The individual nurse practice act may allow for legal or expert members or for election (North Carolina) rather than for the appointment of the members. In all but five states (Texas, Louisiana, West Virginia, California, and Georgia), there is one board of nursing for both professional and practical nursing. The remaining five states have two separate boards.

Boards of nursing have an executive director who is responsible for administering the work of the board and seeing that the nurse practice act provisions, as well as the rules and regulations of the board, are followed. The ANA recommends that boards of nursing:

1. Govern their own operation and administration.
2. Approve or deny approvals to schools of nursing.
3. Examine and license applicants.
4. Review licenses, grant temporary licenses, and provide for inactive status for those already licensed.
5. Regulate specialty practice.
6. Discipline those who violate provisions of the licensure law (American Nurses Association, 1990).

The board is given the authority to set standards by promulgating rules and regulations and has as a charge the enforcement of such rules and regulations. Most state boards of nursing have published standards of professional conduct and guidelines for unprofessional conduct, with enforcement assured by the board's ability to revoke, stipulate, or suspend a previously granted license or to deny licensure.

The board's authority arises from various sources of law. Its authority may be:

1. Legislative, through the promulgation of rules and regulations.
2. Quasijudicial, through hearings.
3. Administrative, through licensure control.

State legislatures may also require that licensure be either mandatory or permissive.

Mandatory Licensure

Mandatory licensure requires that all persons who are compensated as members of a licensed profession obtain licensure prior to practicing actions of the profession. Mandatory licensure regulates the practice of the profession and requires compliance with the statute if an individual engages in activities defined within the scope of that profession (Aiken & Catalano, 1994). Thus both the title of registered nurse and the professional actions are protected.

Several exceptions to mandatory licensure within a jurisdiction usually requiring mandatory licensure are:

1. Performance of nursing actions by unlicensed practitioners in emergency conditions.
2. Practice by nursing students incidental to their current course of study.
3. Nursing actions by employees of the federal government.
4. Practice by graduate nurses for a specific length of time during which licensure is being processed.
5. Nursing care given to patients by qualified nurses during transportation of the patient through a state.
6. Unpaid persons caring for family members or friends.
7. Nurses working for the Red Cross during a disaster.
8. Caregivers who conduct religious services and rites and who do not report to be RNs.

Nurses in the armed services or nurses employed by federal agencies must hold a current state license, but not necessarily from the state in which they are currently employed or assigned.

Permissive Licensure

Permissive licensure (Texas) regulates only the use of the title and does not protect nursing actions. Thus nurses cannot use the title registered nurse (RN) unless duly licensed, but they could perform many or all of the same nursing actions as long as they do not call themselves RNs. For example, in a state with permissive licensure, a licensed practical or vocational nurse (LPN or LVN), working under the supervision or through direct orders of a physician, could perform most of the same actions that an RN performs since only the title is protected, not the nursing actions.

Permissive licensure correlates best with the initial registration acts of the early 1900s. The term "registered nurse" was defined as a person who had graduated from an acceptable school of nursing and had passed an examination, rather than a person engaged in a specific type of practice. These first registration acts provided for permissive licensure.

The state board of nursing may have as its concern only the professional practice of nursing or may incorporate both professional and practical licensed nurses (RNs as well as LPNs or LVNs), and 44 states now have joint boards. If the charge of the state board of nursing is merely professional licensure, then a separate board of nursing for the practical nurse will also exist within the same jurisdiction. Whether one or two separate boards exists, the restriction of mandatory or permissive licensure may vary within the state. For example, professional nurses may have mandatory licensure, while practical nurses may have permissive licensure, or both may have mandatory or permissive licensure.

Institutional Licensure

Institutional licensure is the process by which a state government regulates health institutions. Institutional licensure is the alternative to individual licensure. Most government agencies issue licenses to health care facilities, granting permission for the facility to operate, and the issuing body holds the facility responsible for maintaining sanitation, fire safety, staffing, and equipment. Institutional licensure of individuals gives these facilities the added right to decide who is qualified to perform which tasks and duties, and awards licenses as the facility deems appropriate.

Institutional licensure grants the institution authority to directly regulate staff members' practices as well as the requirements for administration, equipment specifications, fire safety, footage regulations, and minimal nursing staff requirements. Usually the process is implemented, not controlled, by individual state monitoring agencies or national organizations, such as the Joint Commission on Accreditation of Healthcare Organizations (JCAHO). Theoretically, institutional licensure gives nonprofessionals the regulation of a profession without standard criteria for such regulation.

There is a growing impatience by consumers with the seeming indifference of the health care community to individual consumer needs. Many of these consumers feel that the current licensing laws are at fault. The licensing laws have been characterized as more protective of professional jurisdiction than public safety, costly to apply, and too rigid to accommodate the changing needs of the health care delivery system and society at large. Licensing laws are often silent on the more critical issues of competency and quality (Joel, 1995).

Advocates of institutional licensure insist that these issues will be eliminated and rectified by the renewed interest in institutional licensure. The reasons cited include allowing nurses more flexibility in their practices and the opportunity to more effectively expand the practice of nursing. Proponents also claim that institutional licensure will allow professionals to be more responsive to changing needs, that licensure will allow providers to take on and relinquish activities as the situation and their abilities demands, and that it will be more cost-effective, thus saving consumers money.

Perhaps the crucial differences between institutional and individual licensure are more philosophical than practical. Individual licensing reinforces the responsibility of the professional to the individual client rather than to the employer. In an environment that often sacrifices quality in an attempt to lower costs, this would seem a fundamental argument against institutional licensure. Would nurses feel that they could speak against an employer who is also a regulator? And would nursing become lost on a board that has as its charge all regulated areas of practice (Joel, 1995)?

EXERCISE 11-1

List the pros and cons of institutional versus state licensure for nursing. Rewrite the list from the perspective of a consumer rather than that of a professional. Does institutional licensure support or undermine professional nursing? Explain your answer.

NURSE PRACTICE ACTS

Nurse practice acts, which originated to protect the public at large, define the practice of nursing, give guidance within the scope of practice issues, and set standards for the nursing profession. The state nurse practice act is the single most important piece of legislation for nurses because the practice act affects all facets of nursing practice. The nurse practice act is the law, and state boards of nursing cannot grant exceptions or waive its provisions. For example, if licensure can be granted only to individuals who graduate from an approved school of nursing, then the board must refuse licensure to candidates who did not graduate from an approved school of nursing even if they can show evidence of competency and equivalency.

By the early 20th century, the minimum requirements for nursing practice were beginning to take shape. *Nurse registration acts,* permissive precursors to nurse practice acts, were emerging, and in 1901 the state nurses associations adopted proposals supporting commitment to the passage of state laws to control the practice of nursing. North Carolina was the first state to pass a permissive nurse practice act in 1903. By 1923, every state had passed some type of nurse registration act, and in 1938 New York State was the first to enact a mandatory nurse practice act, establishing two levels of nursing practice: licensed RNs and LPNs. Other states followed suit, and by 1952 all states, the District of Columbia, and the United States territories had enacted nurse practice acts.

The early acts mainly regulated registration and fee structures. With the advent of mandatory acts, only licensed professionals could practice nursing. Some states enacted definitions of professional nursing, while other states had no formal definition of professional nursing. In 1955, the American Nurses Association (ANA) approved a model definition for nursing practice and continued through the years to broaden the definition, amending the definition in

1970 to incorporate nursing diagnosis and further allowing for an expanded scope in 1979. To provide for consistency in individual state nurse practice acts, the ANA published a model act for state legislators in 1980 and again in 1990. This latest model nurse practice act incorporates the advanced nurse practitioner as well as the registered nurse (American Nurses Association, 1990).

Individual nurse practice acts continue to be worded differently, with varying concepts of professional nursing. All nurse practice acts are worded in fairly general terms, and there is no laundry list of specific actions to ensure that nurses stay within the given act. Rather, the acts' general provisions should give guidance as to acceptable actions. For example, one reason that specific actions are not listed is that, as statutory law, the nurse practice acts are slow in changing to conform with modern practice and technological advances. If actions were specifically enumerated, one would be required to follow the nurse practice act exactly, even though current practices might have changed.

An example may assist understanding this last statement. Imagine that the state nurse practice act has no provision for nursing diagnosis, yet the JCAHO standards require that nursing diagnoses be written for each patient within hospitals that have JCAHO accreditation. If enumerated actions in the nurse practice act specifically omitted nursing diagnoses as part of the professional practice of nursing within the state, professional nurses would run the risk daily of violating the act or of working in a nonaccredited institution.

Further, suppose that the institution's policies and procedures mandate that nursing diagnoses are part of the assessment due each patient, just as the patient's progress, response to nursing interventions, and nursing care needs are part of the nursing protocol. Now the dilemma would concern the nurse practice act and one's livelihood. Do nurses violate the nurse practice act, or do they ignore the hospital's policy and procedure manual and refrain from making nursing diagnoses? Such a scenario could happen if nurse practice acts were checklists for approved nursing actions.

Thus the acts are not checklists. The practice acts contain general statements of appropriate professional nursing actions. Nurses must incorporate the nurse practice act with their educational background, previous work experience, institutional policies, and technological advancements. If the main purpose of these acts is to protect the public from unsafe practitioners, then their ultimate goal must be to provide competent, quality nursing care by currently qualified practitioners.

EXERCISE 11-2

Read your state's nurse practice act, paying particular attention to the general provisions defining nursing actions. Does the act give enough guidance for nurses to know if their actions are within or outside the scope of the act?

ELEMENTS OF NURSE PRACTICE ACTS

Definition of Professional Nursing

All state nurse practice acts define nursing. As previously stated, some state definitions include nursing diagnoses and speak of collaboration with other professionals. Some nurse practice acts allow for individual treatment, while others specify nursing interventions and therapies. Basically there are three approaches to statutory definitions of professional nursing:

1. The *traditional approach* is based on the ANA's original model definition. This approach does not include diagnosis, treatment, or prescription. Most states currently following this model definition have not addressed expanded practice or advanced practice issues. Some states use a more restrictive definition and then allow for limited expanded roles for nursing by having broad delegatory language in the state medical practice act.
2. The *transitional* approach may also allow some expanded roles beyond those described in the nurse practice act through the use of standing orders and through supervision by a responsible physician. Some states with transitional approaches add an additional act for nurses, such as the legal permission to diagnose and evaluate patients but not to treat them.
3. The *administrative* approach is seen in the majority of states. This approach uses a broader definition of nursing and allows additional acts as may be authorized by appropriate state agencies. Advanced nurse practitioners and expanded nursing roles are incorporated, relying on the authority granted to the state board of nursing to promulgate rules for advanced roles. These rules and regulations are then administered and enforced through the state board of nursing. This approach may also allow for overlap between physician and professional nursing roles and functions. For example, this approach allows both physicians and nurses to diagnose and treat patients within the respective realms of their disciplines.

Requirements for Licensure

Requirements usually center on personal characteristics and educational requirements to ensure that candidates are at least minimally competent to practice professional nursing. These criteria include academic and clinical performance, a passing score on the licensing examination, and personal qualities.

Academic and clinical performance are validated by transcripts from approved schools of nursing. The state board may use their own criteria for approval or may rely on national accreditation agencies such as the National League for Nursing (NLN).

All states administer licensing examinations and use a standardized, nationally normed test. With the advent of computers and the availability of computer-generated examinations, states now allow candidates for licensure to schedule times to take the national examination. Provisions are made for handicapped candidates in accordance with the Americans with Disabilities Act. With the increasing numbers of nurses seeking reciprocity (recognition of licensure from one state to another state) from other state boards, states have adopted or continued the practice of national norms for successful passage of the examinations.

The personal qualifications and attributes screened include citizenship or visa permits, physical and mental health fitness, minimal age requirements, fluency in English requirements, and good moral character references.

Payment of fees is another area to meet licensure requirements. These fees include processing and administration fees for the licensure examination, interim work permit fees, and temporary licensure fees.

Exemptions

Most states allow exemptions from state licensure in very few circumstances. Some of the valid exemptions have previously been enumerated, such as exemptions for professional students in current course work and for graduate nurses during the application process.

Another form of exemption is the *grandfather clause.* This term applies to certain persons working within the profession for a given period of time or prior to a deadline date. These individuals may be granted the privilege of applying for a license without having to meet all the requirements for licensure or without having to take the licensing examination. Such a grandfather clause was used to allow licensure of World War II nurses, or those with on-the-job training and expertise, even though they had not graduated from an approved school of nursing or passed the licensure examination.

The grandfather clause is also projected to be used if the ANA proposal for professional entry into practice for baccalaureate nurses becomes a reality. In 1964, the ANA proposed that the entry level for professional nursing should be the baccalaureate of science in nursing degree (BSN) and that this would be implemented by 1985. Associate degree nurses would be technical nurses, and those previously licensed will be allowed the right to retain the title RN in the proposed new licensing schema. But new graduates will need an earned baccalaureate degree to use the title RN (Hood, 1985).

In 1984, the ANA revised the timetable for implementation and to date little success has been attained in this direction. By 1988, 30 state nurses associations had addressed the issue, and 28 had adopted resolutions advocating the BSN as the professional entry requirement. Today, only two states have succeeded in changing the entry requirements (North Dakota and Maine), and other states are at varying degrees of attempting to achieve this goal (George & Young, 1990). The ANA House of Delegates in 1995 reaffirmed this commitment to the BSN as entry level into professional nursing and voted to assist states in implementing strategies that would make such a goal a reality (American Nurses Association, 1995).

Licensure Across Jurisdictions

Because each state has its own nurse practice act and because most states have mandatory licensure, provisions are included within state nurse practice acts for licensing nurses with valid licenses in other jurisdictions. There are essentially four means of granting licensure across jurisdictions:

1. *Reciprocity* is an agreement by two or more states granting recognition to licensure by other state boards of nursing. For reciprocity, the licensing requirements of the involved states must be equivalent. Such a provision allows licensed nurses to be granted additional licensure merely by application and by payment of required fees. The concept of reciprocity also allows states with similar disciplinary actions to revoke a license in a state based solely on revocation in a sister state (*Schoenhair v. Pennsylvania*, 1983).

2. Under *endorsement*, a similar concept, a state may grant licensure to an already licensed nurse from another state if the two states' qualifications and licensure requirements are comparable. Usually the state granting endorsement requires that similar licensure examinations exist in both states. This means of granting licensure is distinguished from reciprocity in that no prior agreement exists between the two states, and individual nurses must petition for licensure by endorsement. Their cases are decided on an individual basis.

3. *Licensure by examination* is required when the petitioned state does not grant licensure by reciprocity or by endorsement. Essentially *licensure by examination* means that the individual must meet all the state requirements and successfully complete a licensing examination before licensure is granted.

4. *Licensure by waiver* is similar to licensure by examination. If the petitioning candidate meets or exceeds some of the requirements for licensure, the portion previously demonstrated may be waived for the candidate, while other requirements must be demonstrated by the candidate. States may choose to waive educational requirements, experience requirements, or examination requirements while requiring that deficiencies be met.

As with any new graduate within the state, a given state may grant *temporary licenses* to out-of-state nurses, which allow them to practice while permanent licensure is pending or for a limited period of time. For example, the state may grant temporary licensure for a semester or two while the nurse completes graduation requirements for an advanced nursing degree.

Foreign nursing school graduates desiring to practice nursing in the United States must meet the requirements of the state or territory in which they reside and must pass the licensing examination. Each state nurse practice act specifies requirements for foreign nursing school graduates.

The Committee on Graduates of Foreign Nursing Schools (CGFNS), sponsored independently by the ANA and NLN, administers an examination to foreign-educated nurses. This examination addresses their command of the English language as well as knowledge of nursing concepts and skills, and it serves as a guide for their ability to successfully pass the licensing examination. Following successful passage of the CGFNS examination, foreign nurses are allowed to obtain a work permit in the United States. The committee also has a Credentials Evaluation Service (CES) to evaluate transcripts and credentials from foreign countries.

Disciplinary Action and Due Process Requirements

To give credence to the state board of nursing's ability to enforce licensure requirements, the board also has the authority for *disciplinary action.* Various actions may be taken, depending on the severity of the violation. Allowable disciplinary actions include:

1. Private reprimand or warning.
2. Public reprimand.
3. Probation.
4. Suspension of licensure.
5. Refusal to renew licensure.
6. Revocation of licensure.

Not all these measures have the same significance. For minor violations the individual nurse may receive a warning or reprimand. Continued violations may be cause for probation or temporary suspension of licensure. Major violations are dealt with through licensure revocation or refusal to reissue licensure. Some of the possible violations for which disciplinary actions may be instigated include, but are not limited to:

1. *Conviction* of a felony or crime involving *moral turpitude* (an action that is contrary to justice, honesty, modesty, or good moral principles).
2. Use of *fraud or deceit* in obtaining licensure.
3. *Violation* of the provisions of the nurse practice act.
4. *Aiding or abetting* any unlicensed person with the unauthorized practice of nursing.
5. *Revocation, suspension, or denial of licensure* to practice nursing in another jurisdiction.
6. *Habitual use* of, or *addiction* to, alcohol or drugs.
7. *Unprofessional conduct* that is likely to deceive, defraud, or injure the public or patients.
8. *Lack of fitness* by reason of physical or mental health that could result in injury to the public or individual patients.

During licensure suspension or probation, the board of nursing has the authority to impose conditions such as:

1. Obtaining substance abuse rehabilitation and counseling.
2. Obtaining special counseling.

3. Requiring supervision for specific techniques or procedures to validate competency.
4. Requiring satisfactory completion of educational programs.

Disciplinary actions may arise in one of several ways, depending on applicable state law. Generally, a written complaint is filed with the state board of nursing by an individual, a health care agency, or a professional organization. The complaint may be initiated directly by the state board of nursing in some states. The complaint is screened, and an investigation is initiated, if appropriate. A board hearing or hearing before a state hearing officer or judge is then scheduled, and the nurse is entitled to a clear statement of the charges, the right to question and produce witnesses, the right to an attorney, and the right to a fair determination based on the evidence presented. There is increasing pressure on professional boards to delegate the actual hearing authority to an independent administrative judge as a board that hears its own cases can more easily be challenged on due process grounds. In the latter instance, the board serves as the initial investigator, witness, prosecutor, judge, jury, and probation officer. This process is outlined in Table 11–1.

Because state boards of nursing are agencies of state administrative law, nurses are constitutionally allowed due process rights. This means that practicing nurses have the right to adequate notice of the alleged misconduct, an

TABLE 11–1. PROCESS FOR DISCIPLINARY HEARINGS

Filing of the sworn complaint:
  Individual complaint
  Health care agency complaint
  Professional organization complaint
Review of the complaint:
  Notice of hearing to the involved nurse
  Hearing before the board of nursing or state officer/stage judge
  Evidence presented by board and nurse
  Witnesses called by board and nurse
  Decision by the board of nursing
Disciplinary action:
  If found not guilty of misconduct, no action is taken by the board of nursing.
  If found guilty of misconduct, the board of nursing may:
    Issue a reprimand, public or private.
    Place the nurse on probation.
    Deny the renewal of licensure.
    Suspend the nurse's license.
    Revoke the nurse's license.
    Allow the nurse to enter a diversion program.
Court review:
  Review of the board decision and concur with its finding
  Order a new trial
  Appeal to a higher court.

opportunity to present information concerning the alleged misconduct, and the right to appeal the board's action. Some states impose stricter rights; for example, not only do nurses have the right to be heard, they also have the right to call witnesses and to be represented by legal counsel.

During the hearing, both sides are allowed to present witnesses and to be represented by legal counsel. At the conclusion of the hearing, the board of nursing decides if the evidence presented merits disciplinary action or not, and specifies any disciplinary action at this time.

Following the announcement of the disciplinary action to be taken (as warranted), nurses may file a lawsuit to appeal the board's decision. Depending on the jurisdiction, they may file the case in the lowest court of the state or in a special court that handles appeals from state agencies. The appropriate court reviews only the state board of nursing's original decision against the nurse, not the nurse's alleged misconduct. The court's charge is to determine if the board acted properly. Whether the nurse or the state board of nursing prevails, the losing side may further appeal the decision through the court process to the highest court in the given state.

Failure by the state board of nursing to comply with the constitutional rights of due process or of state law may result in the reversal of the board's decision by the judiciary. The court in *Colorado State Board of Nursing v. Hohn* (1954), the landmark case in this area, ordered the nurse's license reinstated, since the hearing was held with less than the full board present and state law mandated a full board hearing.

Typically, state nurse practice acts require that a quorum of the board be present for a disciplinary hearing and for disciplinary decisions. For example, the court in *Stevens v. Blake* (1984) held that a majority of the board of nursing must be in accord for final disciplinary decisions. The court further held that it is not necessary for a majority to be present physically for each step involved in the process.

Adequate notice of an alleged misconduct means more than just 10 to 20 days notice that a hearing will be held by the state board of nursing. Adequate notice encompasses knowledge or reason to have the knowledge that the conduct is prohibited by the state nurse practice act. This means that the wording of nurse practice acts may not be too vague or overly broad. This is usually avoided by a standard of conduct that is widely recognized as unprofessional. For example, the court in *Heinecke v. Department of Commerce, Division of Occupational and Professional Licensure* (1991) upheld the revocation of a nurse's license for having sexual relations with a patient. Contrast that decision with the court in *Hogan v. Mississippi Board of Nursing* (1984), in which the board of nursing could show only that the nurse was guilty of failure to reasonably account for missing narcotics. The court held that the board did not reach the standard of proof required to show misappropriation of controlled substances and therefore ruled that her license could not be revoked.

A 1994 case in Iowa, *Burns v. Matzen*, decided a provision in an Iowa law requiring licensing boards to revoke the licenses of habitually intoxicated health professionals has been upheld by the supreme court of that state. The board of nursing placed a registered nurse on probation in accordance with the statute after finding that the nurse was habitually intoxicated. The nurse challenged the decision and the statute. The nurse argued that the law was unconstitutionally vague because licensees could not sufficiently discern what conduct would constitute habitual intoxication, and they therefore could not avoid violating the statute. The court upheld the statute, ruling that a "person of ordinary intelligence should easily understand what type of conduct is to be avoided." The court concluded that the licensing board could determine whether a nurse violated the statute on a case-by-case basis without developing a specific definition. The nurse's probationary status was upheld.

Fraudulent conduct may be the basis for disciplinary action. In *Derrick v. Commonwealth of Pennsylvania* (1981), a nurse was arrested on the charges that he fraudulently obtained a small amount of a controlled substance from his employer by listing the names of nonexistent patients on the narcotics sheets. He was convicted of theft, tampering with public records, and possession of a controlled substance. After the board revoked his license for "fraud in the practice of nursing," he brought suit against the board. He contended that, because he used nonexistent patients to obtain the controlled substance, his conduct had not affected the health care of any patients. The court, in upholding the revocation of his license, concluded that the statutory prescriptions against fraud in the practice of a health care professional "are not limited to conduct directly affecting patients, but encompass all aspects of professional conduct" (at 287).

This contrasts with the holding in *Rafferty v. Commonwealth, State Board of Nurse Examiners* (1984), a case involving an RN who disconnected a ventilator to assess for spontaneous respirations in a comatose patient. The court, in reinstating the nurse's license, held that, while the actions of the nurse were intentionally done in spite of accepted nursing practices, this one action was not the kind of willful and repeated violation that would support the revocation of licensure.

In 1983, the Texas Court of Appeals upheld the suspension of a nurse's license for "unprofessional and dishonorable conduct . . . likely to injure the public" (*Lunsford v. Board of Nurse Examiners*, 1983, at 391) when the nurse failed to adequately assess a potential cardiac patient. The nurse argued that she had acted according to a direct physician order and could not have allowed admission for the patient to the hospital whether or not she had completed the patient assessment. The board and subsequently the court ruled that her failure to assess and implement appropriate nursing actions was within the adequate notice provision of the state nurse practice act and was within the specific rule promulgated by the Texas Board of Nurse Examiners. Other cases uphold this type of judicial finding, including *Scott v. State of Nebraska, ex rel. Board of Nursing for the State of Nebraska* (1976) and *Ex parte Smith* (1983).

The message for individual nurses seems to be twofold:

1. Nurses must carefully monitor the rules and regulations as they are published by the state board, for, as practitioners, they will be held accountable for the rules and regulations.
2. Nurses must remain knowledgeable about standards of their specific communities because unprofessional conduct is frequently established by expert opinion of nurses as that which falls below the standard of care necessary for the protection of the public interest.

Penalties for Practicing without a License

Most nurse practice acts allow for a fine or imprisonment for practicing without a license. Fines or confinement represent charges that may be pressed against the illegal practitioner. Generally, fines range from $50 to $500, and the term of confinement does not exceed 60 days.

Civil suits may also be filed against the nonlicensed practitioner. Such suits may be filed prior to, concurrent with, or after criminal charges. The civil suits are brought by those harmed by the nonlicensed practitioner and usually concern standards of care.

GUIDELINES: STEPS IN DISCIPLINARY PROCEEDINGS FOR NURSING MISCONDUCT

1. A sworn complaint is filed with the state board of nursing by an individual, a health care agency, or a professional organization, or the complaint may be originated by the board of nursing itself.
2. If there is sufficient evidence, the state board of nursing holds a formal review of the matter, during which both sides may be represented by legal counsel and witnesses are called.
3. Depending on the outcome of the hearing, the board may take disciplinary action.
4. The nurse may appeal the board's decision in state court. The court reviews the actions of the board, not the original act of misconduct by the nurse, and either upholds the board's action or grants a new trial.
5. Whichever side loses at trial level may decide to further appeal the court decision to the next highest court in the state. That court may also uphold the lower court's decision or reverse the decision, and the court may also reinstate the nurse's license if the nurse files the appeal.

DIVERSION PROGRAMS

The nursing profession, through diversion programs, is showing a commitment to the rehabilitation of nurses who are psychologically unable to function or who are addicted to either drugs or alcohol. Rather than being disciplined, these nurses are diverted to rehabilitation programs. Diversion programs also allow the board to protect the public while complying with the Americans with Disabilities Act. See Chapter 17 for a more complete discussion.

Voluntary alternatives to traditional disciplinary actions, *diversion programs* entail attendance at group sessions such as Alcoholics Anonymous, Narcotics Anonymous, or counseling sessions, voluntary submission of urine samples for substance abuse, and special provisions by employers. Facilities that allow diversion program nurses to work within their units must comply with specific guidelines, generally the filing of quarterly reports with the board of nursing, working on general nursing units rather than emergency centers, intensive care units, and postanesthesia care units, working no overtime shifts while in the program, and working during the day hours as opposed to the night shifts. Some programs also forbid recovering employees from assuming charge positions and from administering narcotics to patients.

Nurses may petition the board for reinstatement of full licensure after 12 to 24 months and must show compliance with the provisions of the program and the ability to perform in the workplace. The advantage of the program is that recovering nurses are allowed to fully be rehabilitative and productive in their chosen career as opposed to being denied licensure to work in the nursing profession. If nurses fail to comply with the provisions of the program, the board of nursing institutes more traditional disciplinary provisions.

EXERCISE 11-3

Investigate the existence of a diversion program for substance abuse and/or mental illness within your state. How is the program implemented? What is its success rate? If no program exists, what does the state board of nursing do for nurses who have substance abuse or mental illness issues? Are members of your state working to implement such a program?

ARTICULATION WITH MEDICAL PRACTICE ACTS

Medical practice acts are to physicians what nurse practice acts are to nurses: state laws that allow the individual to practice in a given discipline. Most medical practice acts define medicine as acts of diagnosis, prescription, treatment, and surgery. Some states' acts include only the first three elements.

Incorporated into the language or the intent of medical practice acts is *broad delegatory language,* enabling the physician to delegate to qualified and skilled persons the legal ability to perform certain actions and skills. This broad delegatory language, coupled with standing orders and protocols, has increased the functions of nurses while causing an overlap between nurse practice acts and medical practice acts, *articulation with medical practice acts.* For example, nurses in intensive care units and coronary care units may actually perform some medical acts because of valid standing orders and protocols. When the electrocardiogram rhythm strip shows ventricular fibrillation (a medical diagnosis), the nurse may inject Lidocaine or perform electric cardioversion (a medical treatment).

Not all jurisdictions handle *standing orders* in the same manner. Some states allow standing orders to take precedence if the patient fits a particular classification (eg, because the patient is in the coronary care unit, the coronary care standing orders are immediately valid), while other states mandate that the patient be seen by the physician and the standing orders be signed by a physician before they may be implemented. However a particular state approaches standing orders and protocols, they are a means of expanding the scope of nursing practice.

Another way of incorporating medical practice acts with nurse practice acts is by passing laws that make some functions common to both professions. For example, some state laws allow both nurses and physicians to diagnose and treat patients as long as the nursing diagnosis does not alter the patient's medical regimen. Other states allow nurses to evaluate and diagnose patients but not to treat them. The more modern nurse practice acts are beginning to allow for the treatment and diagnosis of patients by professional nurses.

A third approach to increase nursing's role is by *joint statements* between the disciplines of medicine and nursing. Joint statements are part of an evolving process and, in fact, are stopgap measures until states are able to develop and implement broader definitions of nursing practice. Joint statements thus serve as the basis for expanded nursing practice. There would be no need for joint statements if nurse practice acts were amended at the same time the joint statements were written.

SCOPE OF PRACTICE ISSUES

In recent years, the courts have attempted to settle scope of practice issues and the articulation of medical practice acts with nurse practice acts. As a general rule, negligence issues have caused scope of practice issues to be considered second, rather than first.

Scope of practice issues speak to the actions or duties of a given profession. The phrase "scope of practice" legally refers to permissible boundaries of practice for the health professional, and the scope of practice is defined by statute, rule, or a combination of statute and rule. For example, in a state that statutorily allows nurses to diagnose and treat patients, individual, licensed nurses may diagnose and treat the patients that they encounter. In a state that expressly forbids diagnosis and treatment as a nursing function, nurses would be practicing medicine without a license if they undertook to diagnose and treat patients. In a state in which both nurses and physicians may diagnose and treat patients, the scope of practice issues overlap, and reasonable and customary practice become key issues.

From a legal perspective, scope of practice issues usually arise in one of two instances: (1) A negligent act was associated with the scope of practice issue, or (2) the standard of care owed the patient is increased because of the medical or nursing action. A landmark case that illustrates the first instance is *Cooper v. National Motor Bearing Company* (1955). One of the first cases that mandated nurses to be patient's advocates, the case concerned an occupational health nurse who failed to recognize the patient's signs and symptoms as being indicative of cancer and who further failed to refer the patient to his physician for treatment. The court ruled that occupational health nurses should be able to diagnose sufficiently well to know whether to treat the patient or to refer the patient. Thus diagnosis, outside the scope of nursing practice at that time, was called for in a limited scope. Note that the court failed to question or decide the greater issue of when such diagnoses were outside nursing's scope of practice.

Standards of care issues frequently arise with nurses in expanded roles, such as nurse anesthetists and nurse midwives. In these types of cases, the court usually applies a medical standard of care, reasoning that a greater duty is owed the patient because the nurse is performing actions that physicians typically perform. *Whitney v. Day* (1980) held that nurse anesthetists are professionals with expertise in an area of medicine and as such are held to those higher standards. *Mohr v. Jenkins* (1980) reached a similar conclusion.

One possibility for preventing scope of practice issue differences lies with the hospital or institutional policy and procedure manuals. Since nursing and technology are both fluid and dynamic, up-to-date policies and procedures may ensure that nurses practice within nursing's scope of practice. Policies and procedures accomplish this goal since they tend to be much more narrow than nurse practice acts and give clarity to actions that nurses may or may not perform. For example, the nurse practice act may have a standard that reads as follows: "makes judgments and decisions about the nursing care for the client or patient by using assessment data to formulate and implement a plan of goals and objectives." The hospital policy and procedure manual has a procedure that states, in laundry list fashion, how the patient assessment will be done, when it is to be performed, and specific guidelines for the documentation of the patient assessment. The nurses' assessment data may be inclusive of broad hemodynamic measurements, and the hospital policy and procedure manual should also have a procedure for the performance of hemodynamic measurements and monitoring, arterial lines, thermodilution pulmonary artery catheter lines, and central lines.

Policies and procedures specify the allowable scope of practice within the given setting. They may be more narrow than the scope of practice stated within the nurse practice act, but they may not extend the nurse practice act scope of practice. The professional nurse must choose the nurse practice act over the hospital policy if there is a discrepancy. Professional standards and the nurse practice act mandate quality care for all patients. Professional standards and the state board of nursing's rules and regulations were the central themes reinforced in *Lunsford v. Board of Nurse Examiners* (1983).

To be of maximum value to nurses, the policies and procedures must be current. Ideally they should be developed jointly by medical and nursing committees and should be updated periodically. The policies and procedures should reflect community standards. The committee developing them must be aware of the nursing role within the given community, and policies and procedures written so as to allow nurses to meet and exceed the public standard.

For individual nurses, institutional policies and procedures mandate that they remain current in their practice, either through continuing education classes, in-service education classes, or reading current journal articles. Institutional policies and procedures also help nurses prevent potential liability if they can show how individual nursing actions were within the policies and procedures and thus within the allowable scope of practice.

Other means for preventing scope of practice differences include:

1. Listing accepted procedures in the nurse practice act.
2. Requesting the attorney general's opinions for clarification on allowed or prohibited procedures.
3. Reviewing recent judicial decisions for the definition of roles.
4. Requesting joint statements from professional organizations clarifying roles and practices.
5. Reviewing rules and regulations of the state board of nursing concerning the permitted scope of practice.

A final means of preventing problems with nursing scope of practice is to remember to stay within the scope of one's own profession. A danger in this area is practicing another profession without a license to practice that profession. Seen most often in physicians' offices and some out-patient settings, nurses are sometimes requested to perform ultrasound examinations, apply heat packs, take x-rays, and see patients while the physician is called to an emergency. Such performances are outside the scope of nursing; they tread into the job descriptions of physical therapists, radiation technologists, and physicians. A further issue arises if the patient is billed for the services as if the properly licensed provider had performed the service. The nurse in question may well find himself or herself in three separate arenas and facing three separate charges: (1) the Board of Nursing for practicing outside the scope of nursing practice, (2) other professional boards for practicing without a license, and (3) the insurance board or other third party payor for billing fraud.

Guidelines: Nurse Practice Acts

1. Obtain a current copy of your nurse practice act. This may be done by writing or contacting the state board of nursing, or by contacting the local or state office of the state nurses association. Additionally, copies may be available at a bookstore specializing in medical and nursing literature or at the local medical library.

2. Read the act carefully for the following elements, ensuring that you understand what each element means to you as a professional nurse:

   a. Definition of professional nursing.

   b. Requirements for licensure.

   c. Exemptions.

   d. Grounds for disciplinary actions.

   e. Criteria for out-of-state licensure.

   f. Creation of the state board of nursing.

   g. Penalties for practicing without a license.

3. Know the state board of nursing rules and regulations regarding professional standards of care and dishonorable conduct. As you read the rules and regulations, know what each enumerated rule and regulation means, and apply each to your individual nursing practice.

4. Know whom to contact and what to do if the nurse practice act is violated by licensed or unlicensed practitioners. Remember, you have an obligation to uphold the state nurse practice act and to see that others likewise uphold the act.

UPDATING NURSE PRACTICE ACTS

There are several ways to update individual nurse practice acts:

1. Updating may call for a *simple revision* of the original act or a complete rewriting of the act. Since nurse practice acts are legislative enactments, any changes must be channeled through the state legislative body.

2. *Amendments* add to the nurse practice act or its regulation, usually giving nurses the needed legal permission to perform actions and functions that have become part of the community standard. Amendments have the same force of law as the original act, and many state nurses acts are amended annually by state legislatures.

3. *Redefinitions* involve a rewriting of the definition of nursing and as such automatically change the force of the entire act. An example is to

rewrite the definition of nursing to include diagnosis and treatment or to clarify "diagnosis" to mean nursing diagnosis. The act is thus clarified for the practicing profession, the scope is broadened, and there has been no repeal or piecemeal amendment to the original act.

4. *Application of sunset laws* also aid in keeping nurse practice acts current. Such laws call for a review of the act at a fixed time, such as six to ten years after the enactment of the original act. The purpose of sunset laws is to force a periodic review by legislative bodies and thus prevent an act from becoming hopelessly outdated. The practice act affected automatically expires at the designated date, and most acts are updated during the legislative year immediately preceding the application of the sunset law.

The dynamic process of nursing may also necessitate some needed action before the nurse practice act is actually revised or amended by the appropriate legislative body. Professional organizations, such as the state nurses association and the state board of nursing, may lobby for needed changes in the nurse practice act and thus force redefinition or amendment of the act. Or the state board of nursing may enact new rules and regulations to ensure that the nurse practice act meets the prevailing community standards. Thus practicing professional nurses must do more than just know the original nurse practice act. They must remain current on newly adopted rules and regulations of the state board of nursing and understand the lobbying efforts of the professional organizations, since both may have great impact on individual nurses' scope of practice.

CONTINUING EDUCATION FOR PRACTICING NURSES

Most nurse practice acts speak to *continuing education* for professional nurses. Whether the continuing education is mandatory or voluntary, the concept is crucial for professional nurses. With an expanded and ever-increasing scope of practice and increased accountability for technical nursing skills and functions, nurses need assistance in keeping their practice current and competent. State board of nursing and professional nursing organizations continue to argue for and against mandatory continuing education, but there is no arguing that continuing education is vital for one practicing in today's health care system.

REPORTING PROFESSIONAL VIOLATIONS OF THE NURSE PRACTICE ACT

An important concept for professional nurses concerns the difficulty of knowing how and when to report a co-worker for violations of the state nurse practice act. Reporting may be for unprofessional conduct, extended scope of practice, or substance abuse. Looking the other way may be easier, but all nurse practice acts require the reporting of violations of the act. Failure to report violators is usually grounds for additional disciplinary action. For example, most nurse practice acts also hold the nonreporting nurse in violation of the nurse practice act. Unprofessional conduct includes, but is not limited to, failing to report to the board or the appropriate authority in the organization in which the nurse is working, within a reasonable time of the occurrence, any violation or attempted violation of the nurse practice act or duly promulgated rules, regulations, or orders.

The most obvious means of reporting violations is within the organizational structure. Most nurses have a direct chain of command to hospital or institutional administrations, and the staff nurse should report violations of the act to the immediate supervisor, usually a nurse manager or charge nurse. Reports should be factual and documented in writing. Reports should include as complete a description of the violation as possible, should list other witnesses, and give patient names, as appropriate. The report should be complete so that administrative staff can investigate and gather additional evidence.

Administrative personnel have a duty to act on reported violations. They may insist that the violator receive counseling, further education classes, or supervised demonstrations to ensure quality nursing actions. What the administrative personnel may not do is allow violators to terminate employment, thus allowing them to simply change places of employment without ever seeking help or changing actions. In such cases, the hospital administrator would have a duty to report the violators to the state board of nursing.

Individual staff nurses may also incur the same duty. Suppose an individual nurse reports a nurse for substance abuse or substandard nursing care to the appropriate supervisor. Later the reporting nurse learns that the reported nurse has quit her job and is now working for another hospital within the same city (or state). Upon questioning the supervisor, the reporting nurse learns that no action was taken by the hospital administration. The reporting nurse was merely questioned and voluntarily resigned. To date, the second hospital has not asked for a reference concerning the nurse. If there was sufficient evidence to report the nurse to the supervisor in the first place, then there is sufficient evidence to file the same report with the state board of nursing. An affirmative duty to report the nurse to the state board of nursing exists in such a case.

Reporting a violator of the nurse practice act may be done by writing to the state board of nursing, describing the substance abuse or substandard care, and including all pertinent documentation. Sign the letter, since anonymous complaints are summarily disregarded by most boards of nursing and administrators; in addition, the nurse has not fulfilled the affirmative duty to safeguard nursing practice by an anonymous letter. Most state boards of nursing will preserve confidentiality.

NATIONAL PRACTITIONER DATA BANK

The *National Practitioner Data Bank (NPDB)* was created by the Health Care Quality Improvement Act of 1986 and became operational on September 1,

1990. Although primarily aimed at impacting the practice of medicine, the NPDB also impacts the professional practice of nursing. The NDPB records three types of information relating to:

1. Medical malpractice payments on behalf of health care practitioners.
2. Adverse actions taken against clinical privileges of physicians, osteopaths, and dentists.
3. Actions by professional societies that adversely affect membership.

The information is then available to health care facilities needing the information to verify credentialing of potential practitioners. Failure to report results in fines and penalties if mandatory reporting is identified.

The NPDB affects nursing from the perspective of advanced nursing practice because nurse practitioners, nurse midwives, and nurse anesthetists are subject to credentialing procedures similar to those named in the act as well as the quality of care at facilities that also employ nurses. While far from a perfect system, it is the beginning of a national effort to track and identify professionals who have been found liable of malpractice or who have had professional memberships or professional privileges revoked.

CERTIFICATION

Certification is a form of credentialing that has both legal and professional implications. Certification indicates a level of competence above minimum criteria for licensure and verifies that an individual has met certain standards of preparation and performance.

Certification of an individual awards the certified person with the right to use the title conferred by the certificate. It acts as proof of the special qualifications that the individual has achieved in a defined area of clinical practice.

Many specialty nursing organizations offer certification to professional nurses. Some of the organizations mandate advanced degrees in nursing as prerequisites for certification, while other organizations do not add this prerequisite. The ANA offers a wide variety of certifications, as do other professional organizations. For example, the Emergency Nurses Organization, the American Association of Critical-care Nurses, and the Association of Operating Room Nurses offer specialty certification in their areas of clinical practice.

EXERCISE 11-4

Interview nursing personnel in your facility to see which certificates (if any) are required for various positions. How are staff nurses (eg, critical care or emergency center nurses) urged to attain certification? Is there a pay differential for certification?

SUMMARY

Credentials, which are proof of the qualifications of individuals, include both licensure and certification. The first licensure laws for nurses were, in reality, permissive registration acts. Today, all states and territories have nurse practice acts and administrative boards of nursing that regulate registered and practical nursing practice. Professional nursing organizations and licensing boards offer certification for nurses in advanced clinical practice roles and in advanced nursing practice.

AFTER COMPLETING THIS CHAPTER, YOU SHOULD BE ABLE TO

- Define licensure, including mandatory, permissive, and institutional licensure.
- Describe the process for creating state boards of nursing and their authority, including limitations on their authority.
- Describe the process of how state nursing acts define the professional scope of practice.
- Describe entry into practice in relationship to state nurse practice acts.

APPLY YOUR LEGAL KNOWLEDGE

- How do nurse practice acts provide for consumer protection and for nursing advancement?
- Does the state board of nursing have the authority to change the practice of professional nursing?
- What are the main differences between licensure and credentialing? Is that difference crucial to consumer protection?

REFERENCES

Aiken, T. D. & Catalano, J. T. (1994). *Legal, ethical and political issues in nursing.* Philadelphia, PA: F. A. Davis Company.

American Nurses' Association approves a definition of nursing practice. (1955). *American Journal of Nursing, 55*(12), 1474.

American Nurses' Association. (1980). *The nursing practice act: Suggested state legislation.* Kansas City, MO: Author.

American Nurses' Association. (1990). *Suggested state legislation: Nursing practice act.*

American Nurses' Association. (1995). *Report of the house of delegates: 1995.* Washington, DC: Author.

Burns v. Matzen, #93-100 (Iowa, 1994). In *Hospital Law Manual, 2*(11), 4.

Colorado State Board of Nursing v. Hohn, 129 Colo. 195, 268 P.2d 401 (Colorado, 1954).

Cooper v. National Motor Bearing Company, 136 Cal. App. 2d 229, 288 P.2d 581 (1955).

Derrick v. Commonwealth of Pennsylvania, 432 A.2d 282 (Pennsylvania, 1981).

Ex parte Smith, 435 So.2d 108 (Alabama, 1983).

George, S. & Young, W. B. (1990). Baccalaureate entry into practice. *Nursing Outlook, 29*(8), 41–45.

Heinecke v. Department of Commerce, Division of Occupational and Professional Licensing, 810 P.2d 459 (Utah App., 1991).

Hogan v. Mississippi Board of Nursing, 457 So.2d 931 (1984).

Hood, G. (1985). At issue: Titling and licensure. *American Journal of Nursing, 85*(5), 92–94.

Joel, L. A. (1995). Your license to practice: Variations on a theme. *American Journal of Nursing, 95*(11), 7.

Lunsford v. Board of Nurse Examiners, 648 S.W.2d 391 (Tex. Civ. App.-Austin, 1983).

Mohr v. Jenkins, 393 So.2d 245 (La. Ct. App., 1980).

Rafferty v. Commonwealth, State Board of Nurse Examiners, 80 Pa. Comwlth. 603, 471 A.2d 1339 (Pennsylvania, 1984).

Scott v. State of Nebraska, ex rel. Board of Nursing of the State of Nebraska, 244 N.W.2d 683 (Nebraska, 1976).

Schoenhair v. Pennsylvania, 459 A.2d 877 (Pennsylvania, 1983).

Stevens v. Blake, 456 So.2d 795 (Ala. Civ. App., 1984).

Whitney v. Day, 100 Mich. App. 707, 300 N.W.2d 380 (Ct. App. Mich., 1980).

• twelve

Advanced Practice Roles in Nursing

PREVIEW

During the past few decades, several dynamic factors have shaped and supported the trend away from traditional, hospital-based roles in nursing. Now the focus on advanced practice roles in nursing is even more critical, as the nation wrestles with health care reform and primary health care. The Health Security effort of 1993 emphasized security, savings, simplicity, choice, quality, and responsibility, all components of nursing's advanced practice roles in an environment where a legal system realizes the full potential of advanced practice nursing.

Nurses today require an advanced practice arena that will support advanced education and advanced skills. Increasingly larger numbers of nurses are returning to educational institutions for higher degrees in nursing and are becoming dissatisfied with traditional staff nursing roles. The roles of the nurse anesthetist, nurse midwife, advanced nurse practitioner, and clinical nurse specialist continue to evolve and to expand, improving the quality of health care in a nation that is cost-conscious, yet demanding of access and quality care.

advanced practice roles   prescriptive authority   reimbursement

scope of practice   admitting privileges   direct access

standards of care   antitrust issues

HISTORICAL OVERVIEW OF ADVANCED NURSING PRACTICE ROLES

Early in America's history, women fulfilled the role of autonomous nursing practitioners and midwives (Reverby, 1987). During the late 1800s, physicians assumed the autonomous health care deliverer status that prevails today. This was accomplished through state medical practice acts and the strong organizational structure of the American Medical Association (Stevens, 1971). The modern *advanced practice roles* originated in the late 1960s and early 1970s, when the shortage of primary physicians led to new initiatives to meet America's health care needs.

Today, advanced nursing practice encompasses four distinct practice roles, and there are in excess of 100,000 advanced practice nurses in the United States (American Association of Colleges of Nursing, 1991). The hallmark of these four roles is that nurses have the ability to combine the caring role of the nurse with the more traditional curing role of the physician. Advanced practice nurses are committed to providing basic health care to all people, ensuring health promotion and maintenance, increasing the quality of care, and ensuring the development of better informed consumers (Inglis and Kjervik, 1993).

Interestingly, roles that nurses performed became their occupational titles. While the public is now requiring a specialized body of knowledge rather than a title distinction, advanced practice nurses are still known by these occupational titles.

Nurse Anesthetist

Perhaps the oldest of the expanded roles in nursing is that of the *nurse anesthetist*. In 1878, Sister Mary Bernard was administering anesthesia at St. Vincent's Hospital in Erie, Pennsylvania. Agatha C. Hodgins served as a nurse anesthetist in Cleveland, Ohio, at the turn of the century and was as well-known for her ability to administer anesthesia as she was for teaching doctors and nurses her techniques (Mannino, 1982).

The two world wars, as well as the Korean and Vietnam wars, increased the need for nurses proficient in administering anesthesia. Both at home and at the front, nurses were needed to expand the numbers of medical personnel giving anesthesia. The physician shortage of the early 1960s continued to support the need for this expanded nursing role, and schools of nurse anesthesia quickly opened. The nurse anesthetist currently provides anesthesia for a variety of procedures, including dental, surgical, and obstetrical procedures, many in the rural settings of the United States.

The first legal challenges to this role arose in the mid-1930s. In what has become a landmark decision, the California Supreme Court in 1936 held that the giving of anesthesia by nurses was not "diagnosing nor prescribing by nurses within the meaning of the California Medical Practice Act" (*Chalmers-Francis v. Nelson*, 1936, at 402). Thus nurses could administer anesthesia within the scope of nursing practice.

Nurse-administered anesthesia was the first expanded role in nursing to seek recognition via certification and education. Certification recognizes the attainment of advanced, specialized knowledge and skills beyond that which is necessary for safe practice. The nurse anesthetist may also obtain an advanced degree in nursing such as a master's of science degree in nursing in nurse anesthesia. The professional organization for nurse anesthetists, the American Association of Nurse Anesthetists, will soon require a master's degree as a prerequisite for certification as a CRNA.

Nurse Midwife

The practice of *nurse midwifery* also has its origins in the late 1800s and early 1900s. At that time, midwifery was becoming a regulated, legally recognized profession through state legislative enactments. Prior to these state enactments, the art of midwifery was a lay art, practiced by women who learned about childbirth either by their own experiences or through others trained in the art. After the state enactments, the art of midwifery became more common among nurses. The first nurse midwifery educational program was opened in 1952 by the Maternity Association of New York City.

The practice of nurse midwifery still has some legal uncertainties. Authorization of nurse midwifery may be found in nurse practice acts, medical practice acts, rules and regulations specific to nurse midwives, allied health laws, public health laws, or a combination of any of these. Some states, depending on the jurisdiction, also regulate nurse-midwifery through state agencies.

The practice of nurse midwifery involves the independent management of essentially normal prenatal, intrapartum, postpartum, and gynecological care of women as well as the care of the normal newborns. Usually there is a complex system for medical consultation and collaboration, and in some states all care is given with the understanding that a referral physician is always available. Some states allow the full range of practice, while other states allow more restrictive practices.

As with nurse anesthesia, the earliest cases in nurse midwifery addressed the issue of whether the practice constituted the practice of medicine. The case of *People v. Arendt* (1894) held that the midwife in question was guilty of practicing medicine without a license. Since that time, nurse midwives have worked to develop a clear definition of the status of the role of nurse midwife.

Advanced Nurse Practitioners

Known in some states as nurse practitioners, the role is clarified as *advanced nurse practitioners* for states that refer to all registered nurses (RNs) as nurse practitioners. This role began in 1965 when Drs. Loretta Ford and Henry Silver began a program at the University of Colorado that placed nurses in new practice settings and increased their traditional patient care responsibilities. Goals of the advanced nurse practitioner movement were to prepare nurses with master's and doctorate degrees for independent expert practice, teaching, and clinical research. The advanced nurse practitioner would have a client case load much as a practicing physician carries a client case load. Long-term goals included increased access to quality health care as well as the expanded use of nursing skills in health assessment and maintenance. This increased access to quality health care was mainly seen in rural areas and was used by patients for whom minimal health care was available.

Advanced nurse practitioners may work independently, in a peer relationship with physicians, or dependently under the physicians' standing or direct orders. Depending on the state nurse practice act, nurses may independently diagnose, treat, and prescribe for patients, or they may be limited to managing the care of the patient as a delegated role. The advanced nurse practitioner may also be limited by the state nurse practice act to diagnose and treat, but not prescribe for the patient.

Legal challenges for this role have included scope-of-practice issues, much like those challenges to nurse anesthetists and nurse midwives. One case upheld the suspension of a nurse's license for treating patients without a physician's supervision (*Hernicz v. State of Florida, Department of Professional Regulation*, 1980). Other cases have upheld the right of the nurse to practice as an advanced nurse practitioner (*Sermchief v. Gonzales*, 1983, and *Bellegie v. Board of Nurse Examiners*, 1985).

Idaho was the first state to enact specific legislation defining and promoting the independent role of the advanced nurse practitioner in 1971. Currently advanced nurse practitioners are authorized by their individual state boards of nursing through certification, licensure, official recognition, registration, or approval. Educational requirements vary depending on state requirements, with most states requiring advanced nursing degrees, demonstrated nursing skills, or additional nursing course work. The trend is toward requiring a master's degree for all advanced nurse practitioners.

Certification for the advanced nurse practitioner may be accomplished through the American Nurses Association (ANA). Current nursing practice certification programs offered by the ANA include a wide variety of specialties, such as adult nurse practitioner, family nurse practitioner, school nurse practitioner, gerontological nurse practitioner, and pediatric nurse practitioner (American Nurses Association, 1994). A joint committee of the ANA and the American Association of Critical-care Nurses is developing certification for the acute care nurse practitioner.

Clinical Nurse Specialist

The role of the *clinical nurse specialist,* sometimes known as a *nurse clinician* or *advanced clinical nurse,* also has its origins in the mid-1960s. This role evolved in response to needs expressed by both patients and nurses. Traditionally as nurses advanced in nursing, they moved away from the bedside and entered either administrative or educational roles. Nurses with advanced nursing knowledge and skills who tried to stay within staff positions usually failed due to the economics of the hospital, since it was more cost-efficient to have aides and licensed practical nurses give direct patient care.

Several schools of nursing began to offer curricula that would allow nurses to obtain advanced nursing degrees and to specialize in clinical nursing so that they could continue to work directly with patients, family members, and staff. The specialization also allowed nurses to be proficient in teaching, research methodology, and consultation. This allows the clinical nurse specialists not only to be directly involved with patient care but to be indirectly involved with increasing the quality of nursing care throughout the institution.

In 1974, at the ANA Congress for Nursing Practice, the role was defined as requiring a master's degree in nursing. Ideally, the clinical nurse specialist is a practitioner holding a master's degree with a concentration in a specific area of clinical nursing. The function of the clinical nurse specialists is unique with respect to the use of clinical judgment and skills regarding client care. They serve as advocates when clients are unable to cope with a situation, and they influence for change as necessary in the nursing care and in the health care delivery system (American Nurses Association, 1976). The clinical nurse specialist is also certified through a variety of certification opportunities.

Subroles of the clinical nurse specialist are divided into two broad categories:

1. Direct care functions that include expert practitioner, role model, and patient advocate.
2. Indirect care functions that include change agent, consultant or resource person, clinical teacher, researcher, liaison person, and innovator.

Unlike the other advanced nursing roles, clinical nurse specialists function more as employees than as independent practitioners. Because of this direct employer-employee relationship, clinical nurse specialists are usually not included under legal discussions of expanded nursing roles. However, this more traditional role is being consumed under the general title of advanced nurse practitioner, and there is currently a movement to incorporate these two specialties into a single title and role.

EXERCISE 12-1

Investigate the use of advance practice nurses within your area. Do such roles exist? How are these nurses used in the community and in hospital health care delivery systems? Is the state nurse association and/or other professional organizations working to expand the role of these nurses?

LEGAL LIABILITY OF EXPANDED NURSING ROLES

In some ways professionals practicing in expanded nursing roles have dual legal liabilities:

1. They are licensed to practice by the state board of nursing and are accountable for its rules and regulations.
2. They have assumed advanced standing under the delegatory language of the state medical practice act or have assumed advanced standing under the state nurse practice act, public health laws or other state laws, and are accountable for this independent or interdependent role.

Several legal questions arise when discussing the potential liability of the practitioner in an expanded role. Most of the questions come under the overall classification of scope of practice and standards of care.

SCOPE OF PRACTICE

A major legal issue is the permissible *scope of practice,* which refers to the permissible boundaries of practice for health professionals, as defined by statute, rule, or a combination of statute and rule, and which defines the actions and duties of nurses in these roles. Physicians were the first professionals in virtually all states to define their scope of practice, and by the 1800s had defined medicine to include curing, diagnosing, treating, and prescribing. Physicians also assured against interference in their practice by incorporating provisions that made it illegal for anyone not licensed as a physician to perform acts included in their definition.

Nurses gained legal control of their profession in the early 1900s. By 1930, all states had passed nurse practice acts. *Autonomous practice* was defined as the supervision of patients, the observation of symptoms and reactions of patients, and the accurate recording of patient information. The remainder of the nursing scope of practice was defined as *complementary,* or dependent, to the physician. With the advent of advanced nursing practice, it became apparent that such a definition of scope of practice would prevent independent practice, and several courses of action were undertaken to remedy the situation.

One means of increasing the scope of practice was by amending or totally altering state nurse practice acts. States began to accomplish this by promulgating rules and regulations to expand the scope of practice. In 1971, Idaho became the first state to broaden its definition of nursing to statutorily include diagnosis and treatment as part of the scope of practice of advanced nurse practitioners. Although the intent of the statute was clear, the statute also required that acts of diagnosis and treatment be authorized by rules and regulations jointly developed by the boards of nursing and medicine, and that all institutions employing advanced nurse practitioners develop policies and guidelines for their practice. This latter requirement resulted in constraints in their practice.

Currently, most states have enacted legislation regarding the advanced nurse practitioners' scope of practice. The majority of statutes require that advanced nurse practitioners have sponsoring or supervising physicians, greatly diminishing their scope of practice.

A second means of expanding the legal scope of practice is by court decisions concerning the nature of the advanced nurse practitioners' role. Two significant decisions have been made in this area. *Sermchief v. Gonzales*, a 1983 Missouri Supreme Court decision, held that the Missouri legislature, when it enacted the nurse practice act, had intended to avoid statutory constraints on the evolution of new nursing roles and thereby gave advanced nurse practitioners practice authority through the broad wording of professional nursing. In actuality, the court found that professional nursing in that jurisdiction had the right to practice within the limits of their education and experience.

In *Sermchief*, a group of advanced nurse practitioners were routinely providing gynecological care, including routine PAP smears, pregnancy testing, and birth control measures, pursuant to protocols jointly developed by nursing and supervising physicians. The Missouri Nurse Practice Act did not require direct physician supervision, but defined professional nursing in more general terms, according to specialized education, judgment, and skill. A group of physicians, predominantly those whose practice had declined because of the advent of the advanced nurse practitioners' practice, brought suit claiming that the nurses, rather than practicing nursing, were instead engaged in the illegal practice of medicine. In a lengthy decision, the court held that the advanced nurse practitioners were indeed practicing within the scope of their education and skills and within the scope of nursing as the Missouri legislature had intended.

Sermchief was a significant decision for nursing. A second significant decision was *Bellegie v. Board of Nurse Examiners* (1985). In that case, the Texas Medical Association and the Texas Hospital Association challenged the authority of the Texas Board of Nurse Examiners to promulgate rules and regulations regarding advanced nursing practice within the state. In finding for the Board, the court held that the Board's regulatory authority was not limited to regulating titles, but extended to regulating the activities and education of nursing within their jurisdiction.

These two decisions clearly began the establishment of nursing's legal status as a full-fledged, independent profession. If nursing is to continue to expand as a truly autonomous professional role, then nurses must work at state and national levels to promote the most effective use of the advanced practice nurses.

At the federal level, the scope of practice issues are tied to reimbursement issues. The following issues must be part of nursing's agenda for advanced practice:

1. The elimination of restrictions that allow nurses to practice only in certain geographic settings (for example, rural and underserved areas).
2. The elimination of requirements that make nurses dependent on physician supervision or collaboration.
3. The establishment of requirements that the same services should result in same payments by insurers and third-party payors, regardless of the specialty or profession of the provider.

At the state level, nurses must work to assure that the sole authority for advanced nursing practice is placed within the board of nursing, and that the board has the authority to promulgate rules regarding the practice of advanced practice nurses, passage of statutory definitions of advanced nursing practice, and granting of clinical and admitting privileges to advanced nurse practitioners (Safriet, 1992).

Malpractice Issues

Areas in which advanced practice nurses have incurred liability include:

1. Conduct exceeding the scope of expertise that causes harm (*Gugino v. Harvard Community Health Plan et al.,* 1983).
2. Conduct exceeding physician-delegated authority that results in harm (*Tatro v. State of Texas,* 1983).
3. Independent practice in a state where advanced nurse practitioners must have a sponsoring physician (*Hernicz v. State of Florida, Department of Professional Regulation,* 1980).
4. Failure to refer when the advanced nurse practitioner's skills are exceeded (*Lane v. Otis,* 1982). The failure to refer is the most prevailing cause of action, and advanced practice nurses must refer patients in a timely manner when they see that their expertise will soon be exceeded.

Lawsuits involving advanced nurse practitioners raise inevitable questions about whether the nurse involved was performing an activity that was:

1. Generic to nursing and within the nursing scope of practice.
2. A medical activity that is permitted by law as germane to the advanced practice nurse's scope of practice.
3. A medical activity not within the scope of practice of the advanced practice nurse.
4. A nursing activity that overlaps with a medical activity.

Additional questions center on the elements of malpractice, such as the duty owed the patient, breach of that duty as owed, foreseeability, causation, and damages.

If the activity involved in the lawsuit is purely a nursing function, then nurses will serve as expert witnesses in determining the standard of care owed the patient. If the activity is a medical function not allowed within the nurse scope of practice, the expert witness will testify to medical standards of care. As the next section illustrates, the courts and nursing are still struggling with standards of care when the activity involved is a nursing function that overlaps with a medical function, as opposed to an activity allowable within the scope of the advanced practice nurse.

STANDARDS OF CARE

The question that arises frequently in negligence cases is what legal *standard of care,* or duty of care, is to be applied to nurses in expanded roles? Nurses who perform functions and actions traditionally recognized as medical should be familiar with court decisions concerning standards of professional care. Earlier cases mainly held that nurses in expanded roles are held to the medical standard of care (*Hendry v. United States,* 1969 and *Harris v. State through Huey P. Long Hospital,* 1979). *Whitney v. Day, M.D. and Hurley Hospital* (1981) held that nurse anesthetists are professionals who have expertise in an area akin to the practice of medicine. Because their responsibilities lie in an area of medical expertise, the standard of care is to be based on the skill and care normally expected of those with like education and expertise. A 1925 case disallowed any liability on the part of the physician involved and found that the nurse-midwife was solely negligent (*Olson v. Bolstad,* 1925). While that court also set the medical standard as the standard of care for the midwife, it specifically stated that the physician incurred no liability in relying on the midwife to perform her duties properly.

Fein v. Permanente Medical Group (1985) was one of the first cases to disagree with this line of holdings. In *Fein,* the court set the standard of care for the advanced nurse practitioner. In that case, a patient was misdiagnosed first by an advanced nurse practitioner and subsequently by a physician as having muscle spasms rather than a myocardial infarction. After examining the patient and obtaining a history, the nurse diagnosed muscle spasms and gave the patient a prescription for Valium. The court labored to find that the advanced nurse practitioner was held to the standard of a nurse practitioner performing diagnosis and treatment, not to the standard of a physician performing diagnoses and treatment. Specifically, the court held that "the examination or diagnosis cannot be said—as a matter of law—to be a function reserved to physicians rather than to registered nurses or nurse practitioners" (*Fein v. Permanente Medical Group,* 1985, at 140). Therefore, a physician working with advanced practice nurses or an advanced nurse practitioner functioning in a similar setting would be qualified to establish the standard of care.

A more recent case regarding professional standards of care was *Paris v. Kreitz* (1985), which concerned the standard of care of a physician assistant. The court addressed the liability of the physician's assistant and concluded that "the argument that physicians' assistants are subject to the same standard of care as physicians is without merit" (*Paris v. Kreitz,* 1985, at 244). Citing the standard jury instruction, which states that a health care provider is subject to the standard of practice among members of the same health care profession with similar training and experiences and situated in the same or similar communities, the court concluded that it was clear that a physicians' assistant was not subject to the same standards as a medical doctor. Had the defendant been an advanced nurse practitioner, the conclusion of the court may have been the same: The advanced nurse practitioner is not subject to the same standards as medical doctors.

A final question about advanced nursing practice and standards of care is who may serve as an expert witness in establishing the prevailing standard of care of specific professions. The rule that a medical expert witness must be from the same medical specialty as the physician involved in the case has been eroded (*Samii v. Baystate Medical Center,* 1979). In one California case, an obstetrical nurse practitioner was permitted to establish the prevailing standard of care in a case that concerned an obstetrician. That was because the services provided were the same as those that could be provided legally by an obstetrical nurse practitioner (Marco, 1983). Such findings assist in reassuring the American public that the quality of care of physicians and advanced nurse practitioners is equal.

EXERCISE 12-2

Reread your state's nurse practice act. Does either the act or the board of nursing's set of rules and regulations provide for advanced practice? If neither does, is the board of nursing working on a provision (or rules and regulations) to create such a role? In what ways can the board of nursing strengthen the scope of practice for advanced practice nurses?

PRESCRIPTIVE AUTHORITY

Prescriptive authority is central to independent practice by advanced practice nurses. Only 50 years ago, most drugs not classified as narcotics were available as over-the-counter medications, and nurses worked independently with physicians in recommending such medications (Pearson, 1992). This was changed by the 1938 Federal Food, Drug, and Cosmetic Act. The movement away from consumer control to physician control of education strengthened the medical profession by increasing its social privilege and economic power (Pearson, 1992).

Legal issues in this area involve the extent of professional decision making allowed to advanced practice nurses and the range of drugs from which they may select. States may allow autonomous prescriptive authority while imposing written protocols, or they may mandate formularies that dictate which medications may be prescribed. In states with written protocols, nurses frequently are prevented from prescribing a full range of medications, and the scheduled days of therapy are usually short. In such states, it is not uncommon to see an advanced practice nurse prescribe three days of antibiotic therapy as opposed to the more effective ten-day course of therapy. A written formulary of medications, usually filed with the state board of nursing, is another means of limiting the range of medications that advanced practice nurses can prescribe. Some states further restrict prescriptive authority by requiring physician supervision or direction in the area of medication selection or by restricting prescriptive authority to certain geographical areas (rural or underserved areas) or practice settings (skilled nursing centers).

Today, approximately 43 states allow some degree of prescriptive authority, and 13 give independent authority. Of those 13 states, eight allow nurses to write for controlled substances. Legislation is pending in states without prescriptive authority (Hall, 1993). In states without prescriptive authority, advanced practice nurses frequently provide prescriptions to patients by requesting that the physician write the prescription for them, by calling in the prescription to the pharmacy under a physician's name, or by using existing protocols that have been negotiated among the physician, pharmacist, and advanced practice nurse. From a legal perspective, these practices increase potential legal liability, not only to advanced practice nurses, but also to physicians and pharmacists.

Actions needed at state level to improve prescriptive authority include statutory amendments stating that advanced practice nurses may prescribe scheduled and nonscheduled medications without the necessity of a sponsoring physician and that prescriptive authority is included in the advanced practice nurse's scope of practice, regardless of the practice setting or area. Amendments to state nurse practice acts should eliminate any language on written protocols, because the primary purpose of such protocols is to limit the prescriptive authority of advanced practice nurses.

ADMITTING PRIVILEGES

Admitting privileges, which are granted by individual facilities, may range from allowing the practitioner to visit patients to permitting direct admission and entries in the medical record. Although admitting or hospital privileges are becoming more of an issue, they are facility-controlled, and no state or federal legislation is involved.

Admitting and hospital privileges are an area of major concern to certified registered nurse anesthetists since their practice setting is primarily the hospital setting. Central *antitrust issues* arise when health care professionals seek access to health care facilities controlled by physicians with whom they compete. Because most hospital credentialing committees that vote on extending hospital privileges to qualified practitioners are composed exclusively of physicians, nurse anesthetists must constantly fight this battle.

Antitrust issues arise whenever there:

1. Is exclusion of a class (here nurse anesthetists) from membership on the medical or hospital staff.
2. Are questions about the fair market value of a service.
3. Are attempts by one society or association to restrict its members' use of a second class of practitioners.

The issue that the courts must decide is whether the antitrust laws can eliminate professional group boycotts motivated by anticompetition interests, while preserving legitimate professional self-regulation aimed at maintaining the competence and professional conduct of a particular profession.

The courts are now beginning to help advanced practice nurses secure hospital privileges (*Bahn v. NME Hospitals*, 1987 and *Wrable v. Community Memorial Hospital*, 1987). However, these issues may need to be addressed on the local level rather than on the state and federal levels. Perhaps the biggest hurdle to overcome is the prevailing practice of allowing advanced practice nurses to admit patients to an institution under the name of a supervising physician. This practice decreases the autonomy of advanced practice nurses, while ensuring that only physicians are credentialed by the institution.

REIMBURSEMENT ISSUES

Reimbursement issues and practices are a major stumbling block to expanded practice. Several issues come under this heading, including equal pay for equal services, direct reimbursement by third-party payors, and the range of services for which reimbursement will be paid. Advanced practice nurses will not be able to practice independently until these issues are addressed and solved.

Reimbursement for advanced practice nurses is affected by state and federal regulations. On the federal scene, Medicare and Medicaid dominate reimbursement, and state insurance regulators and private insurance companies generally follow the federal lead. Under current federal acts, specifically the Omnibus Budget Reconciliation Act of 1989, advanced practice nurses are subject to reimbursement at 65% of the physician's fee schedule amount for certified nurse midwives, with a capping of advanced practice nurses' fees and fewer covered services.

To secure equitable reimbursement for advanced practice, nurses must work for change at the federal and state levels. Federal action is needed to expand reimbursement to all services provided by advanced practice nurses, to eliminate regulations that narrowly circumscribe direct reimbursement, and to require that the same services are compensated by the same payment. State regulations are needed to prevent health insurance or health care service plans from discriminating against advanced practice nurses and to extend Medicaid reimbursement to advanced practice nurses' services.

EXERCISE 12-3

In your state:

1. How is reimbursement for advanced practice nurses structured?
2. What is the level of prescriptive authority for advanced practice nurses?

How do these two issues affect the overall ability of nurse practitioners to start their own practices? Which of these two issues has the greater impact on nurses in your area?

DIRECT ACCESS TO PATIENT POPULATIONS

Physicians have traditionally been the gatekeepers of the health care delivery system. *Direct access* to alternate providers, such as advanced practice nurses, has been curtailed by medical practitioners, regulators, and accreditors, including state health departments and the Joint Commission on Accreditation of Healthcare Organizations. Nurses have only recently taken definitive action for discharge planning, including when patients are released from the health care facility.

Some of the current proposals for allowing advanced practice nurses direct access to patient populations concern managed care corporations. Today *managed care corporations* retain the power of the physician as the gatekeeper, but negotiations for advanced practice nurses in these corporations is advancing in some areas of the country. These negotiations are being undertaken in light of the current research on patient outcomes and who provides more optimal services in relationship to cost-containment and patient satisfaction. Such research needs to continue, though, if advanced practice nurses are to be allowed more direct access to patients.

SUMMARY

The major legal challenges involving advanced practice nurses have centered on scope of practice, standards of care, and malpractice issues. If advance practice nurses are to be allowed to fully practice, the legal issues that must be addressed in the future include reimbursement, prescriptive authority, admitting privileges, and direct access to patient populations. For advanced practice nurses to function to their full potential and provide the quality, compassionate care demanded by the American public, they must mount campaigns for change at state and federal levels. Advanced practice nurses must be enabled to deliver independent, health care services to all parts of the United States, rural and urban, in all practice settings, and must be compensated fully for their services. This will ensure that America's underserved and forgotten patients also receive quality health care.

GUIDELINES: NURSING IN EXPANDED PRACTICE ROLES

1. Nurses in an expanded practice role must first recognize that, along with the role's increased autonomy, comes increased accountability and liability. While nurses are always accountable for their actions and omissions, those in an expanded practice role adopt a higher standard of care for the services and actions performed.

2. Accept patients and responsibilities within your field of expertise and within your allowable scope of practice. Review carefully the state nurse practice act, medical practice act, pharmacy act, and public health laws for scope of practice issues. Review and understand the rules and regulations promulgated by the state board of nursing for the allowable scope of practice.

3. Understand the allowable scope of practice if your state requires that you function under the delegatory language of the state medical practice act. Be sure that you do not exceed any physician-delegated responsibilities.

4. Ensure that you have obtained valid informed consent and have obtained such consent from the proper person(s) before proceeding to care for or treat clients. As with physician malpractice suits, this area is frequently cited in nursing malpractice suits.

5. Be sure the client knows of your status as a nurse in an expanded role and understands that you are not a physician. Impersonation of a physician is fraud and opens you to licensure suspension or revocation as well as to other civil lawsuits.

6. Seek assistance from other specialists and physicians when circumstances exceed your scope of knowledge and expertise. Failure to refer the patient to a physician or more qualified advanced nurse practitioner when your skills are exceeded or when complications arise has been the basis of previous lawsuits. The failure to refer in a timely manner may place you in the position of acting beyond the allowable scope of practice for your expanded role.

7. Do not practice independently unless your state recognizes independent practice by advanced nurse practitioners. Many states require a supervising or collaborating physician, and you may not exceed the bounds of that supervision or collaborative role.

8. Maintain your current skills and continue to broaden your knowledge and skills through continuing education and advanced nursing degrees. Maintain your certification, or seek certification through appropriate associations as proof of your qualifications, knowledge base, and skills in a defined functional or clinical area of nursing.

9. Document carefully and accurately any nursing care given. Legible and dependable nursing records are vital if nurses functioning in an expanded nursing role hope to successfully defend a future lawsuit.

AFTER COMPLETING THIS CHAPTER, YOU SHOULD BE ABLE TO

- Define the roles of advanced practice nurses, including nurse anesthetists, nurse midwives, advanced nurse practitioners, and clinical nurse specialists.
- Describe the legal constraints to advanced professional practice encountered by nurses educationally and clinically competent to perform these roles, including:

    Scope of practice.

    Malpractice issues.

    Standards of care.

    Prescriptive authority.

    Hospital or admitting privileges.

    Reimbursement issues.

    Direct access to patient populations.
- Analyze means to overcome these legal constraints.
- Compare and contrast the current status of advanced nursing practice with that role in the future.

APPLY YOUR LEGAL KNOWLEDGE

- How does the state nurse practice act affect the role of advanced nursing practice within a state?
- Is advanced nursing practice making more of an impact in some areas than in others? Does this impact correspond to the primary purposes of advanced nursing practice?
- What must professional nursing do to ensure that advanced nursing practice is fully utilized by persons most needing these professionals' care?

REFERENCES

American Association of Colleges of Nursing. (1991). *Policy statement.* Washington, DC: Author.

American Nurses' Association. (1976). *Congress for nursing practice: The scope of nursing practice. Description of practice: Clinical nurse specialist.* Kansas City, MO: Author.

American Nurses' Association. (1994). *Certification catalog.* Washington, DC: Author.

Bahn v. NME Hospitals, 669 F. Supp. 998 (E.D. California, 1987).

Batty v. Arizona State Dental Board, 57 Ariz. 239, 112 P.2d 1166 (Massachusetts, 1983).

Bellegie v. Board of Nurse Examiners, 685 S.W. 2d 431 (Tex. Ct. App.-Austin, 1985).

Chalmers-Francis v. Nelson, 6 Cal. 2d 402 (1936).

Fein v. Permanente Medical Group, 38 Cal. 3d 137 (1985).

Gugino v. Harvard Community Health Plan et al., 403 N.E. 2d 1166 (Massachusetts, 1983).

Hall, J. (1993). How to analyze nurse practitioner licensure laws. *Nurse Practitioner, 18*(1), 31–34.

Harris v. State through Huey P. Long Hospital, 371 So. 2d 1221 (Louisiana, 1979).

Hendry v. United States, 418 F.2d 744 (2d. Cir., 1969).

Hernicz v. State of Florida, Department of Professional Regulation, 390 So. 2d 194 (Fla. Dis. Ct. App., 1980).

Inglis, A. D., and Kjervik, D. K. (1993). Empowerment of advanced practice nurses: Regulation reform needed to increase access to care. *Journal of Law, Medicine, and Ethics* (21), 193–205.

Lane v. Otis, 412 So. 2d 254 (Alabama, 1982).

Mannino, M. J. (1982). *The nurse anesthetist and the law.* New York: Grune & Stratton.

Marco C. (1983). Can a nurse practitioner testify against a physician? *Legal Aspects of Medical Practice, 11,*(2), 5–6.

Olson v. Bolstad, 161 Minn. 419, 201 N.W. 918 (1925).

Paris v. Kreitz, 331 S.E. 2d 234 (North Carolina, 1985).

People v. Arendt, 60 Ill. App. 89 (1894).

Pearson L. J. (1992). 1992–1993 update: How each state stands on legislative issues affecting advanced nursing practice. *The Nurse Practitioner: The American Journal of Primary Health Care, 11,* 2.

Reverby, S. M. (1987). *Ordered to care: The dilemma of American nursing, 1850–1945.* Cambridge, MA: Cambridge University Press.

Safriet, B. J. (1992). Health care dollars and regulatory sense: The role of advanced practice nursing. *Yale Journal on Regulation* (9), 417–487.

Samii v. Baystate Medical Center, 395 N.E. 2d 455 (Massachusetts, 1979).

Sermchief v. Gonzales, 660 S.W. 2d 683 (Missouri en Banc, 1983).

Stevens, R. (1971). *American medicine and the public interest.* New Haven: Yale University Press.

Tatro v. State of Texas, 703 F.2d 823 (5th Cir., 1983).

Whitney v. Day, M.D. and Hurley Hospital, 300 N.W. 2d 380 (Ct. App.-Mich. 1981).

Wruble v. Community Memorial Hospital, 205 J.J. Super. 428 (1985), aff'd. 517 A. 2d. 470 (October 22, 1986), cert. denied, 526 A. 2d 210 (April 28, 1987).

· thirteen

Nursing in Hospital Settings

PREVIEW

The previous chapter concerned nurses in expanded roles, those nurses recognized by their state nurse practice acts or state boards of nursing to practice within expanded roles. This chapter concerns nurses practicing within hospital and clinic settings, performing daily more highly skilled tasks and having responsibility for increasingly more acutely ill patients. Gone are the days when sophisticated machines were seen only in critical care areas or emergency centers. Patients on general medical and surgical units may have ventilators, central intravenous lines, and chest tubes, as well as a variety of other machines and devices. Thus hospital employees are encountering the need for greater skills as well as facing potentially more liability. This chapter addresses the issues arising within hospital-based nursing, giving guides on competent, quality health care delivery.

KEY CONCEPTS

patient safety	medication errors	failure to adequately assess, monitor, and communicate
suicide prevention	technology and equipment	
restraints		failure to act as patient advocate

HOSPITAL NURSING TODAY

The past 30 years have witnessed dramatic changes within the nurse's role in hospital settings. Three decades ago it was easy to define the practice of medicine and the practice of nursing and to articulate the difference between the two professions. Today, the roles are becoming masked with the advent of:

1. Critical care units.
2. Intermediate care units.
3. Advanced nursing skills within specialized units such as the operating room, postanesthesia care unit, labor and delivery units, and emergency centers.
4. Advanced nursing knowledge, technology, and equipment.

Today's nurses must assume responsibility and accountability for patient care that requires knowledge of complex illnesses and the use of highly sophisticated machinery.

For example, an emergency department nurse may be assigned the role of triage coordinator in patient selection. This role involves performing a thorough assessment of patients, formulating initial nursing diagnoses, and making decisions concerning which patients will be seen by medical personnel immediately and which patients can wait to be seen. Should a patient be misclassified, serious injury could result due to a delay in initiating therapy.

Other examples of increased accountability and responsibility include the use of complex technological skills in labor and delivery units and the postpartum monitoring of maternity patients and newborns. Even psychiatric skills and knowledge have greatly expanded in the past few decades, and patients are returning to home programs and community-based living centers.

Nurses can best avoid potential liability by giving safe and competent nursing care, while recognizing potential problems, identifying the risk areas in individual practice, and remaining current in new technology, nursing diagnoses, and the latest institutional policies and procedures. The following sections list the types of incidents that frequently are encountered in hospital-based nursing.

PATIENT SAFETY

One of the most important responsibilities of nurses today is in ensuring *patient safety*, which includes protecting patients against falls, protecting them from injuring themselves or others in the clinical setting, ensuring that medication errors do not occur, and protecting patients from faulty equipment or unsafe conditions. Examples of how nurses can ensure safety is to inspect siderails to see that they are functional and in the raised position for elderly or confused patients, to foresee risks in the form of slick or wet floors, and to restrain patients as indicated.

SUICIDE PREVENTION

Nurses have obligations related to *suicide prevention.* Not all self-destructive and depressed patients are be hospitalized on psychiatric units, and some patients respond to hospitalization with depression and suicidal thoughts, particularly the elderly, the recently anesthetized, and the postpartum patient. Nurses should listen carefully to comments spoken by patients, since nearly all suicidal patients have some ambivalence and give warning clues before engaging in self-destructive behavior. Once a patient is identified as a potential suicidal or self-destructive patient, the duty of care increases, since the foreseeable consequences of not meeting the duty of care required is obvious. Identification of such patients offers nurses the opportunity to counsel the patient, alert psychiatric clinical nurse specialists or psychiatric intervenors that a patient is at risk for self-destruction, and implement precautions while the patient is recovering. Above all, nurses should treat this patient and family with concern, consistency, and caring behaviors.

The nurse should understand which patients are more likely to become self-destructive. Older patients are more likely to commit suicide than younger patients, although younger patients may be more verbal. Women make more suicide attempts, but men, by a two-to-one ratio, are more likely to be successful in their attempts. Most successful suicide patients have a previous history of suicide attempts or prior hospitalization for self-destruction.

Should the nurse identify such a patient or potential patient, several nursing interventions might be initiated. Although not an exhaustive list, some of the more obvious nursing interventions include:

1. Close supervision of the patient by staff or family members.
2. Removal of potentially dangerous objects from the patient's bedside and room.
3. Ensuring that the patient takes all medications when given so that there can be no accumulation of medications to be taken all at once.
4. Transferring the patient closer to the nursing station or to another unit, as needed, for closer observation and more frequent checks.

5. Transferring a rooming-in infant back to the nursery since postpartum depression may become manifest not in self-destruction, but as destructive behaviors aimed at neonates.
6. Ensuring that windows in the patient's room cannot be opened or opened only partially.
7. Notifying the physician promptly of changes in that patient's condition and administering medications as needed to prevent further depression or self-destruction.
8. Restraining the patient as indicated.

RESTRAINTS

Restraints, both physical and chemical, are used daily in many hospital settings, from the critical care unit to the psychiatric unit. While used, restraints should be the last option to be considered when caring for confused and/or hostile patients. Options that should first be considered include better communications with patients and families, use of lighting in patients' rooms, the transfer of patients to rooms nearer to the nurses' station or in clearer view of the nurse, and extra time spent with the patient. Only when these measures fail, should restraints be considered a viable option.

Physical restraints assist in preventing patient falls, discourage patients from disconnecting vital equipment or intravenous and feeding lines, and prevent patients from harming either themselves or others. *Chemical restraints* also prevent patients from disconnecting vital, life-sustaining equipment, assist in preventing hostile and impaired patients from hurting themselves or others, and allow the staff to care for all patients on a given unit.

But restraints are not without serious side effects and harm. Physical restraints can cause skin injury, impaired respiration, strangulation, neurological damage, and death. Chemical restraints may result in increased drowsiness, respiratory distress, hemodynamic instability, decreased competency and judgment, and confusion.

All hospitals have policies and procedures outlining when and how restraints are to be used and the nursing care that must be documented on restrained individuals. Because of the inappropriate use of restraints, many hospitals insist on securing a physician's order before applying restraints, and federal law prohibits chemical restraints in certain nursing home patients.

Yet case law has several examples of patients harmed because they were not properly restrained, educated, or a combination of the two. For example, in *Reifschneider v. Nebraska Methodist Hospital* (1986), a patient was allowed to fall because the siderails on a stretcher had been raised, even though the patient was not belted or restrained in any other way and there was no hospital employee in attendance with the patient. Her cause of action was failure to restrain and negligent failure to provide adequate supervision.

Contrast the preceding court case with the following one. In *Melley v. Penater, M.D., and Gnaden Huetten Hospital* (1991), a patient jumped from a hospital window, incurring numerous fractures. The family brought suit for failure to restrain, noting that a nurse had previously assessed the patient as delusional and had recommended that the patient be closely watched, with a possibility of applying restraints. The patient was seen by the physician and he spoke with her, noting she was less anxious, and left without ordering any type of restraint. Soon after the physician's visit, the patient squeezed through a 13-inch window opening and fell. The physician testified that he had ordered no restraints since he felt that would only increase the patient's agitation and that he had not considered the possibility that this obese patient could squeeze through the 13-inch window. The jury returned a verdict for the defendants. A similar holding was reached in *Estate of Clotilde Roman v. St. Elizabeth Hospital, et al.* (1994), with the court holding that patients must display a need for restraints before health care personnel will consider their application. In the latter case, the patient fell, striking his head and causing a subdural hematoma and death. The defendant's contention was that the patient was greatly improved prior to the fall and that restraints were not indicated; thus no restraints were applied.

When using restraints, it is vital to follow hospital policy and procedure, documenting adequately why patients were restrained, how they were restrained, how patient safety needs were met during the time restraints were used, and the removal or continuance of restraints. In documentation, record what type of patient behavior necessitated the restraints, including ineffective methods of restraint that may have been used and the exact type of restraint finally applied, such as soft wrist restraints, Kerlix hand restraints, or a posey belt. The date and time of application of restraints should be noted, as well as the patient's response to the restraints. Patient safety needs, such as skin integrity, circulation in the restrained extremities, respiratory status, nutrition and elimination needs, and elevation of the patient's head prior to feeding should be noted according to the hospital policy. Also document the need for continued restraint and periodic assessments to ascertain when restraints may be removed.

If restraints as applied are not effective, chemical restraints may augment the physical restraints. For example, the ventilator-dependent patient with adult respiratory distress syndrome may be physically restrained to prevent the accidental dislodgement of an endotracheal tube and chemically restrained to allow the ventilator to regulate respiratory rate and tidal volume. Or chemical restraints may be used without physical restraints, as in patients in whom sedation alone is effective.

A newer trend in restraints is to use a bed occupancy monitor or similar device so that personnel are alerted immediately when a patient is no longer in bed. While it may not prevent the patient from falling, the device assures that assistance is provided immediately. Since some patients can successfully free themselves from all restraints, courts look to how quickly and effectively the patient was treated after falling. Bed occupancy monitors greatly aid in early intervention and assistance.

GUIDELINES: CHEMICAL AND PHYSICAL RESTRAINTS

1. Involve the patient and family in the decision about the need for restraints as possible and practical. This allows the nurse to explain the purpose of the restraints, why they are needed, and care given while the person is restrained.
2. Document the reason for the restraint, any explanation given to the patient and family, and measures undertaken to assure the continuing safety of the patient. This includes circulation checks, range of motion exercises, meeting nutritional and hydration needs, and assessing frequently for the continuing need for the restraint.
3. Document a thorough assessment of the extremity to be restrained before applying the restraining devices. This protects you against allegations that the restraint caused physical harm to the patient if your assessment shows that the skin was bruised or broken prior to applying the restraint.
4. Document your continuing assessment of the restrained extremity according to hospital policy and the removal of restraints for short periods of time, if that is part of your policy.
5. Document the continuing need for restraints and the elimination of reasons necessitating the restraints, if possible. For example, if a certain medication is causing the patient confusion, document the discontinuance of the medication.

EXERCISE 13-1

Review your institution's policies and procedures for documenting the use of chemical and physical restraints. How does the current policy requiring documentation adhere to the preceding Guidelines recommendations? Are there separate forms for documenting the continuous assessment of restrained patients? If not, develop a form that assists nurses in accurately documenting such patient care. If there is a form, does it allow for accurate and continuous charting? How would you alter the form?

MEDICATION ERRORS

A significant number of lawsuits result from *medication errors* (Globis, 1995). Medication errors are difficult to defend because they are easily averted. Take the time needed to recheck the patient, the medication, the time and route of administration, the dosage amount, and the desired effects as well as potential side effects. Most medication errors fall into one of the following categories.

Incorrect Patient

Institution policy and procedure manuals insist that nurses check patient identification bands frequently, even if they are sure of the patient's identification. Such policies exist to prevent giving a medication to anyone other than the patient for whom the medication is intended and to prevent harmful side effects of the medication in the patient. In *Demers v. United States* (1990), the plaintiff's husband was admitted to the hospital for the implantation of a pacemaker. Subsequent to the procedure, the patient was administered Cardizem, a medication intended for another patient in the unit, resulting in his premature demise.

Incorrect Time of Administration

Giving medications at wrong time intervals may cause patients serious injury. In an old case illustrating this point, a Utah nurse failed to give an antipsychotic medication as ordered, and the patient subsequently jumped from the hospital window and was permanently paralyzed. In finding for the plaintiff, the court stressed the importance of timely giving ordered medications and the need to understand the actions and desired effects of such medications so that timely administration would occur (*Farrow v. Health Services et al.*, 1979).

Incorrect Dosage or Route of Administration

More commonly, nurses administer medications in wrong doses or by routes other than those ordered. Such errors can stem from the nurses' lack of knowledge about the medication. For example, a decedent suffered a cardiac arrest when a nurse administered an overdose of Lidocaine (*Dessauer v. Memorial General Hospital*, 1981). In that case, the nurse, who normally worked on the obstetrical unit, had been floated to the emergency room, where she gave a dosage of 800 mg of IV Lidocaine rather than the ordered 50 mg. More recent case-law in this area of incorrect dosage includes:

1. *Wingstrom v. Evanston Hospital* (1992) where two grams of IV Lidocaine were substituted for a 100 mg dosage.
2. *Van Hyning v. Hamilton Hospital* (1994), where a solution of 99% acetic acid was substituted for a 5% solution during surgery to remove genital warts.
3. *Gallimore v. Children's Memorial Hospital* (1992), where the nurse substituted 200 mg of IV Gentamycin for an ordered 30-mg dosage.
4. *Sharrow v. Archer* (1983), which again concerned an overdosage of IV Lidocaine. In this latter case, the nurse also altered the patient's record at the direction of the attending physician and the plaintiffs recovered damages for both malpractice and fraud.

Improper Injection Technique

Biggs v. United States (1987) illustrates this cause of action. In *Biggs*, the patient claimed that the nurse had used incorrect technique in administering an IM injection. The injection, if given 3–4 inches above the knee as was claimed, could have resulted in nerve damage and would have been contrary to nursing standards of care. Since the patient exhibited signs and symptoms of nerve damage, the court remanded the case to trial level on the issue of nursing malpractice.

Standards of care require nurses not only to be able to administer medications correctly, but to understand the pharmaceutical actions of the medications, potential side effects, and contraindications. Nurses must understand the interactions of medications, since most patients receive more than three medications during a 24-hour period, and they must properly question the prescribing physician before administering the medication. Nurses should also reverify orders for medications if the order is illegible or if any portion of required information is omitted, such as the route of administration. A final responsibility of the nurse is to educate patients about possible side effects and ensure that the patient consents to the medication.

EXERCISE 13-2

You are the medication nurse for a busy medical surgical unit. After properly giving a patient her medication, the patient complains of itching and slight shortness of breath. You notice obvious signs of an allergic reaction on her skin. Should the patient decide to later file suit (and name you in the case), could you be held liable for the allergic response and subsequent harm to the patient? What would be your best defense against liability in such a suit?

TECHNOLOGY AND EQUIPMENT

Advances in **technology and equipment** have created special problems of liability for nurses. In addition to assessing and monitoring patients, nurses must also know the capabilities, limitations, hazards, and safety features of numerous machines and devices. As Aiken (1994) notes, most equipment injuries occur not because of unfamiliarity with the equipment, but because of carelessness or misuse. Thus nurses should carefully follow manufacturer's recommendations for the use of equipment and refrain from making modifications to it.

Nursing negligence associated with the improper use of equipment can arise in a variety of ways. First, after learning the correct usage of machinery, nurses are expected to conform with the manufacturer's recommendations and hospital policy and protocols (Killian, 1990). In *Stark v. Children's Orthopedic Hospital and Medical Center* (1990), the nurse mistakenly plugged heart monitor leads into a live power cord rather than the heart monitor. Luckily, the child survived. Liability was averted because of extenuating circumstances with the child's parents. In a 1991 Minnesota case, a nurse disconnected the oxygen hose from the ventilator and reconnected it improperly, causing the patient to become hypoxic. Depositions in the case also showed that the same nurse had disconnected the ventilator alarms, so that a warning alarm did not sound when the oxygen was disconnected (*Mele v. St. Mary's Hospital of Rochester, Minnesota, and Mayo Foundations,* 1991).

Liability can result from using defective or unsafe equipment, and nurses have a duty to make a reasonable inspection of equipment and refrain from using equipment that is defective or not working properly (Tammelleo, 1990). In *Beltran v. Downey Community Hospital* (1992), a patient recovering from disc surgery reported that her bed folded into a V, causing her pain and necessitating a second surgical procedure. In investigating the patient's complaint, counsel discovered that the previous patient to have used the bed stated that the same thing had happened to her and that the nursing personnel had refused to change the bed or have the bed repaired. While this case was settled in favor of the hospital because it could be shown in court that the bed could not move in the way described, the case indicates that nurses could be found liable for failure to reasonably inspect equipment and refrain from using defective equipment. The *Beltran* case may have been avoided had the nursing personnel alerted maintenance when the first patient complained of the bed.

Nurses are also expected to give quality, competent care despite equipment failures and faulty equipment. An older case illustrates this point. In *Rose v. Hakim* (1971) an infant, who had sustained a cardiac arrest during surgery, required the use of a hypothermia unit in a pediatric intensive care unit. The continuous read-out thermometer on the hypothermia unit was faulty. The nurse caring for the child failed to verify the thermometer's accuracy or use ancillary cooling measures such as medications, ice packs, or alcohol sponge baths. The infant suffered a grand mal seizure and a respiratory arrest, and was placed on a ventilator for respiratory assistance. When the infant showed signs of poor air exchange on the ventilator, the nurse corrected an obvious kink in the ventilator tubing, but failed to check oxygen concentration and tidal volume delivery. The court held that the infant's subsequent injuries were due first to negligent actions and omissions by the nursing personnel and secondly to the defective equipment.

FAILURE TO ADEQUATELY ASSESS, MONITOR, AND COMMUNICATE

Nurses are frequently told that their most important duty is that of communication, whether to physicians, other staff members, or through written documentation. Communication is vital, but one must have something to communicate. Perhaps equally important are nurses' roles first in assessing and monitoring patients, then in communicating to others.

Failure to adequately assess, monitor, and communicate can occur in all aspects of nursing and in all hospital units. And this same failure can occur with all types of nursing procedures and skills, from the simplest to the complex.

Failure to Monitor

Failure to monitor blood pressure and respirations was the cause of action in *Barton v. AMI Park Place Hospital et al.* (1992). In that case, a high school student was involved in automobile accident and admitted the hospital with right upper quadrant pain. Over a course of seven hours, he bled to death, and his parents brought suit for negligence in monitoring his deteriorating condition and for failure to provide necessary care to stop the bleeding.

Failure to monitor for compartment syndrome in orthopedic cases is a common malpractice allegation. In *Pirkov-Middaugh v. Gillette Children's Hospital* (1991), a 4-year-old developed compartment syndrome following hip surgery. Evidence at trial showed that:

1. The nurses had not monitored for compartment syndrome, and did not have the equipment needed to test quickly for compartment syndrome.
2. They did not know what equipment was needed.
3. Neither the nurses nor the physicians even knew where the needed equipment was located.

Too often nurses fail to monitor adequately because of lack of knowledge of potential complications or fail to notify physicians when the patient's condition changes.

Failure to Assess and Monitor

The failure to assess and monitor is a frequent holding in obstetrical cases. In *Fairfax Hospital System, Inc. v. McCarty* (1992), a labor and delivery nurse was found liable for failure to monitor during a 10-minute period after fetal distress had become apparent. A similar cause of action occurred in *Dobrzenieck v. University Hospital of Cleveland* (1984), when a 36-week preeclampsia patient was admitted for observation. Within two hours, a monitor indicated fetal distress, which went undetected by the nurse and was therefore not reported to the attending physician. Four hours later the infant was delivered by cesarian section and resuscitated.

Failure to Communicate with Patients

Obstetrical nurses must also be attentive to communication of relevant patient data. In *Bryant v. John Doe Hospital and John Dee, M.D.* (1992), the patient had two hours of late decelerations, but the nurse failed to communicate these late decelerations to anyone. Sometimes, though, the physician fails to listen to the nurse. In a separate case that same year, the nurses notified the physician of fetal distress on the monitor, and one nurse even begged him to do an immediate cesarian section to no avail. The physician continued to order drugs to further induce labor and was absent when the woman finally delivered a profoundly retarded neonate (*Herron v. Northwest Community Hospital*, 1992).

The importance of nursing communications cannot be overemphasized since treatment decisions may be made based on communication or the lack of communication. In *Lopez v. Southwest Community Health Service* (1992), a woman, 28 weeks pregnant, experienced pain at home and called the physician's office. She was instructed to go to the hospital. The physician's nurse called the hospital to inform them of the impending admission and to tell them that the patient was in labor. Two nurses worked with her in the hospital. The first nurse failed to examine her, and the second nurse, after doing a pelvic examination, determined that she was 10 cm dilated and that the membranes were bulging. Upon being notified of these results, the physician ruptured the membranes and delivered the baby, who is now a quadriplegic, deaf, blind, and brain-damaged.

Neither of the nurses questioned the patient or her mother when they arrived at the hospital, and neither did a history of the patient, nor must they have talked with her. If they had, they would have known that neither the patient nor her mother believed that she was in labor, but were concerned about her persistent pains. And the physician would not have delivered the child had he not listened to the nurses.

Other cases reflect this failure to listen to patients and what they are trying to tell the staff. In *Parker v. Bullock County Hospital Authority* (1990), the patient fell while taking a shower in the hospital. The patient had had surgery, and she told the nurse who helped her to the shower that she was dizzy and lightheaded. The nurse left her unattended to take her shower, obviously ignoring her statement.

Failure to Communicate Pertinent Data

What the nurse fails to communicate is equally important. Several cases have held nurses directly liable for the failure to communicate pertinent patient data, or for not informing the primary health care provider in a timely manner. In one case, a 6-year-old boy lost the use of his hand because the nurse had written an accurate assessment in the nursing notes, but failed to bring that same data to the attention of the attending physician before permanent injury occurred (Mandell, 1993).

Nor is the duty to communicate directly exclusive to nurses. In *Rixey v. West Paces Ferry Hospital, Inc.* (1990), the court held that a physician has a duty to alert nurses to the fact that they should anticipate a significant change in the patient's condition and a possible medical emergency. In this case, a 24-year-old patient was admitted for shortness of breath and chest tightness. The x-ray indicated air in the subcutaneous neck tissues and mediastinum, and the patient was intubated and placed on a ventilator. The physician, though, failed to tell the staff about the air seen on the x-ray and about the possibility of a tension pneumothorax developing. The physician left the facility, and the patient subsequently arrested and could not be successfully resuscitated.

In the postanesthesia care unit (PACU), the primary responsibility of nurses is to monitor patients. Cases such as *Torbert v. Befeler* (1985) and *Sanchez v. Bay General Hospital* (1981) show the tragedy that can occur rapidly when patients are not adequately assessed in the PACU environment. In *Torbert*, a patient began having premature ventricular contractions (PVCs) after anesthesia was started, but before the surgical procedure was begun. A consulting cardiologist was called. The patient was given IV Lidocaine and cleared for surgery. While in the PACU, the patient continued to have PVCs, and she arrested three hours after surgery, suffering hypoxic brain damage and death. The family brought suit for failure to closely monitor the patient. The patient had been given Lidocaine approximately 45 minutes before her arrest, but the primary nurses caring for her were assisting another patient and the arrest went undetected for some 10 minutes.

In *Sanchez*, the patient had undergone an elective laminectomy and had vomited upon admission to the PACU. Even though the patient's vital signs were taken and recorded every 15 minutes, the various nurses caring for her failed to note the obvious changes in her vital signs or that she was having difficulty breathing. The patient then went into cardiac arrest, and none of the PACU nurses were able to perform cardiopulmonary resuscitation. On review of her record, the court noted that:

1. There was no suctioning equipment ordered for the patient, even though she had been vomiting on admission and during her stay in the PACU.
2. No comparison was made of vital signs in the recovery room, although there had been a significant change in vital signs between admission and the time of the arrest.
3. Vital signs were not taken more frequently after the arrest.
4. No neurological examination of the patient had been performed.
5. No physician was notified of deteriorating vital signs.
6. The nurses failed to note that she had an atrial catheter, although they had used it as an IV.
7. No report was made to the oncoming shift of the patient's deteriorating condition.

A third case in this area had similar results. A 27-year-old male, following gallbladder surgery was taken to the PACU. He was conscious, thrashing about, and attempting to remove his oral airway. Upon admission to the PACU, the anesthesiologist requested that the admitting nurse monitor the patient frequently since he had just received a sufentanil, a potent respiratory depressant. The admitting nurse immediately asked a second nurse to monitor the patient, neglecting to tell the second nurse about the sufentanil injection, and she then left the PACU. When the admitting nurse returned, the patient was alone and his respiratory rate was 8 or less. Shortly after the nurse's return, the anesthesiologist returned, asked about the patient, and was assured the patient was fine. However, when the anesthesiologist approached the patient's bedside, the patient was in a full respiratory arrest. The court found that the sole negligence and cause of the respiratory arrest was the nurse's failure to monitor (*Eyoma v. Falso*, 1991).

Assessment and monitoring allow nurses to use the nursing assessment of the patient to prevent harm or deterioration of the patient's status, while notifying the physician, and to make appropriate nursing diagnoses based on the assessment. One of the better case examples in this area is *Lunsford v. Board of Nurse Examiners* (1983). Ms. Lunsford was a registered nurse who failed to fully assess a potential heart attack patient and thereby failed to initiate appropriate nursing interventions. No medical diagnosis of a myocardial infarction, pulmonary embolism, or pulmonary edema was needed for Lunsford to take vital signs, to listen for cardiac and breath sounds, and to assess for diaphoresis, shortness of breath, and an abnormal cardiac rhythm. Had such steps been taken, she could have communicated and intervened with the hospital physician and seen that the patient received proper care. Ms. Lunsford was the triage nurse on the day of this occurrence. Because of her failure to follow acceptable standards of care, assess and monitor the patient, her license was suspended, and she settled out of court in the subsequent civil lawsuit.

Communicating with the Culturally and Ethnically Diverse

Some of the issues concerned with communication involve working with culturally and ethnically diverse patients and health care workers. The fact that English is not the primary or first language for many Americans today may create communication difficulties. There is some limited case-law to support not hiring personnel because of their inability to communicate effectively with the public, an essential requirement of jobs involving individual interfaces with people daily (*Fragante v. City and County of Honolulu, et al.*, 1989) and in refusing to allow nurses to converse in their native language, as opposed to English (*Dimaranan v. Pomona Valley Medical Center, et al.*, 1991). In *Dimaranan*, the hospital prohibited nurses on a maternity unit from conversing in their native Filipino dialect, because such conversations had created differential treatment for the nurse who spoke the dialect and adversely affected worker morale and supervision. The court further stated that this language restriction did not violate the nurses' civil rights because it was motivated by a desire to eliminate dissension that could have compromised patient safety and quality health care delivery.

Because of this diversity, state laws, JCAHO standards, and the American Hospital Association Bill of Rights for Patients have included provisions for ensuring that patient rights include being able to meet their communication needs, particularly if patients do not speak English or speak it so brokenly that they are unable to express themselves or understand what is said to them. To prevent such a happening, most institutions now provide interpreters for non-English–speaking patients, and nurses must make reasonable efforts to ensure that patients understand care issues and discharge education and instructions.

Nurses should document who was used as the interpreter, whether the interpreter was a family member or hospital-provided, what instructions were given, and what means were used to assure that the patient understood the instructions or conversations. Means that may be employed to assure comprehension include having the patient repeat the material to the nurse or asking questions and requiring that the patient respond. As more non-English–speaking patients enter the health care delivery system, the profession may see additional causes of action based on their noncomprehension and failure to follow instructions because they never understood the instructions.

A patient, admitted for minor surgery, tells you that he is having chest discomfort and shortness of breath. The patient, with a known cardiac condition, had nitroglycerine prescribed for chest pain. You give him the ordered medication, and go back to the task you were doing when he called for assistance. You do not notify the physician of the chest discomfort, nor do you check back with the patient to see if the medication eased the pain or had any effect at all. Later in the day, during a preoperative visit by the nurse anesthetist, the nurse anesthetist asks about the patient's status and recent cardiac history. Again, you say nothing. If the patient suffers a massive heart attack during surgery the next morning, could liability for failure to assess, monitor, and communicate be found against you? What would you plead as your best defense in such a case?

FAILURE TO ACT AS A PATIENT ADVOCATE

As the nursing profession has developed, nurses have come to owe a higher duty to patients than merely following physicians' orders. Professional nurses serve in the role of patient advocate, developing and implementing nursing diagnoses, and exercising good patient judgment as they monitor the care given to patients by physicians as well as peers. The failure to function in this independent role has long been recognized by the courts as a *failure to act as patient advocate,* and court decisions continue to emphasize this vital nursing function.

The professional nurse has a duty to report medical care or medical orders that jeopardize the care of patients. In *Catron v. The Poor Sisters of St. Frances* (1982), a patient was admitted for an unintentional drug overdosage. While in the hospital, the patient had been intubated via a nasotracheal tube for several days before its removal. He then had a tracheostomy to prevent respiratory failure. The patient brought this cause of action due to his inability to speak in a normal voice after removal of the endotracheal tube and tracheostomy.

The hospital defended the case by asserting that it was medical judgment when to remove an endotracheal tube and how long one could remain in place without causing the patient harm. In finding against the hospital and nursing staff, the court held that, while a hospital is usually not liable for nurses following physicians' orders, an exception exists when the nurses know that the practice does not follow usual procedure. The nurses had an affirmative duty to report this deviation to their supervisors.

Thus, nurses have a duty to question not only incomplete and illegible orders, but also orders that deviate from the usual standards of practice. They have the duty to inform hospital administration, via nursing supervisors and midmanagement nurses, of such deviations. Fiesta (1994) suggests that this affirmative duty involves not only questions of competence or inappropriate medical decisions, but also the reporting of "bizarre and disruptive behavior or conduct which may be a symptom of impairment" (p. 15).

But contrast the preceding case with *Dixon v. Freuman* (1991). In this case, the physician ordered the removal of a Foley catheter, and the nurses removed the catheter per hospital policy. When the patient brought suit that the catheter should not have been removed, the court held that in the absence of proof that the order to remove the catheter was "clearly contraindicated by normal practice," the nurses and hospital could not be held liable for the subsequent fistula.

The duty to serve as a patient advocate may also require nurses to directly disobey physicians' orders. In *Cruzbinsky v. Doctor's Hospital* (1983), a circulating nurse was ordered by the physician to leave the operating room before the patient had ben sent to the PACU. While the nurse initially questioned the order, she finally left at the doctor's insistence. After her departure, the patient arrested, suffering significant permanent damage. The patient then brought suit against the hospital and nurse for abandonment.

The court held that the nurse had a duty to remain with the patient, following the hospital policy and procedure manual, even if the physician was insistent and "yelling at her." The court further concluded that this abandonment was so obvious that no expert witness was needed for the jury to conclude that abandonment had occurred.

Premature patient discharge is another area in which nurses have a duty to be the patient's advocate. Court cases such as *Wickline v. California* (1986) and *Wilson v. Blue Cross of Southern California* (1992) speak to the harm that can befall patients if discharged from acute care settings before they are sufficiently improved or stabilized. In the first case, the patient lost her leg due to infection, and in the second case a psychiatric patient committed suicide after his early discharge. While these two cases were directed at physicians and utilization reviewers, there seems little doubt that the courts would also extend such holdings to nurses who failed to serve as patient advocates, speaking directly to the involved physicians and to nursing supervisors, when patients are discharged inappropriately. In *Koeniquer v. Eckrich* (1988) that was the court's holding. Nurses have a duty to question physician's discharge orders or to delay the discharge if they believe that the discharge violates acceptable standards of care.

GUIDELINES: ACTING AS A PATIENT ADVOCATE

1. Nurses should be aware of hospital policies and protocols, as well as acceptable standards of care. Question physicians when orders are contrary to the acceptable standard of care or when you believe following the order could cause a patient harm. Do not be intimidated into following orders; use your independent judgment. If physicians persist or refuse to change the order, consult nursing supervisory personnel.

2. In emergency situations where you believe that following the physician's order could result in harm to the patient, disobey the order, assure the patient's safety and the administration of appropriate nursing care, and then notify nursing supervisors and administrative supervisors.

3. If a patient is discharged early and the early discharge could cause direct harm to the patient, voice your concern to the attending physician and nursing supervisor. Remember that you have a duty to attempt to prevent early discharges.

4. Discharge planning and instruction must begin early, when the patient is admitted, and be completed before the patient's discharge. Include in your teaching potential complications for which the patient/family member must be alert and what to do if signs and symptoms of complications arise. Give the patient written instructions, if available, and document carefully your instructions in the patient's medical record.

5. The patient is your priority concern and nurses have an affirmative duty to serve as patient advocates.

The issue of early discharge also addresses the crucial need for early and ongoing discharge planning and education of patients. In a home health care case, *Ready v. Personal Care Health Services* (1991), a child was discharged from home health care services, developed pneumonia, and died. The parents brought suit, in part, for the failure of the nurses to adequately address potential complications and to educate the parents about the possibility of such life-threatening conditions.

Nurses have a duty to protect patients, to question orders that are inappropriate or likely to cause harm to the patient, and to provide adequate, early discharge education. If directly speaking with the attending physician does not result in the desired outcome, then nurses have a duty to inform their supervisors and midmanagement personnel so that other means of providing safe and competent health care may be obtained. Communication is vital, and interventions taken on behalf of patients should be promptly and adequately charted in the patient record.

EXERCISE 13-4

Mr. Jones, a newly diagnosed insulin-dependent diabetic is to receive discharge planning about his condition. You are the diabetic coordinator for the hospital and have developed a wonderful diabetic teaching protocol. Dr. Smith, one of the good old boys, tells you not to teach his patient anything. "He's my patient and I'll teach him what he needs to know. I do not want you interfering in my patient's care, now or ever." How would you proceed in this instance? Does Dr. Smith have the final say about his patients in all aspects of their care? If Mr. Jones does not receive proper discharge planning and suffers significant harm as a result, could you be held liable?

SUMMARY

Potential lawsuits for nursing malpractice can arise from almost any act or failure to act that results in injury to a given patient. This chapter has stressed the more commonly occurring areas of nursing liability, giving guidelines, nursing interventions, and current case-law examples for nurses to implement and understand in avoiding future litigation in these areas. As the acuity of inpatient care increases, so will the potential for liability. The growing trend of courts in assessing nurses liable for malpractice will also continue as standards of care are redefined and professional autonomy is recognized.

AFTER COMPLETING THIS CHAPTER, YOU SHOULD BE ABLE TO

- Describe the changing health care environment that has created increased responsibility among staff nurses.
- Differentiate two types of restraints, and describe the difference between them, including nursing management of the restrained patient.
- Describe the nurse's responsibility in medication errors and five means to avoid the errors.
- Analyze the potential liability for nurses when using technological advances and specialized equipment.
- Compare and contrast the nurse's responsibility for assessing, monitoring, and communicating in clinical settings.
- Describe the role of the nurse as a patient advocate.

APPLY YOUR LEGAL KNOWLEDGE

- If a patient falls and suffers injury, is the nurse always liable? What defenses could nurses argue in their support?
- What can nurses do to prevent medication errors?
- In which areas of the hospital are the potential liabilities of a staff nurse greater than in others? What can the staff nurses on those units do to prevent potential lawsuits?
- How do communications prevent lawsuits? What must be communicated and to whom?

REFERENCES

Aiken, T. D., & Catalano, J. T. (1994). *Legal, ethical, and political issues in nursing.* Philadelphia, PA: F. A. Davis Company.

Armstrong v. Paoli Memorial Hospital, 633 A. 2d 605 (New Jersey, 1994).

Barton v. AMI Park Place Hospital et al., No. 909-066318 (Texas, 1992).

Beltran v. Downey Community Hospital. (1992). *Medical Malpractice Verdicts, Settlements, and Experts,* 8(5), 30.

Biggs v. United States, 655 F. Supp. 1093 (W.D. Louisiana, 1987).

Bryant v. John Doe Hospital and John Doe, M.D. (1992). *Medical Malpractice Verdicts, Settlements, and Experts,* 8(1), 35.

Catron v. The Poor Sisters of St. Francis, 435 N.E. 2d 305 (Indiana, 1982).

Ciarlo v. St. Francis Hospital. (1994). WL 713864 (Del Super).

Cruzbinsky v. Doctors' Hospital, 188 Cal. Rept. 685 (Cal. App., 1983).

Demers v. United States. (1990). *Medical Malpractice Verdicts, Settlements, and Experts,* 6(3), 34.

Dessauer v. Memorial General Hospital, 628 P. 2d 337 (N. M. Ct. App., 1981).

Dimaranan v. Pomona Valley Medical Center et al., 775 F. Supp. 338 (C. D. Cal., 1991).

Dixon v. Freuman, 573 N.Y.S. 2d (New York, 1991).

Dobrzenieck v. University Hospital of Cleveland, #17843 (Cyahoga City Ct. of Common Pleas, May 22, 1984).

Estate of Clotilde Roman v. St. Elizabeth Hospital et al. (1994). #89L-9835 *Medical Malpractice Verdicts, Settlements, and Experts,* 10(9), 23.

Eyoma v. Falso, 589 A. 2d 653 (New Jersey, 1991).

Fairfax Hospital System Inc. v. McCarty, 419 S.E. 2d 621 (Virginia, 1992).

Farrow v. Health Services et al., 604 P. 2d 474 (Utah, 1979).

Fiesta, J. (1994). Failing to act like a professional. *Nursing Management, 24*(7), 15–17.

Fragante v. City and County of Honolulu et al., 888 F. 2d 591 (9th Cir., 1989).

Gallimore v. Children's Hospital Medical Center, WL37742 (Ohio App. 1 Dist., 1992).

Gobis, L. A. (1995). Medication errors: Learn from your colleagues' mistakes. *RN, 58*(12), 59–63.

Herron v. Northwest Community Hospital. (1992). Emergency Medical Associates, et al., *Medical Malpractice Verdicts, Settlements, and Experts 8*(10), 33.

Killian, W. H. (1990). Equipment mishaps may result in lawsuits. *The American Nurse, 22*(3), 34.

Koeniquer v. Eckrich, 422 N.W. 2d 600 (South Dakota, 1988).

Lopez v. Southwest Community Health Service, 833 P. 2d 1183 (New Mexico, 1992).

Lunsford v. Board of Nurse Examiners, 648 S.W. 2d 391 (Tex. Civ. App.-Austin, 1983).

Mandell, M. (1993). What you don't say can hurt you. *American Journal of Nursing, 93*(8), 15–16.

Mele v. St. Mary's Hospital of Rochester, Minnesota, and Mayo Foundations. (1991). CV-3-87-818. *Medical Malpractice Verdicts, Settlements, and Experts, 7*(10), 32.

Melley v. Penater, M.D. and Gnaden Huetten Hospital, No 90.666 (Pennsylvania, 1991).

Parker v. Bullock County Hospital Authority. (1990). A9OAO 762 *Medical Malpractice Verdicts, Settlements, and Experts, 6*(10), 28.

Pirkov-Middaugh v. Gillette Children's Hospital, No. C9-91-526 (Minnesota, 1991).

Ready v. Personal Care Health Services, #842472 (California, 1991).

Reifschneider v. Nebraska Methodist Hospital, 387 N.W. 2d 486 (Nebraska, 1986).

Rixey v. West Paces Ferry Hospital, Inc., 916 F. 2d 608 (Georgia, 1990).

Rose v. Hakim, 335 F. Supp. 1121 (D.C.C., 1971).

Sanchez v. Bay General Hospital, 172 Cal. Rept. 342 (Cal. App., 1981).

Sharrow v. Archer, 658 P. 2d 1331 (Alaska, 1983).

Sloan, A. (1995). When language is an obstacle. *RN, 22*(6), 55–57.

Stark v. Children's Orthopedic Hospital and Medical Center. (1990). #87-2-12416-9, *Medical Malpractice Verdicts, Settlements and Experts, 9*(10), 28.

Tammelleo, D. (1990). Who's to blame for faulty equipment? *RN, 17*(5), 67–72.

Torbert v. Befeler, No. L-17463-81, Union Cty. Sup. Ct. (April 25, 1985).

Van Hyning v. Hamilton Hospital. (1994). *Medical Malpractice Verdicts, Settlements, and Experts* 10(9), 24.

Wickline v. State of California, 192 Cal. App. 3d 1630, 239 Cal. Rept. 810 (1986).

Wilson v. Blue Cross of Southern California, 222 Cal. App. 3d 660, 271, Cal. Rept. 876 (1992).

Wingstrom v. Evanston Hospital, WL 97934 (ND Ill., 1992).

· fourteen

Employment Laws: Corporate Liability Issues

PREVIEW

Whenever nurses are employed by another, be it a hospital, clinic, or physician, the employing entity accepts potential liability for the nurse-employees. The nurses become the employer's representatives and, because of their special legal status, convey potential liability to the employer. Never, though, do nurses convey all liability to the employer. Individuals are ultimately responsible for their actions. This chapter discusses theories of corporate liability and a variety of employment laws.

KEY CONCEPTS

vicarious liability

respondeat superior

borrowed servant doctrine

dual servant doctrine

corporate liability

negligent hiring and retention

ostensible authority

independent contractor

personal liability

indemnification

Equal Employment Opportunity Commission (EEOC)

1964 Civil Rights Act

Federal Tort Claims Act of 1946

Age Discrimination in Employment Act of 1967

affirmative action

Equal Pay Act

Occupational Safety and Health Act of 1970 (OSHA)

employment at will

wrongful discharge

collective bargaining (or labor relations)

National Labor Relations Act

Family and Medical Leave Act of 1993

THEORIES OF VICARIOUS LIABILITY

Vicarious liability, or substituted liability, is the term used to describe the instance in which one party is responsible for the actions of another. The law allows substituted liability to prevent further injustice to the injured party and to encourage employers to maintain employee competence. If injured parties could sue only the nurse who harmed them, they might not be able to be fully compensated monetarily, unless, of course, the nurse is independently wealthy. Making the employer liable increases the chances that money will be available to cover the damages incurred. It also encourages the employer to hire and retain safe practitioners.

Vicarious liability is not a shift in liability but an extension of liability to allow justice to be fairly distributed. Vicarious liability extends liability to include the employer but never to the extent that personal and individual liability is lost.

Respondeat Superior

Respondeat superior—"let the master respond" or "let the master answer"—is the old common law principle of substituted liability based on a master-servant relationship. While nurses may disagree with the master-servant aspect of the relationship, the courts have found similar elements: (1) The employer controls the actions of the employee, and (2) substituted liability applies only to actions within the scope and course of employment. The effect of this doctrine is that the employer is given responsibility and accountability for an employee's negligent actions and that the injured party may recover damages from the employer or employing institution.

The rationale for such recovery lies in a benefit burden analysis. Employers, standing to reap the benefits of their employees' activities, must also bear the burden of the employees' errors. Employers have an obligation to see that those whom they hire perform duties and tasks in a safe and competent manner. As the court said in *Hunter v. Allis-Chambers Corporation, Engine Division* (1986), "An employer is directly liable for torts caused by his employees against others. The employer could have prevented these torts by reasonable care in hiring, supervising, and, if necessary, firing the tortfeasor" (at 1419).

The leading case for respondeat superior in health care is *Duling v. Bluefield Sanitarium, Inc.* (1965). In that case, a 13-year-old was admitted to the hospital with a diagnosis of rheumatic heart disease. At 7:00 PM on the evening of her admission, Nancy Duling was seen by the attending physician, who told her mother that the child could easily develop heart failure. The physician explained to Mrs. Duling signs and symptoms to be alert for and to notify the nursing staff immediately if she observed any of them.

Shortly after the physician left, Nancy began exhibiting signs of failure and Mrs. Duling notified the staff. The nurses did not check Nancy and, in spite of frequent pleas for help and an obvious deterioration in Nancy's condition, the nurses waited over six hours before adequately assessing the patient. By that time, her condition was so serious that subsequent treatment failed to save her life.

The issue at court was whether the hospital was liable for the negligence of the nursing staff for failure to provide competent nursing care. The court enumerated the hospital's standard of care thusly: "A private hospital, conducted for profit, owes to its patients such reasonable care and attention for their safety as their mental and physical condition, if known, may require. The care exercised should be commensurate with the known inability of the patient to care for himself" (at 759). Thus, the court found that the hospital was liable for the care provided (or not provided) by its employees.

This reliance on the doctrine of respondeat superior stems from the nurses' responsibility to act according to standards of care and from the employment relationship with the hospital in which the nurse provides care and meets not only legal standards, but also hospital mandates.

Scope and Course of Employment

Two hurdles that the injured party must pass before the principle of respondeat superior is allowed are: (1) The injured party must show that the employer had control over the employee, and (2) the negligent act occurred within the course and scope of the employee's employment. The first element is fairly straightforward and is usually shown by proving employment status. The second element is more difficult, since the injured party must show that the actions were those for which the nurse was hired and that they occurred during the course of work.

Courts tend to decide scope and course of business on a case-by-case basis. The first factor that courts of law consistently determine is foreseeability of the action. Should the employer have been able to foresee that an employee could perform a certain action as he or she did? Various case decisions indicate that most activities undertaken by employees will be held foreseeable for the purpose of finding employer liability. For example, the court in *Robertson v. Bethlehem Steel Corporation* (1990) held that if the employee acted within the scope of his employment and his actions were in connection with the employer's business, the plaintiff could recover. *Biconi v. Pay 'N Pak Stores, Inc.* (1990) extended the scope and course of employment to intentional torts as well as negligent torts.

Some of the other factors consistently analyzed by courts include:

1. Usual place of employment.
2. Whether the act's purpose, in whole or in part, was in furtherance of the employer's business.
3. The extent to which the act was similar or different from authorized acts of the employer.
4. The extent to which the act was a departure from the employer's customary methods.
5. The extent to which the employer should have expected such an act to occur (*American Jurisprudence*, 1992).

Two examples may help. In the first example, Nurse A allows Mr. Jones to fall as she is assisting him back to bed. Mr. Jones is a patient in the intensive care unit who had hip surgery two days prior to this incident. Liability would flow to the hospital, as the hospital policy and procedure manual mandates that she properly assess the patient and obtain adequate help before assisting the patient either to or from his bed. Note, however, that if Nurse A failed to assist Mr. Jones in the manner prescribed by hospital policy, the hospital would have cause to argue that this action was not performed according to the master-servant doctrine.

In the second example, Nurse A is in the hospital for the sole purpose of collecting her paycheck. Nurse B, a co-worker in the intensive care unit, asks Nurse A to put Mr. Jones back to bed so that Nurse B can finish her charting and then join Nurse A for lunch. Mr. Jones subsequently falls. Nurse A would be solely accountable for her actions, as she was not within the course and scope of her employment at the time of Mr. Jones' fall. The hospital may still be held accountable, however, through the actions of Nurse B, also a hospital employee.

Actions that would be outside the course and scope of employment include the rendering of voluntary health services, either at the scene of an accident or as part of a community health drive, and the giving of health-related advice on a voluntary basis, for example, to a neighbor or friend. Additionally, performing actions that are reserved for physicians or advanced practice nurses are not considered within the scope of employment for staff nurses.

Note that the nursing supervisor is also acting as an employee of the hospital, not the employer. While the nursing supervisor may be liable if an employee of the hospital commits a negligent act, the supervisor's liability is incurred because of a failure to perform the supervisory duties in a competent manner, for example, as a reasonably prudent nursing supervisor would.

The doctrine of respondeat superior applies equally to acts of omission as well as those of commission. In the landmark decision of *Darling v. Charleston Community Memorial Hospital* (1965), the nurses and thus the hospital were found liable for their failure to notify the medical staff or the chief of the medical service when the attending physician failed to deliver proper medical care to James Darling.

In *Darling,* the patient had undergone a cast procedure to set a broken leg bone. The nurses assigned to care for Mr. Darling subsequent to the cast application assessed his recovery accurately: The circulation to his casted extremity was sluggish, he continued to require ever increasing amounts of pain medications, and there was a foul odor coming from the cast site. Numerous nurses charted their observations and continued to apprise the attending physician of the patient's symptoms. The attending physician responded to their assessments by ordering increased amounts of pain medications and increasing the antibiotic therapy. Ultimately, James Darling was transferred to a second hospital, and, despite aggressive therapy, the physicians were unable to save the leg.

The court, in finding against the nurses and the hospital, stated that it is not sufficient to merely apprise the attending physician of a deterioration in a patient's condition. Hospital staff have a further duty to inform others in authority positions so that the patient may receive competent care. In the preceding case, for example, the chief of staff or the hospital medical committee could have intervened had they known of James Darling's substandard medical care.

When a lawsuit is filed using the master-servant or respondeat superior doctrine, both the hospital and the nurse are sued. To avoid liability, often the hospital will attempt to claim that nurses were acting outside the scope of their employment. Thus nurses must first show that they were within the scope of employment at the time of the incident. Also, some suits are filed against the employer without naming the nurse as a defendant. The employer may still be held liable because of the employer-employee relationship.

EXERCISE 14-1

Judy Jones, an employee of Doctor Doe, and Beth Smith, an employee of Doctor Roe, are friends, and both their offices are in the same building. One day, as the nurses were leaving the building for lunch, they noticed an elderly lady in the building lobby, in obvious respiratory distress. Judy recognized the lady as a patient of Doctor Doe and immediately ran back to the office to get him. Meanwhile, Beth Smith, in an attempt to help the patient, injures her. The patient subsequently dies and her estate sues Doctor Doe and Doctor Roe, claiming negligence on the part of Beth Smith. Are the physicians negligent under the doctrine of respondeat superior? Who, if anyone, is at fault? Will the family be able to recover damages?

Borrowed Servant and Dual Servant Doctrine

The *borrowed servant doctrine* is a special application of the doctrine of respondeat superior. A *borrowed servant* is one who, while in the general employment of another, is subject to the right to direct and control the details of the servant's activities. This right to direct and control must be more than a mere cooperation with the suggestions of an authority figure. The borrowed servant doctrine applies when one employer lends completely the services or skills of an employee to another employer, and the key to this doctrine is the right or manner of control.

The borrowed servant doctrine's usual application in nursing is seen when nurse-employees come under the direct supervision and control of a physician, and the employer hospital would not be liable for negligent or intentional torts of nurses while they are under the direct control and supervision of the directing physician. The directing physician becomes liable under the doctrine of respondeat superior if the injured party can prove exclusive control and course and scope of employment. The right to control, said the court in *Harris v. Miller* (1994), is not presumed because the surgeon is in charge during the operation, but it must be proven during the course of the trial.

Traditionally the borrowed servant doctrine applies to situations within the operating room or to cardiopulmonary resuscitation, and it is sometimes referred to as the *captain of the ship doctrine.* The name and application refer to situations in which one person and only one person has command, and any negligence incurred will be imputed back to the person in command. The captain of the ship doctrine was first used in a medical malpractice context in 1959 (*McConnell v. Williams*).

The trend in national case law is away from the captain of the ship doctrine. This is reflected by the landmark decision made by the Texas Supreme Court in *Sparger v. Worley Hospital, Inc.* (1977), which concluded that the captain of the ship doctrine is a false application of a specific rule of agency and that one must first determine if the nurses are borrowed servants in deciding liability issues. Recent case law in Kansas, Colorado, and Washington, though, shows that the captain of the ship doctrine is still used in some jurisdictions (*Oberzan v. Smith*, 1994; *Spoor v. Serota*, 1992; *Van Hook v. Anderson*, 1992). In the *Van Hook* case, a mistake was made in the sponge count, and the court held that the physician was not liable under the captain of the ship doctrine for the nurse's error in counting the sponges. In fact, the court noted that counting sponges entailed following written hospital policy and procedures and that there was no showing in this case that the surgeon gave orders how or when to count sponges.

For the hospital to be relieved of liability, the nurse must be totally following the physician's order. If the nurse is merely taking a short-cut and violating hospital policy, then the hospital usually retains its responsibility and liability. Some courts prefer to enact a dual servant doctrine, since this doctrine allows for vicarious liability to flow to both the employer hospital and to the physician (*Holger v. Irish*, 1993). A *dual servant* is one who can be shown to be serving both entities at the same time. For example, circulating nurses in the operating room remain hospital employees, yet strictly follow the orders of the surgeon in charge. In *Holger*, the injured plaintiff had to show that the operating nurses were negligent, *and* that the nurses were the surgeon's employees or agents, *or* that other facts established the surgeon's supervision and control over the nurses at the time of the incident. As with all vicarious liability situations, the nurse who does not act in a reasonably prudent manner may be held individually negligent along with the employer.

CORPORATE LIABILITY

The courts have slowly created what is now known as **corporate liability,** a doctrine that evolved as hospitals became more profitable and competitive. The *Darling* case is the landmark case for corporate liability, placing certain nondelegable duties regarding patient care directly on the hospital corporation. Prior to the *Darling* ruling, hospitals bore no liability for the provision of health care since the facility was considered to be a facility where others provided care.

Under this new doctrine, corporations have a direct duty to the public that they serve, ensuring that competent and qualified practitioners will deliver quality health care to consumers. A later court case interpreted *Darling* to include the duty to make a reasonable effort to monitor and oversee the treatment that is prescribed and administered by physicians and nurses practicing within the institution (*Bost v. Riley*, 1990).

All of the hospital's corporate duties have a direct impact on the provision of patient care. The emphasis on the hospital's responsibility for adequate care is apparent. Most of the early case-law dealt with the hospital's responsibility to select and delineate clinical privileges of physicians. The hospital, though, has duties to the patient outside of clinical privileges, which include adequate staffing, supervision for education and training of staff members, maintaining the premises in a reasonably safe manner, provision of properly functioning and reasonably updated equipment, reasonable care in the selection and retention of employees, and the duty to meet a national standard of care.

Negligent Hiring and Retention

The doctrine of **negligent hiring and retention** of employees is often used by injured parties when respondeat superior cannot be applied to the current fact situation. Examples are when nurses are not acting within the course and scope of employment or are acting solely for personal reasons. This doctrine essentially means that the employer can still be held liable if the injured party can show that the employee was incompetent or unsafe for the position and that the employer knew or should have known this fact.

Like respondeat superior, negligent hiring and retention is based on the master-servant relationship. An employer is under a duty to exercise reasonable care so as to control employees while they are acting outside the scope of their employment and to prevent them from intentionally harming others. Hospitals are under an affirmative duty to provide adequate numbers of staff as well as adequately educated and skilled staff members.

The hospital's obligation under this doctrine is to monitor or supervise all personnel within the facility, ensuring quality care to patients within the facility. The institution would be liable for substandard care or injury incurred by patients if personnel fail to perform in accordance with acceptable standards of care. Institutions must also periodically review staff competency (*Park North General Hospital v. Hickman*, 1990). A second obligation that institutions have under this doctrine is to investigate the credentials of physicians and advanced practice nurses before allowing them admitting privileges. Most importantly, the doctrine requires that the hospital terminate unqualified practitioners or make available to these practitioners the education and skills needed to competently deliver quality health care to patients.

OSTENSIBLE AUTHORITY

Ostensible authority, an application of agency law, allows a principal to be liable for acts and omissions by independent contractors working within the principal's place of business or at the direction of the principal and a third party misinterprets the relationship as employer–employee. In health care law, hospitals have been held responsible for actions by independent contractors in suits where reasonable patients argued that they could not distinguish the hospital employees from the independent contractors.

Ostensible authority is also known as *agency by estoppel.* While there is no true agency authority and no agency has been created, with respect to an unknowing third party the court will allow the principal to be held liable to the injured third party (*Corpus Juris Secundum,* 1984). The courts employ four criteria to establish ostensible authority:

1. Subjective.
2. Inherent function.
3. Reliance.
4. Control.

Subjective

This criterion speaks to the extent that third parties see the person as a hospital employee, and it is subject to their interpretations of the relationship. In hospitals where the emergency center or urgent care physician is an independent contractor working in the hospital facility, the court would look to the subjective interpretation of a patient in assuming that the physician is indeed a hospital employee.

Inherent Function

Here the courts center their arguments and interpretations on whether the independent contractor is furthering the primary function of the corporation or has a role easily seen as distinguishable from the corporation's primary function. For example, the emergency center physician is contracted to serve the primary function of the hospital by providing emergency and other treatment to persons in need in the hospital setting. This type of subcontractor is easily distinguished from a food vendor that the hospital contracts to provide food while the hospital cafeteria is renovated.

Reliance

Reliance, akin to the subjective criterion, involves the faith that the patient places in the hospital's judgment. If the hospital contracted with Dr. Jones, then the patient assumes that his credentials and skills have been investigated and that he is competent to perform the role of an emergency center physician.

Control

To determine who had greater control—the independent contractor or the hospital—the court ascertains the following factors:

1. The extent to which the employer determines the details of the work and work setting.
2. Whether the work is supervised by the employer or the independent contractors are free to perform the work in the manner they see fit.
3. Who supplies the instruments, equipment, and supplies needed to perform the work.
4. The actual worksite.
5. The method of payment.

The more control that the corporation has in determining these factors, the more likely the court will find ostensible authority.

THEORIES OF INDEPENDENT LIABILITY

Several legal theories and dictates refer specifically to one's personal responsibilities and liabilities. Such theories serve to make one continually accountable for one's own actions.

Independent Contractor Status

An *independent contractor* is one who arranges with another to perform a service but who is not under the control or right to control of the second person.

In nursing, the independent contractor status usually applies to private duty nurses and to selected advanced practitioner roles. As with ostensible authority, the key issue is control, and neither party may terminate the contract at will. Termination should be a provision of the expressed contract, as should length of contract, dispute resolution, relationship of the parties, duties and responsibilities of the independent contractor, payment schedule, and professional liability insurance (Aiken & Catalano, 1994).

In theory, the classification of this status makes nurses solely liable for negligent or intentional torts and should relieve the hospital or employer of liability. In application, however, many hospitals have been assessed liability by courts under the doctrine of corporate liability or nondelegable duty. One such case was *Zakbartchenko v. Weinberger* (1993). In that case, a rabbi was held negligent in the performance of a bris. The court ruled that the hospital would be held liable if the child's parents established that they had relied on the availability of the hospital's facility and personnel in deciding to perform the bris at the hospital. Since they could establish reliance, the hospital was also liable to the parents.

The hospital owes certain legal duties to the patient—duties completely independent of any derivative liability such as liability for (1) inadequate facilities, (2) inadequate institutional policies, and (3) improper enforcement of rules and regulations of the Joint Commission for Accreditation of Healthcare Organizations (JCAHO) and other licensing and accrediting bodies.

Personal Liability

Stated simply, the doctrine of *personal liability* makes individuals responsible for their own actions. The law does not impose liability on a third party or entity, and allows the person primarily at fault to avoid responsibility and accountability; one cannot negate one's responsibility merely because a second or third party also has responsibility.

Neither does the law impose liability on the competent practitioner. The mere fact that a second or third party has liability does not necessarily convey the liability back to the first individual. For example, a team leader assigns a new staff member to care for an uncomplicated patient. The staff member draws a blood sample from the patient in a negligent manner or fails to monitor the patient's vital signs accurately. Both tasks should be capable of being performed competently by the new staff member. The court finds the staff member negligent and therefore liable in a subsequent lawsuit that is filed. The team leader would not share in the liability even though he or she was the person who directly assigned the patient's care to this nurse. As a team leader, one has a right to expect that staff members are capable of performing functions normally assigned to staff members. The example changes, however, if the staff member expresses, at the time of the assignment, an inability to competently perform the tasks. Then both the team leader and the assigned nurse could incur liability.

Indemnification

Closely akin to personal liability is the principle of *indemnification,* which allows the employer to recover from the individual personally responsible any damages paid under the doctrine of respondeat superior for the negligent act. Nurses' personal liability for negligent actions make them subject to this principle after the hospital, via respondeat superior, has paid damages to the injured party. The key to applying this principle is twofold: (1) The employer is at fault in a liability suit only because of the employee's negligence, and (2) the employer incurs monetary damages because of the employee's negligence. The employer can then institute a lawsuit against the negligent employee and recover the amount of damages that the employer paid to the injured party.

Prior to the 1980s, employers seldom instituted such lawsuits. Today it is more commonplace to see such lawsuits filed, although it is hardly a trend.

EXERCISE 14-2

Jose, an 8-year-old boy, is admitted to your hospital in extreme pain late one evening. About 10:00 that evening, while playing basketball with his friends, he fell, dislocating his shoulder. He is seen by the emergency center physician. After what seems forever, an x-ray is done. The physician tells Jose's parents that surgery will be done "first thing in the morning," since there is no anesthetist on call, and that he will be there about 8:00 AM. Jose is sedated and spends a long and painful night at the hospital. Following surgery, he develops a permanent disability of his shoulder and arm due to the delayed surgery. His parents bring suit against the hospital, the emergency center physician, and the anesthetist. What are their grounds for liability? Who will be found liable for Jose's injury?

EMPLOYMENT LAWS

The federal and individual state governments have enacted a cadre of laws regulating employment. To be effective and legally correct, nurses must be familiar with these laws and how individual laws affect the institution and labor relations. Many nurses have come to fear the legal system because of their personal experience or the experiences of colleagues. Much of this concern may, however, be directly attributable to uncertainty about the law or partial knowledge it. By understanding and correctly following federal employment laws, nurse managers may actually lessen their potential liability by complying with both federal and state laws. Table 14–1 gives an overview of key federal employment laws.

TABLE 14–1. SELECTED FEDERAL LABOR LEGISLATION

Year	Legislation	Purpose and Effect
1935	The Wagner Act; National Labor Act	Established many rights in unionization; NLRB established.
1947	The Taft-Hartley Act	Resulted in more equal balance of power between unions and management.
1946	Federal Tort Claims Act	Permitted the U.S. government to be sued for torts of its employees.
1962	Executive Order 10988	Allowed public employees to join unions.
1963	Equal Pay Act	Made it illegal to pay lower wages to employees based solely on gender.
1964	Civil Rights Act	Protected against discrimination due to race, color, creed, national origin, etc.
1967	Age Discrimination Act	Made it illegal for employers to discriminate against older men and women.
1974	Wagner Amendments	Allowed nonprofit organizations to join unions; opened unionization in nursing.
1990	Americans with Disabilities Act	Sweeping legislation against discrimination against disabled individuals in the workplace.
1991	Civil Rights Act	Specifically addresses sexual harassment in the workplace; overrides and modifies previous legislation in this area.
1993	Family and Medical Leave Act of 1993	Allows men and women to take medical leaves from their employment to care for a child, spouse, or parent with a serious medical condition, and for the birth or adoption of a child.

Source: *Adapted from Marquis and Huston (1994, p. 319). Used with permission.*

EQUAL EMPLOYMENT OPPORTUNITY LAWS

Several laws have been enacted federally to expand equal employment opportunities by prohibiting discrimination based on gender, age, race, religion, handicap, pregnancy, and national origin. These laws are enforced by the *Equal Employment Opportunity Commission (EEOC)*. Additionally, states have enacted statutes that address employment opportunities and that the nurse manager should consider both when hiring and assigning nursing employees.

The most significant legislation affecting equal employment opportunities today is the amended *1964 Civil Rights Act* (43 Fed. Reg. 1978). Section 703 (a) of Title VII makes it illegal for an employer "to refuse to hire, discharge an individual, or otherwise to discriminate against an individual, with respect to his compensation, terms, conditions, or privileges of employment because of the individual's race, color, religion, sex, or national origin." Title VII was also amended by the Equal Opportunities Act of 1972 so that it applies to private institutions with 15 or more employees, state and local governments, labor unions, and employment agencies.

In 1991, the Civil Rights Act was signed into law. This act further broadened the issue of sexual harassment in the workplace and supersedes many of the sections of Title VII. Sections of the new legislation define sexual harassment, its elements, and the employer's responsibilities for harassment in the workplace, especially prevention and corrective action. The Civil Rights Act is enforced by the EEOC as created in the 1964 act; its powers were broadened in the 1972 Equal Employment Opportunity Act. The primary activity of the EEOC is the processing of complaints of employment discrimination. There are three phases: investigation, conciliation, and litigation. Investigation focuses on determining whether Title VII has been violated by the employer. If the EEOC finds "probable cause," an attempt is made to reach an agreement or conciliation between the EEOC, the complainant, and the employer. If conciliation fails, the EEOC may file suit against the employer in federal court or issue to the complainant the right to sue for discrimination.

The EEOC also promulgated written rules and regulations that reflect its interpretation of the laws under its auspices. Included in these written rules and regulations are those relating to staffing practices and those relating to sexual harassment in the workplace. The EEOC's definition of sexual harassment is broad, and it has generally been upheld in the courts. Nurse managers must realize that it is the duty of employers (management) to prevent employees from sexually harassing other employees. The EEOC issues policies and practices for employers to implement for both sensitizing employees to this problem and preventing its occurrence; nurse managers should be aware of these policies and practices and seek guidance in implementing them if sexual harassment occurs in their units.

Employers may seek exceptions to Title VII on a number of bases. For example, it is lawful to make employment decisions on the basis of national origin, religion, and gender (never race or color) if the decisions are necessary for the normal operation of the business, although the courts have viewed this exception very narrowly. Promotions and layoffs based on bona fide seniority or merit systems are permissible (*Firefighters Local 1784 v. Scotts,* 1984) as are exceptions based on business necessity.

FEDERAL TORT CLAIMS ACT OF 1946

The *Federal Tort Claims Act of 1946* was enacted to allow patients and persons with claims against federal workers to be able to sue the Unites States government. Prior to that time, the government was immune, even if negligent actions of its employees caused injury or loss of property to nongovernmental individuals. After the enactment of this law, the government is substituted as the defendant in civil actions filed to recover damages against federal employees, and the Federal Tort Claims Act is the sole remedy available to patients injured by a federal employee providing health care.

Under this act, the court first establishes whether the individual was an employee or an independent contractor with the government. This is done since greater liability exposure occurs with employees than with independent contractors. For example, in *Broussard v. United States* (1993), the court held that no negligence had occurred on the part of the defendant since the physician was an independent contractor at the time of the injury. There was a contract between the government facility and the physicians that the physicians would assume full responsibility and accountability for their own actions. In *Bird v. United States* (1991), the ruling had been just the opposite, and a nurse anesthetist was considered a government employee because the nurse was under the same control and supervision as a regularly employed governmental employee.

AGE DISCRIMINATION IN EMPLOYMENT ACT OF 1967

The outcome of the **Age Discrimination in Employment Act of 1967** is that it became illegal for employers, unions, and employment agencies to discriminate against older men and women. The law, in a 1986 amendment, prohibits discrimination over the age of 40. The practical outcome of this act has been that mandatory retirement is no longer seen in the American workplace.

As with Title VII, there are some exceptions to this act. Reasonable factors, other than age, may be used when terminations become necessary; such reasonable factors would be a performance evaluation system and some limited occupational qualifications, such as tedious physical demands of a specific job.

AFFIRMATIVE ACTION

The policy of **affirmative action (AA)** differs from the policy of *equal employment opportunity (EEO)*. AA centers enhance employment opportunities of protected groups of people, while EEO is concerned with utilizing employment practices that do not discriminate against or impair the employment opportunities of protected groups. Thus, AA can be seen in conjunction with several federal employment laws; for example, in conjunction with the *Vietnam Era Veteran's Readjustment Act of 1974*, the AA requires that employers with government contracts take steps to enhance the employment opportunities of disabled veterans and other veterans of the Vietnam era.

EQUAL PAY ACT OF 1963

The *Equal Pay Act* makes it illegal to pay lower wages to employees of one gender when the jobs:

1. Require equal skill in experience, training, education, and ability.
2. Require equal effort in mental or physical exertion.
3. Are of equal responsibility and accountability.
4. Are performed under similar working conditions.

Courts have held that unequal pay may be legal if based on seniority, merit, incentive systems, and a factor other than sex. The main cases filed under this law in the area of nursing have been by nonprofessionals.

OCCUPATIONAL SAFETY AND HEALTH ACT

The *Occupational Safety and Health Act of 1970 (OSHA)* was enacted to assure healthful and safe working conditions in the workplace. Among other provisions, the law requires isolation procedures, the placarding of areas containing ionizing radiation, proper grounding of electrical equipment, protective storage of flammable and combustible liquids, and now the gloving of all personnel when handling bodily fluids. The statute provides that, if no federal standard has been established, state statutes prevail. Nurse managers should know the relevant OSHA laws for the institution and their specific areas. Frequent review of new additions to the law must also be undertaken, especially in this era of AIDS and infectious diseases, and care must be taken to ensure that necessary gloves and equipment as specified are available on each unit.

EMPLOYMENT-AT-WILL AND WRONGFUL DISCHARGE

Historically, the employment relationship has been considered as a *free will relationship.* Employees were free to take or not take a job at will, and employers were free to hire, retain, or discharge employees for any reason. Many laws, some federal and predominantly state, have been slowly eroding this at-will employment relationship. And evolving case law provides at least three exceptions to the broad doctrine of *employment-at-will.*

The first exception is a public policy exception, which involves cases in which an employee is discharged in direct conflict with established public policy (Twomey, 1986). Examples are discharging an employee for serving on a jury, for reporting an employers' illegal actions (better known as "whistle blowing"), and for filing a worker's compensation claim.

The second exception involves an implied contract and the concept of *wrongful discharge.* The courts have generally treated employee handbooks, company policies, and oral statements made at the time of employment as "framing the employment relationship." In *Toussaint v. Blue Cross and Blue Shield* (1980), the court held that a statement in the company's policy handbook that stated an employee would be discharged only for "good cause" provided an enforceable contract between the employer and employee.

The third exception is a "good faith and fair dealing" exception. The purpose of this exception is to prevent unfair or malicious terminations, and the exception is used sparingly by the courts. In *Fortune v. National Cash Register* (1977), an employee was discharged just before a final contact was signed between his employer and another company for which the employee would have received a large commission. The court held that he was discharged by National Cash Register, in bad faith, solely to prevent paying the commission.

Nurses are urged to know their respective state laws concerning this growing area of the law. Midlevel management nurses and those in higher management positions should also review institution documents, especially employee handbooks and recruiting brochures, for unwanted statements implying job security or other unintentional promises. Managers are also cautioned not to say anything during the preemployment negotiations and interviews that might be construed as implying job security or other unintentional promises to the potential employee.

COLLECTIVE BARGAINING

Collective bargaining, also called *labor relations*, is the joining together of employees for the purpose of increasing their ability to influence the employer and improve working conditions. Usually, the employer is referred to as *management* and the employees, even professionals, as *labor*. Persons involved in the hiring, firing, scheduling, disciplining, or evaluating of employees are considered management and may not be included in a collective bargaining unit. Those in management could form their own group, but are not protected under these laws. Nurse managers may or may not be part of management; if they have hiring and firing authority, then they are part of management.

Collective bargaining is defined and protected by the *National Labor Relations Act* and its amendments. The National Labor Relations Board (NLRB) oversees the act and those who come under its auspices. The NLRB ensures that employees are able to choose freely whether they want to be represented by a bargaining unit, and it serves to prevent or remedy any violation of the labor laws.

Collective bargaining is relatively new to nurses. *Executive Order 10988* in 1962 made it possible for public employees to join collective bargaining units, and nonprofit health care organizations have only been subject to these laws since 1974 with an Amendment to the Wagner Act. The American Nurses Association has long supported the right of nurses to bargain collectively. Since 1946, the American Nurses Association, through its state constituent associations, has collectively represented the interests of nurses within the individual states. Two of the main reasons proposed for this support are that (1) collective bargaining allows for achieving the basic elements of professional status, and (2) collective bargaining allows a mechanism for nurses to resolve conflicts within the workplace setting, thereby enhancing quality of care to patients.

Collective bargaining is a power strategy based on the premise that there is increased power in numbers. Collective bargaining assists in the following areas:

1. Basic economic issues as salary, shift differentials, overtime pay, length of the work day, vacation time, sick leave, lunch breaks, health insurance, and severance pay.

2. Unfair or arbitrary treatment such as scheduling, staffing, rotating shifts, on-call, transfers, seniority rights, and posting of job openings.
3. Maintenance and promotion of professional practice as acceptable standards of care, other quality of care issues, and adequate staffing ratios.

Issues against collective bargaining by professionals include the charges of unprofessionalism, unethical behavior especially when faced with a strike situation, divisiveness, and the endangerment to job security posed by the closed shop (the requirement that everyone must join the union). Most health care unions are open shops, allowing nurses to either join the union or not. All these issues have many sides that can be argued; many nurses now acknowledge that they have progressed because of collective bargaining and unionization.

The process of unionization is a complex one. Table 14–2 highlights some of the terms used in unionization and collective bargaining. Organizing is the first phase and a labor organization is formed, called an *organizing council.* This proceeds to NLRB-supervised elections when enough written interest has been expressed to warrant the formulation of a recognized union. This election period is normally tense, and both management and union officials attempt to influence the vote in their favor.

If the election is successful for the union and the bargaining agent is certified by the NLRB, a contract negotiation period is begun. Each side appoints a spokesperson and good faith bargaining is mandated by law for both sides. During this phase, there may be stalemates, mediation, and binding arbitration. The *arbitrator* is a neutral party whose purpose is to be fair to both sides. Since the arbitrator's solution and recommendations are binding to both sides, often the two sides are likely to negotiate for small favors.

If the two sides cannot agree and are unwilling to call for arbitration, work stoppages by employees and lockouts by management can occur. With ten days' notice, the union can then proceed to a strike. Usually, ratification of the agreement is reached since no side wants a strike, and negotiations take on added fervor during work stoppages and lockouts.

Once ratified, collective bargaining does not end, but enters the enforcement stage. Grievances can be brought by either management or employees if there are disputes and complaints. Grievances typically can be solved without further steps being taken, but there are specific provisions for resolution, including arbitration.

From a management position, nurse managers and upper-level management can do several things to prevent unionization. Since most unions form because of real or perceived disagreement with management, a well-rounded, high-quality, effective leadership team is needed to prevent dissatisfaction from becoming rampant. Some suggestions for management include:

1. Provide opportunity for participation in organizational decision making; a participative approach may extend to unit self-governance.
2. Maintain salaries in relationship with the education required and the responsibility given.

TABLE 14–2. COLLECTIVE BARGAINING TERMS

Arbitration	The terminal step in the grievance process during which an impartial third party attempts to come to a reasonable solution taking into consideration both management and labor issues; may be either a voluntary or a government enforced compulsory process; this person has the final power of decision-making in the dispute
Closed shop	Synonymous with union shop
Collective bargaining	The relations between employers and labor; employers act through their management representatives and labor acts through its union representatives
Conciliation and mediation	These are synonymous terms describing the activity of a third party to assist the disputants reach an acceptable agreement; this individual has no final power of decision-making as does the arbitrator
Free Speech	Under Public Law 101, Section 8, the "expression of any views, argument, or dissemination thereof, whether in written, printed, graphic, or visual form, shall not constitute or be evident of unfair labor practice under any provision of this Act, if such expression contains no threat of reprisal or force or promise of benefit"
Grievance	Process undertaken when the perception exists on the part of a union member that management has failed in some way to meet the terms of the labor agreement
Lockout	Consists of closing a place of business by management in the course of a labor dispute for the purpose of forcing employees to accept management terms
National Labor Relations Board	Formed to implement the Wagner Act and serves to 1) determine who should be the official bargaining unit when a new unit is formed and who should be in the unit and 2) adjudicate unfair labor changes.
Open shop	Also known as an agency shop; employees are not required to join a union, although they may if they so desire and one exists within the workplace
Professionals	Have the a right to be represented by a labor union; cannot belong to a union that also represents nonprofessionals unless a majority of the professionals vote for inclusion into the nonprofessional unit
Strike	A concerted withholding of labor supply in order to bring economic pressure upon management and force management to grant employee demands
Supervisors	Someone who has the authority to hire, fire, transfer, and promote employees; supervisors are excluded from protection under the Taft-Hartley Act and cannot be represented by a union
Union shop	Also known as a closed shop; all employees are required to join the union and to pay dues

GUIDELINES: TIMETABLE FOR CALLING A STRIKE

1. Make sure that you are following the most recent federal guidelines. Check the current status of the law before proceeding, and be sure to comply with all procedural requirements of the act.

2. The party wishing to end or modify a contract must notify the opposition 90 days prior to the contract expiration date.

3. If within 30 days of notification the two sides cannot agree, notification of the dispute must be given to the Federal Mediation and Conciliation service and its corresponding state agency.

4. This federal agency appoints a mediator within 30 days and, if needed, an inquiry board.

5. The mediator or inquiry board makes its recommendations within 15 days after appointment.

6. Fifteen days after these recommendations, if the parties still cannot agree, the employees may plan to strike, and a strike vote by union members is conducted.

7. With the majority of employees voting to strike, the union must give ten days' notice of the scheduled strike, giving to management the exact day, time, and place of the strike. (Note: No strike may be scheduled before the contract actually expires.)

3. Treat professionals as true professionals; this entails affording respect, trust, and value to all professionals in the organization.

4. Develop, implement, and refine a grievance procedure. This ensures that staff members have direction when they feel dissatisfied and prevents dissatisfaction from becoming so overwhelming that unionization is the only foreseeable answer.

5. Conduct timely and regular surveys and meetings to allow staff an opportunity to express their feelings and views. Open channels of communications are crucial in maintaining positive working relationships.

Once the contract has been accepted and nurse managers are managing and leading within a union framework, there are some things that they must know and remember. First, know and understand the contract provisions. A thorough understanding and following of the contract can prevent most grievances. Second, treat all supervised persons with equal respect and consideration, both union and nonunion members. This prevents a charge of discrimination and should serve to maintain morale. Third, should an issue arise, perform as a professional, be nondefensive, and do not crumble under the pressure. Admit wrong statements or decisions, and negotiate a better solution to the problem, assuring that the institution goals will be upheld. If necessary, seek assistance from upper management, especially if the conflict cannot be immediately resolved. Fifth, continue to expand personal knowledge of management principles either through formal education or through continuing education, and practice those principles.

CASE-LAW AND THE NATIONAL LABOR RELATIONS BOARD IN THE 1990s

On March 10, 1993, the sixth circuit court held that staff nurses, including licensed practice nurses (LPNs) at a nursing home facility, were supervisors under the definition of the NLRA and therefore were not entitled to the act's protections (*National Labor Relations Board v. Health Care and Retirement Corporation of America*, 1994). The case was granted review by the Supreme Court to determine whether the duties of nurses in directing the activities of lesser-skilled employees qualify the nurses as supervisors.

The facts of the case are relatively uncomplicated. The LPNs had brought action, alleging that they were disciplined by the nursing home for engaging in protected conduct for the purpose of collective bargaining. The four LPNs involved in the initial action were staff nurses whose primary responsibilities involved monitoring the work of nurses aides, evaluating the aides' performances, and resolving their grievances. Based on the LPNs' job description, the corporation asserted that these nurses were supervisors and therefore not within the protection of the NLRB since employers cannot be compelled to negotiate with representatives of supervisors. The act defines *supervisor* as "any individual having authority, in the interest of the employer, to hire, transfer, suspend, lay off, recall, promote, discharge, assign, reward, or discipline other employees, or responsibility to direct them, or to adjust their grievances, or effectively to recommend such action, if in connection with the foregoing the exercise of such authority is not of a merely routine or clerical nature, but requires the use of independent judgment" (29 *USCA*, section 152[11]).

The nurses (through the NLRB) argued that, since the primary focus of staff nurses is to exercise their professional skills to care for patients, they do not operate in the interest of the employer's interests. They further argued that the direction of the nursing assistants' work by staff nurses is given routinely in connection with the treatment of patients to ensure that quality care is provided to all patients within their care units. There is no evidence that the staff nurses' direction of employees' work goes into personal authority, which more directly promotes the interests of the employer and is not motivated by patient care needs. The administrative law judge who heard the case initially agreed with this statutory argument and held that the protective provisions of the act covered staff nurses.

But, on May 23, 1994, the Supreme Court disagreed. Justice Kennedy, writing for the court, criticized the NLRB's insistence on the interest of the employer as the test for determining whether staff nurses are supervisors. He concluded that, when staff nurses exercise professional responsibilities by caring for a patient, they act in the interest of the nursing home, whose business is patient care.

The NLRB further argued that the health care profession should be treated differently from other professions because the concern over divided loyalty between supervisors and subordinate employees played no role in health care professions. Nurses, the Board argued, would not divide loyalty between subordinates and the employer, but nurses would place their professional responsibility to care for patients above any loyalty. The court also rejected this argument.

The court's decision is most important in treating the health care profession as other professions. Interns, residents, salaried physicians, and nurses can be classified as supervisors in the future, overturning the longstanding precedents of the NLRB, which held that health professionals were covered by the NLRA. Professionals who use independent judgment and who are employed by employers subject to the NLRA could be exempted from the protections of the act because of their supervisory status.

Ultimately, the court concluded that it was "up to Congress to carve out an exception for the health care providers, including nurses, should Congress not wish for such nurses to be considered supervisors" (*National Labor Relations Board v. Health Care and Retirement Corporation of America*, 1994, at 1556). Indeed, the court further stated, Congress had made no attempt to carve nurses or health care professionals out of the NLRA's definition of supervisor in the 1974 amendments. Perhaps Congress did not specify this action because it was satisfied with the NLRB's careful avoidance of applying the definition to health care professionals whose activities were directed at quality patient care. If nurses and other health care professionals wish to change this current status, new legislation will have to be enacted in Congress.

Interestingly, a further decision by the National Labor Relations Board, reached in late February, 1996, once more serves to confuse the issue. The decision reached in the *National Labor Relations Board v. Providence Hospital* recognizes that the judgment used by registered nurses in monitoring and assessing patients is part of the professional role, rather than part of any statutory supervision as defined by the National Labor Relations Act. This decision paves the way for nurses of Providence Hospital to organize and to be represented by the Alaska Nurses Association as the bargaining agent.

This decision and its companion decision, ruling that licensed practical nurses in a New York nursing home oversee the work of certified nursing assistants in a routine manner, without using the independent type of judgment necessary to be a statutory supervisor, has implications for a number of cases currently before the NLRB (Ketter, 1996). The final outcome of these two decisions will almost assuredly be played out in court in the years to come.

FAMILY AND MEDICAL LEAVE ACT OF 1993

The *Family and Medical Leave Act of 1993* was signed into law in February 1993, becoming effective upon its enactment. The law was passed due to the large number of single- and two-parent households in which the single parent or both parents are employed full-time, placing job security and parenting at odds. The law was also passed due to the aging population of the United States and the demands that aging parents place on their working children. The act attempts to balance the demands of the workplace with the demands of the family, allowing employed individuals to take leaves for medical reasons. Such medical reasons include the birth or adoption of a child, and the care of a child, spouse, or parent who has a serious health problem. Essentially, the act provides job security for unpaid leave while the employee is caring for a new infant or other family health care needs. The act is gender-neutral and allows both men and women to the same leave provisions.

EXERCISE 14-3

A staff member requests vacation for the next two weekends. She has a family wedding out of state on the first weekend. On the Friday of the second week, her mother is having surgery, and she has promised to help take care of the mother that weekend. Do you schedule the staff member for vacation? Explain your reasoning. What if the contract is silent as to how many weekends a worker can work during a four-week period?

DUTY OWED THE EMPLOYER

Professional nurses owe the employer and themselves the highest standards or qualities of the profession, including:

1. Maintaining the standards of their state nurse practice act.
2. Continuously upgrading their skills and education through mandatory or voluntary continuing education.
3. Being a patient care advocate, as needed, to assure quality care to all patients.
4. Recognizing and applying legal principles as they apply to all areas of patient care.

SUMMARY

A variety of legal issues arise when one employee supervises others in a corporation. Issues of direct corporate liability, through negligent hiring and firing, ostensible agency, and borrowed servant doctrine, as well as various liabilities, may overwhelm nurses in management positions. This chapter has reviewed these concepts and employment laws. The next chapter explores more thoroughly how these concepts directly impact nurses in management roles.

AFTER COMPLETING THIS CHAPTER, YOU SHOULD BE ABLE TO

- Describe the doctrines of respondeat superior, ostensible authority, corporate negligence, and direct corporate liability.
- Describe federal and state employment laws that affect the delivery of health care in the United States.
- Define and discuss the role of individual contractors in the health care delivery system.
- Define and describe indemnification from a corporate perspective.
- Describe the employer's obligation to nurse employees and the professional nurses' obligations to the employing agency.

APPLY YOUR LEGAL KNOWLEDGE

- How are hospitals liable for acts of individual nurses, even if no lawsuit is brought against the nurses?
- Can an institution be held liable for the actions of independent contractors?
- On employment questionnaires or during employment interviews, what questions should never be asked and the nurse not answer?
- How does the doctrine of indemnification further the concept that individuals are ultimately responsible for their own actions?

REFERENCES

Aiken, T. D. & Catalano, J. T. (1994). *Legal, ethical, and political issues in nursing.* Philadelphia, PA: F. A. Davis Company.

American Jurisprudence (1992). 4A Agency.

Bird v. United States, 949 F. 2d 1079 (10th Cir., 1991).

Biconi v. Pay 'N Pak Stores, Inc., 746 F. Supp. 1 (D. Oregon, 1990).

Broussard v. United States, 989 F. 2d 171 (Texas, 1993).

Bost v. Riley, 262 S.E. 2d 391 (N.C. App., 1980), 51 *ALR* 4th 235 (1990).

Civil Rights Act, 43 *Fed. Reg.* 1978, Sec. 703 et. seq., 1964.

Corpus Juris Secundum (1984). 2A Agency, Sections 1–59.

Darling v. Charleston Community Memorial Hospital, 211 N.E. 2d 253 (Illinois, 1965), cert. den'd, 383 U.S. 946 (1966).

Duling v. Bluefield Sanitarium, Inc., 142 S.E. 2d 754 (West Virginia, 1965).

Executive Order 10988 (1962).

Firefighters Local 1784 v. Scotts, 467 U.S. 561, 34 FEP Cases 1702 (1984).

Fiesta, J. (1990). The nursing shortage; whose liability problem? Part II. *Nursing Management, 21*(2), 22–23.

Fortune v. National Cash Register Company, 272 Mass. 96, 264 N.E. 2d 1251 (1977).

42 *USC* sec. 12101 et. seq., 1990.

Harris v. Miller, No. 345A91, 1994 N.C. LEXIS 16 (January 28, 1994).

Holger v. Irish, 851 P.2d 1122, 316 Or. 402 (Oregon, 1993).

Hunter v. Allis-Chambers Corporation, Engine Division, 797 F.2d 1417 (Cir. App. 7, 1986).

Ketter, J. (1996). Nurses score victory in NLRB decision. *The American Nurse, 28*(1), 1 and 6.

McConnell v. Williams, 361 Pa. 355, 65 A. 2d 243 (1959).

National Labor Relations Act. (July 5, 1935), chapter 372, 49 Stat. 449.

National Labor Relations Board v. Health Care and Retirement Corporation of America, 987 F.2d 1256 (6th Cir., 1993), cert. granted 62 U.S.L.W. 3244 (U.S., Oct. 5, 1993), 114 S. Crt. 1178 (1994).

Oberzan v. Smith, 869 P.2d 682, 254 Kan. 846 (Kansas, 1994).

Park North General Hospital v. Hickman, 703 S.W. 2d 262 (1985) 51 *ALR* 4th 235 (1990).

Public Law 93-360 (1974), Sec. 2(5) 88 Stat. 395.

Public Law 103-3 (February 5, 1993).

Robertson v. Bethlehem Steel Corporation, 912 F.2d 184 (Cir. App. 7, 1990).

Sparger v. Worley Hospital, Inc., 547 S.W. 2d 582 (Texas, 1977).

Spoor v. Serota, 852 P.2d 1292 (Colorado, 1992) cert. den'd.

Toussaint v. Blue Cross and Blue Shield, 408 Mich. 579, 292 N.W. 2d 880 (1980).

29 *USCA* Section 152[11], 1935.

Twomey, D. P. (1986). *A concise guide to employment laws: EEO and OSHA.* Cincinnati: South-Western Publishing Company.

Van Hook v. Anderson, 824 P.2d 509, 64 Wash. 353 (Wash. App., 1992).

Zakbartchenko v. Weinberger, 605 N.Y.S. 205 (New York, 1993).

• fifteen

Nursing Administration and the Nurse Manager

PREVIEW

The role of the professional nurse has expanded to include increased expertise, specialization, autonomy, and accountability. Paternalistic attitudes of the past, with which physicians and hospitals assumed responsibility for the action of employees, are no longer the norm. Though respondeat superior still exists, more and more individuals are being held accountable for their actions. Nurses in nursing administration must increase their understanding of the changing legal climate and of their responsibilities. This chapter explains key concepts underlying nursing management, including supervision of others, the temporary reassignment of nurses to units other than those with which they have primary expertise, unlicensed assistive personnel issues, and the recent change in supervisory status of nurses according to the National Labor Relations Board.

LIABILITY: PERSONAL, VICARIOUS, AND CORPORATE

Personal liability defines each person's responsibility and accountability for individual actions or omissions. Even if others can be shown to be liable for a patient injury, each individual retains personal accountability for his or her actions. The law sometimes allows other parties to be liable for certain causes of negligence. Known as *vicarious or substituted liability,* the doctrine of *respondeat superior* (let the master answer) makes employers accountable for the negligence of their employees. The rationale underlying the doctrine is that the employee would not have been in a position to have caused the wrongdoing unless hired by the employer and that the injured party will be allowed to suffer a double wrong merely because most employees are unable to pay damages for their wrongdoings. Nurse managers can best avoid these issues by ensuring that their staff members know and follow hospital policy and procedure and that they deliver competent nursing care.

Often nurses believe that the doctrine of vicarious liability shields them from personal liability, that the institution may be sued, but not individual nurses. Patients injured due to substandard care have the right to sue both the institution and the nurse. The institution has the right under indemnification to sue the nurse for damages paid an injured patient. The principle of *indemnification* is applicable when the employer is held liable based solely on the actions of the negligent staff member and when the employer pays monetary damages because of the employee's negligent actions.

Corporate liability, a newer trend in the law, essentially holds that the institution has the responsibility and accountability for maintaining an environment that ensures quality health care delivery for consumers. Corporate liability issues include negligent hiring and firing issues, a duty to maintain safety in the physical environment, and maintenance of a qualified, competent, and adequate staff. Nurse managers play a key role in assisting the institution to avoid corporate liability. For example, the nurse managers are normally delegated the duty to ensure that staff remain competent and qualified, that personnel within their supervision have current licensure, and that incompetent, illegal, or unethical practices are reported to the proper persons or agencies.

CAUSES OF MALPRACTICE FOR NURSE MANAGERS

Nursing managers are charged with maintaining a standard of competent nursing care within the institution. Several potential sources of liability for malpractice among nurse managers may be identified. These causes of action include negligent hiring, negligent retention of incompetent or impaired employees, inappropriate assignment of staff, failure to delegate wisely, failure to supervise and train staff, and failure to warn prospective employees of past problems with previously employed staff. Once identified, guidelines to prevent or avoid these pitfalls can then be developed.

Delegation and Supervision

Nursing management involves the supervision of various personnel who directly provide nursing care to patients. The nurse manager remains personally liable for the reasonable exercise of delegation and supervision activities. The failure to delegate and supervise within acceptable standards of professional nursing practice may be seen as malpractice. Additionally, in a newer trend in the law, the failure to delegate and supervise within acceptable standards may extend to direct corporate liability for the institution. Remember that *delegation* involves the transfer of responsibility for the performance of tasks and skills without the transfer of accountability for the ultimate outcome. Nurse managers may delegate duties to staff nurses, but they retain some accountability for the adequate completion of the delegated duties.

Note, though, that nurse managers are liable not merely because they have a supervisory function. The degree of knowledge concerning the skills and competencies of those supervised are of paramount importance. The doctrine of "knew or should have known" becomes a legal standard in delegating tasks to the individuals supervised. If it can be shown that nurse managers delegated tasks appropriately and had no reason to believe that the assigned nurse was anything but competent to perform the task, then they have no personal liability. But the converse is also true. If it can be shown that nurse managers were aware of incompetencies in an employee or that the assigned task is outside the employee's capabilities, then they become potentially liable for the subsequent injury to a patient.

Nurse managers have a duty to ensure that staff members under their supervision are practicing in a competent manner. In a recent case with implications for discrimination under the Americans with Disabilities Act, a nurse, suffering from uncontrollable epilepsy, was hired to work in an institution's burn unit. Subsequently, nursing management was notified that the nurse continued to suffer unpredictable seizures while at work, compromising staffing levels and patient care, and was a potential danger to patients. Because she was unable to meet the requirements for her position on the burn unit, the court held that the hospital did not act with prejudice, nor was it unfair in removing her from her nursing duties (*Journal of Health and Hospital Law*, 1991).

The nurse manager must be aware of nurses' knowledge, skills, and competencies and that they maintain their competencies. Knowingly allowing a staff member to function below the acceptable standard of care opens both nurse managers and institutions to liability. Some means of ensuring continued competency are continuing education programs and assigning staff members to work with other staff members to improve technical skills. Another method is to require the nurse in question to attend additional courses at area institutions of higher education. This latter means of increasing nursing proficiency may be used to improve nurses' knowledge of pharmaceutical agents or to increase their knowledge and skills in health and physical assessment techniques.

Duty to Orient, Educate, and Evaluate

Most health care facilities have continuing education departments whose function is to orient nurses new to the institution and to supply in-service education for new equipment, procedures, and interventions. Nonetheless, nurse managers have a *duty to orient, educate, and evaluate.* They are responsible for the daily evaluation of whether nurses are performing competent care. The key to meeting this expectation is *reasonableness.* Nurse managers should ensure that they promptly respond to all allegations, whether by patients, staff, or other health care personnel, of incompetent or questionable nursing care. Nurse managers should thoroughly investigate, recommend alternatives for correcting the situation, and include follow-up evaluations in nurses' records, showing that the nurses are competent to care for patients within clinical settings.

A recent Texas case, *St. Paul Medical Center v. Cecil* (1992), concerned allegations that the hospital was negligent in retaining, supervising, and assigning a nurse. In that case, a term obstetrical patient presented at St. Paul Medical Center, stating that her "water had broken." The nurse checked the patient by means of a pelvic examination and assessed the patient's vital signs, fetal heart tones, and contractions.

An hour later, the patient was again assessed, this time by a resident, who determined that the membranes had ruptured and that meconium was present. After another hour passed, the nurse attached an external fetal monitor and recorded the printout. During the third hour after admission, the resident attached an internal fetal monitor, whose printout showed severe fetal hypoxia and bradycardia, and more meconium was observed. Telling the nurse to alert the attending physician of the need for an immediate cesarian section, there was still an hour delay before a severely brain damaged infant was delivered.

One issue that arose in the defense of the nurse-defendant concerned evaluations that had been written about the nurse's performance three months before this incident arose. At that time, the nurse had been rated as an unsatisfactory employee who sometimes fell asleep while on duty, had difficulty in using electronic fetal monitors, and was reluctant to seek the supervisor's advice or consult with the supervisor when problems arose concerning labor and delivery issues. No subsequent evaluations could be found to support that any of these problems had been addressed or that any had been resolved. The court found the hospital and the nurse both liable to the patient. Liability was averted on the part of the physician by settling out-of-court prior to the start of the trial.

One of the many lessons to be learned from this case is the importance of following through on incompetent staff members, either by reassigning the nurse to less critical areas of the institution, by retraining the nurse to safely perform staff nursing skills and intervene in an appropriate and timely manner, or by discharging the nurse. The second lesson is the importance of reevaluation and ensuring that current evaluations show the improved competency of the nurse in question.

Failure to Warn

A new area of potential liability for nurse managers is the *failure to warn* potential employers of staff incompetence or impairment. Information about suspected addictions, violent behavior, and incompetency of staff members is of vital importance to subsequent employers. If the institution has sufficient information and suspicion on which to discharge an employee or force a letter of resignation, then subsequent employers should be aware of those issues.

One means that courts have used to address this issue is that of *qualified privilege* to certain communications. As a general rule, qualified privilege concerns communications made in good faith between persons or entities with a need to know. Most states now recognize this qualified privilege and allow previous employers to give factual, objective information to subsequent employers (Trudeau, 1992). Chapter 7 should be reviewed for more information on this defense.

Hiring Practices

Nurse managers participate in the hiring of new employees. To avoid potential liability in this area, the nurse manager must be conversant with effective *hiring practices* and aware of potential pitfalls. One such pitfall is any representation made about the position during the interview that may later lead to a breach of express or implied contract claims. Such representations usually occur in prehiring interviews, contract negotiations, in letters offering the position to an individual, or in employee handbooks. Representations may be made about future wages, benefit increases, terms of employment, or cause for termination standards.

Employee handbooks frequently create enforceable rights about specific disciplinary procedures. In *Daldulav v. St. Mary Nazareth Hospital Center* (1987), the court ruled that an employee handbook or other policy statement creates enforceable contractual rights if the traditional requirements for contract formation are presented. These elements include a policy statement containing a promise clear enough for the employee to reasonably believe it to be an offer, with acceptance of the employee's beginning or continuing to work after learning of its existence. In a later case, *Karnes v. Doctors Hospital* (1990), the court disagreed with this ruling, stating that the employee handbook did not create an express or implied contract. In that case, the employee stated that she was aware of the at-will employment and had not read the handbook. The lesson seems to be ensuring that language in the handbook does not constitute expressed conditions or the court will treat it as contractual.

Oral comments made during the interview may also be seen as binding on the employer, particularly those promising continued employment. Thus, during oral negotiations, the nurse manager should:

1. Avoid making promises about career opportunities.
2. Use words such as "possible," "potential," and "maybe" when describing career opportunities.
3. Refrain from predicting future pay raises or benefits, and refer to past pay raises as merely guides.
4. Use words like "now" and "presently" when referring to benefits.
5. Note that all employee benefit plans are subject to change.

EXERCISE 15-1

Does your institution offer an employee handbook? If so, is it given either to new employees or to all employees during a calendar year? Does the handbook contain specific enough terms that could create a duty on the part of the institution? For example, "The employee will be given three disciplinary warnings before termination" could be seen as creating such a duty. Are there other examples? How would you change the handbook so that language creating a duty is completely eliminated?

STAFFING ISSUES

Three different issues arise under the general term *staffing*:

1. Adequate numbers of staff members in a time of advancing patient acuity and limited resources.
2. Floating staff from one unit to another.
3. Using temporary or "agency" staff to augment hospital staffing.

Adequate Staffing

Accreditation standards, namely the Joint Commission for the Accreditation of Healthcare Organizations (JCAHO), the Community Health Accreditation Program (CHAP), as well as other state and federal standards, mandate that health care institutions must provide *adequate staffing* with qualified personnel. This incudes not only numbers of staff, but also the legal status of the staff member. For instance, some areas of the institution must have greater percentages of RNs than LPN/LVNs, such as critical care areas, postanesthesia care areas, and emergency centers, while other areas may have equal or lower percentages of RNs to LPN/LVNs or nursing assistants, such as the general floor areas and some long-term care areas. Whether short staffing or understaffing exists depends on a careful, objective analysis of the number of patients, the amount of care required by each patient, and the number and classification/type of staff members (Fiesta, 1994). Courts determine whether understaffing indeed existed based on an individual case-to-case determination.

While the institution is ultimately accountable for staffing issues, nurse managers may also incur some potential liability as they directly oversee numbers of personnel assigned to a unit on a shift. Courts have traditionally looked to the constant exercise of professional judgment rather than relying on concrete rules in times of short staffing. This means that using judgment to ensure patient safety and quality care is more important than ensuring that each unit has the exact nurse-to-patient ratio. For nurse manager liability to occur, it must be shown that the resultant patient injury was directly due to the "short staffing" and not due to the inappropriate or incompetent actions of an individual staff member. Remember that staffing problems never cancel the institution's obligation to maintain a reasonable standard of care.

In a Georgia case, a hospital was sued for negligence to provide adequate staffing. The case concerned the ability of the emergency center staff members to adequately diagnose and intervene appropriately with a patient who suffered a myocardial infarction. The court concluded that the hospital was required to provide staff competent to exercise a reasonable degree of care and skill when delivering health care to patients (*Harrell v. Louis Smith Memorial Hospital*, 1990).

Short staffing guidelines for nurse managers include alerting hospital administrators and upper level managers of concerns. First, though, nurse managers must have done everything under their control to alleviate the circumstances, such as approving overtime for adequate coverage, reassigning personnel among the areas they supervise, and restricting new admissions to the area. Second, remember that nurse managers have a legal duty to notify the chief operating officer, either directly or indirectly, when understaffing endangers patient welfare. One way of notifying the chief operating officer is through formal nursing channels, for example by notifying the nurse manager's direct supervisor. Upper management must then decide how to alleviate the short staffing, on either a short-term or a long-term basis. Appropriate measures could be closing a certain unit or units, restricting elective surgeries, or hiring new staff members. Once nurse managers can show that they acted appropriately, used sound judgment given the circumstances, and alerted their supervisors of the serious nature of the situation, then the institution becomes potentially solely liable for staffing issues.

If the hospital has no collective bargaining contracts, the employment is considered to be at-will employment. The hospital is free to set the terms and conditions of employment, including the numbers of hours worked and when the hours are worked. The federal Fair Labor Standards Act, which governs employment conditions, and most state labor laws do not restrict the number of hours that nurses can work in a given pay period or week. Additionally, under employment at will, workers can be terminated at any time and for any reason, including failure to follow a direct order, such as mandatory overtime.

One means that nurse managers in employment-at-will states use is insisting that nurses work mandatory overtime as a means of alleviating short staffing. A recent New York licensure case illustrates what can happen when such mandatory overtime is requested. In *Husbert v. Commissioner of Education* (1992), a nurse was notified by the supervisor that one of the day shift nurses would be required to work an extra shift due to staff shortage. Under the hospital's mandatory overtime policy, the nurse with the least seniority was required to stay. The RN informed the supervisor that she would stay but left after an hour, informing no one that she was leaving. Twenty-nine patients were left with no RN supervision, though there were nurse's aides and orderlies. Many of the patients were elderly, suffering from multiple illnesses, and requiring multiple intravenous injections. Three of the patients were intubated and ventilator-dependent.

The case was brought before the hearing panel, who found that the policy was appropriate, that the nurse was aware of the policy, and that a true emergency understaffing issue existed on the day of the occurrence. The panel found that the nurse had abandoned the patients and suspended her license for one year. Since there had been no reasonable notice given to the nursing supervisor, the supervisor had no opportunity to find a replacement nurse. When she left the floor, the RN had informed the staff that she was going to see the supervisor and that she should be paged if an emergency arose.

The case illustrates nurses' responsibility to the hospital for assisting in times of short staffing by providing reasonable patient care in as safe a manner as possible. For a variety of reasons, management is reluctant to resort to such mandatory overtime, because it is demoralizing to staff and can lead to increased absenteeism, burnout, and turnover of staff. More importantly, mandatory overtime may also be dangerous from a patient perspective, because mistakes and oversights occur more often when one is overworked and tired.

Float Staff

Float staff, or staff that is rotated from unit to unit, raises the second issue concerning overall staffing. Institutions have a duty to ensure that all areas of the institution are adequately staffed. Units temporarily overstaffed, either due to low patient census or a lower patient acuity ratio, usually float staff to units less well staffed. Floating nurses to areas with which they have less familiarity and expertise can increase potential liability for the nurse manager, but to leave another area understaffed can also increase potential liability.

Before floating staff from one area to another, nurse managers should consider staff expertise, patient care delivery systems, and patient care requirements. Nurses should be floated to units as comparable to their own as possible. From a legal perspective, the nursing care delivered by the float staff need not be perfect, but it must be consistent with that provided by a reasonably prudent nurse with similar skills and expertise under similar circumstances. This requires the nurse manager to match the nurse's home unit and float unit as much as possible or to consider negotiating with another nurse manager to cross-float the nurse. For example, a manager might float a critical care nurse to an intermediate care unit and float an intermediate care unit nurse to the floor unit. Or the manager might consider floating the general floor nurse to the postpartum floor and floating a postpartum floor nurse to labor and delivery. Open communications regarding staff limitations and concerns, along with creative solutions for staffing, can alleviate some of the potential liability and create better morale among the float nurses. A newer option is to cross-train nurses within the institution so that they are familiar with two or three areas and can competently float to areas in which they have been cross-trained.

Staff nurses have a responsibility to the employer to float to other units in times of need or overstaffing on their primary unit. This includes taking advantage of the opportunity to orient to other units in the institution so that, when floated to that unit, they already know unit policies, procedures, and are more apt to give quality nursing care. A recent case reiterates the employee's responsibility. In *David W. Francis v. Memorial General Hospital* (1986), an intensive care nurse refused to float to an orthopedic unit because he did not feel qualified to act as charge nurse on that unit. The hospital offered to orient him, but he declined and was later terminated at the institution. The court sided with the employer, noting that the employee's unwillingness to orient or even try working with hospital administration undermined his case.

Agency Personnel

The usage of *agency* (or *temporary*) *personnel* has created increased liability concerns among nurse managers. Until recently, most jurisdictions held that such personnel were considered to be independent contractors and that the institution was not liable for their actions, although their primary employment agency retained potential liability. Today, courts have begun to hold the institution liable under the principle of apparent agency or ostensible authority (whereby a principal becomes accountable for the actions of an agent). Apparent agency is created when a person (agent) holds himself or herself out as acting on behalf of the principal. In issues concerning agency nurses, the patient is unable to ascertain if the nurse works directly for the hospital (has a valid employment contract) or for a different employer. At law, lack of actual

GUIDELINES: FLOAT NURSES

Responsibilities of a nurse temporarily assigned to another unit are as follows:

1. Before accepting a patient assignment, state any hesitancy that you might have about it to appropriate persons (direct supervisor, nurse manager, or team leader). Make your objections clear and specific. Follow your verbal hesitancies with a written memo to your supervisor, and make a photocopy of the memo for your records. In the written memo, state how you would feel more comfortable in the reassignment, such as requesting a formal orientation period or more specific knowledge of the nursing routine for the new unit.

2. State your qualifications and skills concerning assessment skills, performance of routine procedures, and the like to the appropriate charge person. Thoroughly understand the patient assignment before accepting it, for, once you accept it, you are legally accountable for the nursing care of the patients and could be charged with abandonment if you choose to leave before the next shift of nurses arrives.

3. Identify your immediate resource person, and ask any questions you might have about the assignment, orders, routine procedures, and the like. Resource persons might be the charge nurse, a physician, a team member, or an interdisciplinary staff person.

4. Recognize and give yourself credit for your strengths as well as enumerating your weaknesses. Ask for help only if you truly need it, remembering that you are capable of routine nursing procedures and assessments.

5. Remember that much of the case-law involving float nurses concerns the broad area of medications. Double check references, call the pharmacist, or contact your direct supervisor prior to administering any medication about which you are unsure. If there are numerous unfamiliar medications to be given to several patients, arrange to perform more routine nursing procedures for the patients while another nurse who is familiar with the medications, unit, and patients administers all the medications.

The responsibilities of the charge nurse to whose unit a nurse is temporarily reassigned are as follows:

1. Thoroughly assess the qualifications of the reassigned nurse. Ask specific questions so that you may competently make patient assignments. Offer to orient the assigned nurse to the unit and start with the more critical policies and procedures first.

2. Make the patient assignments carefully. Refrain from taking advantage of float nurses (such as overloading them or by assigning difficult patients) merely because they are not permanent members of your staff. Float nurses may later decide to ask for permanent assignment to your unit based on your fairness and management style.

3. Continue to reassess reassigned nurses. Offer assistance as needed and follow behind them as much as possible to reassure yourself that competent patient care is being delivered.

4. Keep your immediate supervisor apprised of changes within the unit or in patient status. Whether additional help is available or not, you may escape potential liability as you correctly assess the situation and ask for help when it is needed.

5. Reassign patients as dictated by changes in their status or in the number of patients because of admissions to the unit.

6. Run interference as much as possible to assure all the nurses on the unit that you are continually balancing the needs of the patients with the individual demands and needs of the nursing staff.

7. Be aware that much of the case-law in this area involves medication errors. Be constantly available as a resource person, and ask questions to ascertain that the float person understands proper dosages, administration routes, and potential side effects. Alternately, give the medications yourself, and allow the float nurse to assume other responsibilities of direct and indirect patient care.

authority is no defense. This principle applies when it can be shown that the reasonable patient believed that the health care worker was an employee of the institution. If it appears to the reasonable patient that the worker is an employee of the institution, then the law will consider the worker an employee for the purposes of corporate and vicarious liability.

This newer trend of the law makes it imperative that the nurse manager consider temporary workers' skills, competencies, and knowledge when delegating tasks and supervising their actions. If there is reason to suspect that the temporary worker is incompetent, the nurse manager must convey this fact to the agency. The nurse manager must also either send the temporary worker home or reassign the worker to other duties and areas. The same screening procedures as those used with new institution employees should be performed with temporary workers.

Additional areas that nurse managers should stress when using agency or temporary personnel include assuring that the temporary staff member is given a short but thorough orientation to institution policies and procedures,

Guidelines: Staffing Issues

1. When you first realize that a unit will be understaffed, try to get qualified help immediately. Options include asking nurses to work overtime, coming in on a day off, floating nurses from other units, and employing temporary agency nurses.

2. Keep a record of all requests for additional staffing in a log or journal. This ensures an accurate record of what transpired should litigation develop as a result of staffing. While such a record may not prevent some liability, it will show what steps were taken and how you attempted to address the problem.

3. Make frequent visits to the understaffed unit, assessing the situation, and working with the charge nurse to set priorities. Transferring patients to other units may be a viable option, depending on the specialty of the understaffed unit and staffing in other units.

4. If you use agency nurses, assign them to fully staffed units and float one of that unit's staff to the understaffed unit. Staff RNs will probably be more help for the understaffed unit, particularly since they know the hospital policies and procedures and need to ask fewer questions.

5. Pitch in and help as you can. This includes both nursing as well as clerical tasks. Reassign ancillary personnel also to assist with clerical and non-nursing tasks, further freeing nursing staff to meet high-priority tasks.

6. Plan ahead for potential understaffing. When hiring new personnel, ascertain if they can assist with additional work time. Even four hours would be an assistance in times of short staffing, and nurses may be willing to help if they are not required to work a full 8- or 12-hour shift. Orient new employees to a least two units, so that you have more leverage in times of short staffing on one unit.

7. Talk to management about establishing a nursing resource pool or per diem nursing staff. These nurses would be knowledgeable about the hospital's policies and procedures, could be oriented to a variety of units, and are then available for just such emergencies.

is made aware of resource materials within the institution, and is briefed on documentation procedures. It is also advisable that nurse managers assign a resource person to the temporary staff member. This resource person serves in the role of mentor for the agency nurse and serves to prevent potential problems that could arise merely because the agency staff member does not know the institution routine or is unaware of where to turn for assistance. This resource person also serves as a mentor for critical decision making for the agency nurse.

EXERCISE 15-2

Terry Sanchez, an agency nurse floated to labor and delivery, was informed that a patient of Dr. Kwan, a 38-week pregnant patient, was on her way to the hospital. Dr. Kwan had a standing order that all his patients were to have fetal monitors. After placing the monitor on the patient, Terry failed to note that the patient indicated a pattern consistent with fetal distress. Dr. Kwan, arriving 45 minutes later, looked at the monitor and ordered an immediate cesarean section, but the child was born severely brain damaged. In the subsequent suit against the hospital, Dr. Kwan, and Terry Sanchez, who would be found liable and why? Which of the defendants could show absence of liability and why?

UNLICENSED ASSISTIVE PERSONNEL

As management struggles to become more cost-effective and provide for better patient outcomes, the issue of alternative patient care providers has been addressed by health care facilities. Many institutions have now employed individuals called *unlicensed assistive personnel (UAP)*, persons not authorized under respective nurse practice acts to provide direct patient care. Legal concerns about these UAPs abound.

One of the first questions that arises concerns licensure questions of RNs and LPNs/LVNs. Remember, only licensed persons are granted that license, and only they can lose it. A variety of unlicensed personnel have functioned in health care institutions for years without this question arising, including orderlies, nursing aides, nursing students from a variety of programs, and clerical workers. These persons work under the auspices and license of the institution, not the professional nurse.

Secondly, there should be an institution mechanism for the consistent and adequate orientation and training of UAPs. This will be established by nursing administration, taking into consideration how these persons will be used by the institution and where their services are most needed. Patient care responsibilities should be well delineated and UAPs must be taught when to inform other personnel of patient data (for example, vital signs) or untoward happenings. Additionally, nurses should know that they have a responsibility to inquire about expected outcomes, such as asking about the blood pressure readings for a patient scheduled to receive potent vasopressor medications or the heart rate in a patient being treated for cardiac palpitations.

Should untoward patient outcomes occur and a lawsuit be filed for negligence against the health care providers, issues that arise include the responsible delegation and supervision of UAPs. Once UAP workers are trained in the skills and tasks needed, professional nurses are responsible for the safe delegation of tasks, including follow-up to ensure that the tasks are performed, and the adequate supervision of UAPs. These are the same issues that professional nurses face daily and are not exclusive to UAPs.

A second issue is that professional nurses must ensure that the tasks delegated to UAPs are within a delegable scope of practice and that tasks requiring licensure are not delegated to UAPs. Once a task is delegated, the nurse must ensure that the action was performed and performed correctly.

As health care attempts to restructure and contain cost, it is conceivable that a variety of nurses will be used in new and innovative ways. In a recently reported pilot project, LVNs, working in consultation with RNs, were found to be capable and competent in giving selected routine, low-risk telephone instruction in an ambulatory care setting (Buccini and Ridings, 1994). Such creative, innovative ideas may be used with UAPs. The important points to be remembered are that UAPs are not to be delegated tasks requiring a license and that the UAPs are to perform the delegated tasks in a competent manner.

When deciding to use UAPs in patient care units, nursing management should consider the following factors:

1. The type of UAP support being planned and whether it is primarily supportive or patient care delivery.
2. Previous experience and the credentials the UAPs need to be eligible for employment.
3. Who is responsible for supervising the UAPs, and whether each of these potential supervisors understands both the role and the limitations of UAPs.
4. The type of staff mix to be used in the institution.
5. How professional and nonprofessional staff have been included in the work redesign efforts.
6. The specific tasks or responsibilities that will be delegated.
7. Whether the institution's policies, procedures, job descriptions, and performance evaluations match the revised roles and expectations.
8. How these changes are announced to other health care providers in the institution.
9. What types of communications are available for staff to make their concerns known.
10. What types of evaluations will be done to assess the effectiveness of UAPs (Blouin & Brent, 1995A).

HIV CASES AND NURSE MANAGER CONCERNS

The rise of HIV and AIDS has impacted the role and responsibility of nurse managers. Failure to monitor and recognize potential problems can lead to issues of liability for both the individual nurse manager and the institution. There are also ramifications for patients and the nursing staff.

Courts have consistently recognized legally protected interests in antidiscrimination, privacy and confidentiality, and workplace safety in deciding these cases (Blouin & Brent, 1995B). Appellate courts continue to wrestle with conflicting interests in deciding these cases, and many involve health care settings and staff. Nurse administrators must remain alert to potential for conflicts and weigh the varying interests carefully. If a threat to patient safety emerges, the first concern should be patient safety.

Two cases have arisen in the past few years that have direct implications for nurse managers. Both cases involved workplace safety and discrimination issues, but from very different perspectives.

In *Armstrong v. Flowers Hospital* (1994), a pregnant nurse held that she had been terminated for refusal to care for an HIV-positive patient and that this was unlawful discrimination, forcing her to choose between her unborn child and her nursing position. The case had been granted summary judgment at the trial level in favor of the defendant hospital, and the nurse appealed. The appellate court concurred with the trial court, but the analysis of the case by the court may assist nurse managers.

The nurse in this suit was a home health care nurse, with previous nursing experience in a newborn nursery. She was assigned approximately 25 patients, visiting them in their homes and providing nursing care to them. After being employed by the home health care division for about four months, she was informed that she was being assigned an HIV-positive patient, recently diagnosed with crypotococcal meningitis. The patient would require approximately four hours of care per day. He had problems with nausea and vomiting, and it would be necessary for her to draw blood work. She was to be provided sharps containers for used needles and special bags for contaminated materials.

This new patient assignment came at a time when she had just learned of her pregnancy and she had never before, to her knowledge, taken care of an HIV-positive patient. Part of her concern came from her diagnosis of gestational diabetes, which she believed would cause her immune system to be weakened, and part of her fear was because she was in the first trimester of her pregnancy, the most vulnerable time for the fetus. The nurse voiced her concerns to her supervisor and was told that she was in the best position to care for this patient. There was also a division policy stating that refusal to care for a patient could be grounds for termination. After the administrator met with the supervisor, the nurse decided that she would refuse this assignment and chose to be terminated rather than resign.

The hospital and the home health care division shared some policies, and some were different. The AIDS-universal precautions policies were identical, but a number of written policies pertained only to the hospital such as those restricting pregnant nurses from working with hepatitis B patients, patients with active herpetic lesions, or patients receiving bronchial or interstitial irradiation. After talking to a nursing supervisor at the hospital, the nurse also maintained that the hospital had an unwritten policy of assigning or at least attempting to assign isolation patients to nonpregnant nurses.

The nurse argued that her termination was based on her pregnancy, a direct violation of the Civil Rights Act of 1964, with its 1978 amendment pertaining directly to pregnancy discrimination. The purpose of the act was to ensure that employees who provided disability benefits to their employers also provided these benefits to pregnant employees unable to work because of their pregnancy and to prevent differential treatment of the pregnant employee.

Using a *disparate treatment claim,* the nurse first tried to show that she, as a pregnant employee, suffered from differential application of work or disciplinary rules. This she tried to show because of the different policies at the hospital and the home health care division. Intent to discriminate must be shown by the plaintiff. The court rejected that argument as the nurse was treated no differently than other pregnant nurses in the home health division.

The second theory, *disparate impact,* involves employment policies that appear to be neutral, but fall more harshly or disproportionately on one group of employees and cannot be justified by a business necessity. Intent to discriminate is not necessary with this cause of action. The emphasis is on the effect of the policy, not its intent.

The nurse's argument under this approach was that she was placed in the difficult position of choosing between her fetus and her job, a choice placed only on pregnant employees. The court was unsympathetic with this approach. The court acknowledged that the nurse had offered evidence that a pregnant employee is more susceptible to contagious diseases than the nonpregnant employee and that contagious diseases may be communicated by the mother to her fetus. However, the court could find no evidence presented that these risks were comparable to any risk for which the hospital or the home health care division made an accommodation to the pregnant employee.

The plaintiff also argued that an employer must make the decision easier by offering alternative work. To the contrary, held the court, an employer normally is prohibited from deciding what course of action is best for pregnant employees. The court further contended that the plaintiff was, in reality, arguing for the preferential treatment of pregnant workers. The preferential treatment would consist of accommodation of the pregnant employee's concerns with respect to the risks for herself and her unborn child through rescheduling of nursing assignments at the expense of nonpregnant workers who would have no right to refuse the assignment. The Pregnancy Discrimination Act does not require preferential treatment.

This case is unusual in its application. Previous discrimination suits had dealt with health care workers and patients who are HIV-positive, and this appears to be the first case in which a person had argued that the requirement to attend an HIV-positive individual constitutes discrimination. Because of the widespread fear of HIV and AIDS, individuals who are concerned about exposure to virus in the workplace are expected to bring future lawsuits.

This case should be helpful to nursing managers and administration for a number of reasons. One is the policy that the hospital and home health care division did not discriminate against pregnant workers. A reverse policy would have been almost impossible to defend from a discrimination perspective. As the court said, "Title VII [of the Civil Rights Act] does not require employers to treat employees with kindness" (*Armstrong v. Flowers Hospital,* 1994, at 1317).

Second, the policies of the two entities were identical with respect to the treatment of patients who are HIV-positive. If the policies had differed, the court might have looked more closely at the accommodation of the pregnant worker by one entity and not the other. At it was, there was no discrimination or differential treatment of the pregnant worker by either entity.

Third, the home health care division was consistent in its application of the rule regarding the treatment of all patients. Additional factors that allowed the hospital to prevail were the timely introduction of materials relating to universal precautions during the nurse's orientation and the rationale for assigning the HIV-positive patient to her care. She was the most available to care for the patient at the present time. Lastly, the supervisor and administrator discussed with the nurse her options and left the decision to her. There was no appearance of callous indifference in this instance.

Interestingly, the court seemed to take note of the fact that the nurse had not consulted her primary physician about the increased risk of infection to herself or her fetus, nor did she inquire about the availability of gowns, masks, and other items that would further protect her while caring for the patient. This lack of inquiry served to show the court that she had already made up her mind and was not open to alternative approaches.

Nurse managers should hesitate before making assignments that accommodate pregnant nurses and serve to single them out as a class. Preferential treatment of pregnant nurses may not pass legal scrutiny and may place the hospital in a discrimination suit by male nurses, since this opens the way for a gender-based discrimination charge.

The second case that affects this area of the law is *Ramirez v. Oklahoma Department of Mental Health* (1994). In that case, an HIV-positive mental health aide was accused of roughly treating a mental patient. Specifically, the aide had grabbed her tightly and dug his fingernails into her skin, causing contusions and abrasions. The patient was examined and the injuries noted. The examining psychiatrist and other team members were all aware of the HIV status of the aide and that the patient was now at risk of infection. The team members filed a patient grievance with their superiors in the Department of Mental Health (DMH).

Less than two months later, all members filing the grievance received notices of proposed adverse personnel actions against them for failure to follow the DMH policies regarding discrimination against individuals with AIDS and for misconduct in using the wrong form to report the alleged misconduct. Two members of the team were either terminated (the psychiatrist) or transferred (the nurse), with the transfer affecting her seniority and promotion prospects.

These two members of the team brought this action against the DMH, claiming that the defendants wrongfully took personnel actions against them in retaliation for their having exercised their freedom of speech to report an incident of patient abuse and possibly lethal infection. They requested monetary damages and reinstatement to their prior positions. The lower court granted the defendants' motion to dismiss and the appellate court reversed that decision.

The court first addressed the issue of governmental immunity, rejecting that in part because the aide was not a governmental official and in part because the attorneys and hearing officers for the defendant violated clearly established rights. The court then addressed the first amendment freedom of speech contention, concluding that the nurse and psychiatrist correctly expressed their first amendment rights consistent with their professional duties and ethics. The court then stated that the issue of the right of a public employee as a citizen to express comments on matters of public concern and the right of a governmental entity to ensure the efficiency of the public services it performs had to be balanced. This latter concern included the retaliation cause of action brought by the two members of the mental health team. The court found that the timing of the adverse personnel actions, plus the giving of seemingly inconsequential reasons for disciplinary action (the filing of the wrong grievance form), and a secret agreement between the attorney for the DMH and the aide to discipline the team members in exchange for the aide not filing suit supported the inference of a retaliatory action.

Although the major concern of the hospital seemed to be liability to the aide, and the concern is understandable given the various legal protections given to individuals who are HIV-positive, the court concerned itself with workplace safety issues in general and with the safety of patients in particular. In the event that the two collide, the court clearly believed that patient safety should prevail. And in this case the threat was an actual one since the patient had suffered abrasions and contusions at the hands of an HIV-positive aide. Had the danger to the patient been only a potential one, such as with the handling of a patient who did not pose a risk for the transfer of the HIV virus, the court might well have found in favor of protecting the employee against possible discrimination. The lesson for the nurse manager seems to be to err on the side of safety, particularly in the face of clear-cut danger.

Personnel actions should still be handled carefully, with impartial investigation and confidentiality. Personnel matters must be handled with tact, impartial procedures, and rationales given for actions taken.

EXERCISE 15-3

Does your institution have personnel policies concerning HIV-positive status? If so, are they written? Do they outline need for confidentiality, grievance procedures, and procedures for refusing patient assignments if such assignments will potentially harm the HIV-positive worker?

POLICIES AND PROCEDURES

Risk management is a process that identifies, analyzes, and treats potential hazards within a setting. The object of risk management is to identify potential hazards and to eliminate them before anyone is harmed or disabled. Written *policies and procedures* fall within the scope of risk management activities, and they are a requirement of JCAHO. These documents set standards of care for the institution and direct practice. They must be clearly stated, well delineated, and based on current practice. Nurse managers should review the policies and procedures frequently for compliance and timeliness. If policies are outdated or absent, request the appropriate person or committee either to update or to initiate the policy.

SUMMARY

Nurse managers are both employees and employers. As managers, they have an obligation to be aware of pertinent laws and litigation that impact what managers may or may not do. As employees, they have many of the same rights as staff nurses. Effective managers balance these two concepts to enhance patient care delivery.

AFTER COMPLETING THIS CHAPTER, YOU SHOULD BE ABLE TO

- Compare and contrast the doctrines of respondeat superior, vicarious liability, and personal liability from a nursing management perspective.
- Define three separate issues concerning temporary staffing from the aspect of legal liability.
- Define and evaluate the role of unlicensed assistive personnel in relationship to professional accountability.
- Describe the significance of the recent National Labor Relations Board changes in defining supervisory personnel and its effect on professional nursing.
- Describe the goals of risk management.

APPLY YOUR LEGAL KNOWLEDGE

- What are the most common potential legal liabilities for nurse administration and nurse managers in health care settings?
- How can these areas of potential liability be minimized or avoided?
- Is there a role for ancillary personnel within the current health care delivery system?
- By what mechanisms can professional nursing minimize the impact of the recent National Labor Relations Board's definition of supervision in nursing? Can nursing make a difference?

REFERENCES

Armstrong v. Flowers Hospital, 33 F.3d 1308 (11th Cir., 1994).

Blouin, A. S., & Brent, N. J. (1995A). Unlicensed assistive personnel: Legal considerations. *Nursing Management, 23*(11), 7–8, 21.

Blouin, A. S., & Brent, N. J. (1995B). Legal concerns related to workers with HIV or AIDS. *Nursing Management, 25*(1), 17–18.

Buccini, R., & Ridings, L. (1994). Using licensed vocational nurses to provide telephone patient instructions in a health maintenance organization. *Journal of Nursing Administration, 24*(1), 27–33.

Daldulav v. St. Mary Nazareth Hospital Center, Docket No. 62737 (Illinois, 1987).

David W. Francis v. Memorial General Hospital, 726 P.2d 852 (New Mexico, 1986).

Fiesta, J. (1994). Legal update for nurses. Part II: assigning, delegating, and staffing. *Nursing Management, 24*(2), 14–16.

Harrell v. Louis Smith Memorial Hospital, 397 S.E.2d 746 (Georgia, 1990).

Husbert v. Commissioner of Education, 591 N.Y.S. 99 (New York, 1992).

Journal of Health and Hospital Law. (1991). 5(12), 380.

Karnes v. Doctor's Hospital, 555 N.E.2d 280 (Ohio, 1990).

Ramirez v. Oklahoma Department of Mental Health, 10 IER Cases 102 (10th Cir., 1994).

St. Paul Medical Center v. Cecil, 842 S.W.2d 809 (Texas, 1992).

Trudeau, S. (1992). *Hospital Law Newsletter.* March.

· sixteen

Contract Principles

PREVIEW

Nurses are becoming entrepreneurs, freelancing as consultants and educational special-ists, and entering into partnerships with other health care providers. As they become more independent of the hospital setting, understanding and knowing aspects of contract law be-come imperative. Some hospital nurses have had formal, written contracts, although the majority of nurses working in noncollective bargaining states and institutions are truly bet-ter classified as at-will employees. This chapter outlines contract law, defining the various aspects of formal and informal contracts, and concludes with a discussion of legal issues in-volved in contract law.

contracts	contract termination	mediation
statute of frauds	breach	arbitration
formal contract	monetary damages	fact finding
oral contract	injunctions	summary jury trial
expressed contract	specific performance	contract negotiation
implied contract		

CONTRACT PRINCIPLES

A *contract* is a legally binding agreement made between two or more persons to do or to refrain from doing certain actions. Every contract, to be enforceable by law, has the following features:

1. There must be *promises* or *agreements* made between two or more persons or entities for the performance of an action or for restraint from doing certain actions. Most nursing contracts specify the conditions and performances that nurses will undertake, but contracts may also be made to prevent certain actions.
2. There must be *mutual understanding* of the terms and meaning of the contract by all parties to the contract.
3. There must be *compensation*, something of value, in exchange for the action or inaction expressed by the contract terms. Usually this compensation is monetary, such as a specified salary or dollar-per-hour earned wage, but other items of value may be seen as compensation.
4. The contract must fulfill a *lawful* purpose. There can be no enforceable contract for illegal acts or fraud.

Legal Elements of a Contract

Legally, a contract has four elements:

1. *Offer:* The person or the entity (a hospital or home health care agency) extends an offer to someone to be hired or with whom it will have a contractual relationship. The person extending the offer is the *offeror*, and the person to whom the contract is extended is the *offeree.*
2. *Acceptance:* The actual accepting or agreeing to the terms and conditions of the contract creates the contract. Acceptance may be done in

written form, or it may be verbally accepted. Contracts may also be accepted by the beginning performance of the offeree, such as when the nurse shows up promptly on the first day of work in a new position.

Exceptions to verbal acceptance have been created by the law. The *statute of frauds* is the legal principle stating that a contract does not need to be written to be enforceable. Exceptions to this statute include agreements involving marriage, the sale of land or interests in land, the sale of goods over a certain dollar figure, suretyship (agreements to pay or perform actions in the event that the principal is unable to meet his or her obligations), and agreements that cannot be performed within a 12-month period.

3. *Consideration:* This element concerns the economic costs of an agreement. Consideration is what is negotiated between offeror and offeree. Often consideration is seen as the salary figure or dollar figure per hour worked, but consideration may also include a set fee per unit of work or other objects of value.

4. *Consent* (sometimes referred to as *mutuality of agreement and obligation*): This element involves the mutual assent to the agreement, or actions that lead the parties to the contract to reasonably believe that an agreement has been reached. As with acceptance, the beginning performance by the offeree would indicate consent to the contract to both parties.

Consent also involved the competency of the parties to the contract to enter into a valid contract. Issues that courts of law evaluate in determining competency include the age of the parties (adults versus those under the age of majority) and the mental capacity to understand the terms and meanings of the contract.

Additional issues that may be considered include the *legality* or *lawful purpose* of the contract. Courts of law do not enforce contracts made for other than lawful purposes. Contracts that provide for criminal or tortious actions or actions opposed to public policy will not be enforced. Thus the entire range of criminal and tort law is incorporated into this element.

TYPES OF CONTRACTS

A *formal contract* is one that is required by law to be in writing. To prevent fraudulent practices, all states have statutes of fraud requiring certain contracts to be in written form. Some formal contracts also require that they be written under seal, stamped with an official seal, or written on a special imprinted paper. All other contracts are considered *simple contracts,* whether written or oral.

An *oral contract* is as equally binding as a written contract, though the terms of the contract may be more difficult to prove in courts of law. The terms of the contract are subject to memory and interpretation, and often there is a change in personnel during the term of the contract, causing new interpretations of the contract. For these reasons, most contracts are written and include language that they survive the employment of the original signers.

An *expressed contract* concerns terms and conditions that were specifically negotiated or discussed during the creation of the contract. These expressed terms may be either oral or written, and both parties to the contract must have the opportunity to either question or renegotiate the expressed terms at the time of entering the contract. An *implied contract* concerns terms or conditions of the contract that each side anticipated were a part of the contract, but were never actually expressed or discussed. Most expressed contracts have some implied provisions as well. For example, the nurse is expected to perform quality, safe nursing care and to follow the policies and procedures of the hospital even though such expectations are not explicitly written or verbalized, and the employer is expected to provide a safe work site for the employee and to have the necessary supplies and equipment to ensure competent nursing care.

Individual contracts are negotiated between a single individual and the offeror, while *collective contracts* are negotiated by collective bargaining units for the benefit of the unit. Most individual contracts are informally offered and accepted, while collective contracts are negotiated formally, specifying all particulars of the contract, and accepted in writing.

EXERCISE 16-1

Obtain a copy of the contract used in your health care facility, if one exists. Which terms are expressed? Which terms affecting nursing practice are silent? If you were the nurse who was to sign the contract, how would you attempt to negotiate the contract differently?

TERMINATION OF A CONTRACT

Contract termination signifies that the terms of the contract have been fulfilled or that the parties to the contract agree to the contract's end. Sometimes the term "released" from a contract is used to indicate its ending point. A release implies that the contract had not been completely fulfilled, but that there has been no breach. In individual employment contracts with health care agencies, the offeree traditionally writes a letter of resignation, and the employer-offeror releases the employee from any further obligations under the terms of the contract.

A second means of terminating a contract is by *breach,* which is essentially the failure of one or both of the parties to abide by the agreement and to meet the contractual obligations. For example, if an employee agrees to work at a health care facility for a period of no less than 12 months in return for a sign-on bonus and leaves the institution after eight months, the employee has breached the contract. Remedies for breach of a contract include monetary damages, injunctions, and specific performance.

Monetary damages are the usual remedy for breach of contractual obligations. Because the underlying goal in breach of contract suits is to place damaged or injured parties in as good a position as they would have been if the provisions of the contract had been fulfilled, the court allows injured parties to be compensated monetarily. In the preceding example, the nurse may be required to pay back the entire sign-on bonus previously received or a prorated portion of it.

If the employer breaches the terms of the contract, the employee wrongfully discharged may bring suit for lost salary and other economic benefits that had been agreed on by the terms of the contract. The injured employee may also ask for reinstatement as well as monetary damages.

The injured party may request *injunctions,* which are court orders requiring a person to refrain from doing a specific act. The hospital in the preceding example may ask the court to issue an injunction against the nurse, preventing him or her from working at another health care facility for the remainder of the contract term. Although injunctions are not often requested, injured parties may seek injunctive relief, particularly if the business concerns a specialty trade or craft. Injunctions may also be obtained preventing a former employee from contacting individuals served by the business. In a company that has spent years building an established clientele, the company may seek an injunction preventing the former employee from contacting, either directly or indirectly, any of the persons doing business with the previous employer.

Specific performance is enforcement by the court to comply with the terms of the contract. The court could force the breaching employee to work the remainder of the four months of the contract, having already received the sign-on bonus. Again this is seldom sought as a remedy by the injured party since morale and work performance become problematic when workers are forced to stay in jobs or positions after they have either left or announced their decision to leave.

ALTERNATIVE DISPUTE RESOLUTIONS

Nurses are frequently reluctant to challenge contract disputes in courts of law because of the harm they perceive to their reputation and the time that such suits take from their personal and professional lives. Because of such concerns, there are now alternative means of resolving contract disputes. The contract as signed should have a provision that alternative dispute resolution processes will be used as needed.

Mediation

Mediation allows the disputing parties to resolve differences while maintaining a professional relationship. Mediators are neutral third parties who facilitate disputes by assisting both parties to identify their specific needs and concerns and to work toward an agreeable solution. Costs of using mediators are usually shared by the parties, and several consultants offer this service.

Arbitration

Arbitration involves the selection of a neutral third party arbitrator who is knowledgeable in the area of contention and who renders a decision and award. Often used in employment contract disputes, the neutral third parties are knowledgeable about working conditions, terms of employment contracts, and factors leading to such disputes. They are empowered to make final decisions, and their decisions are usually binding to both sides of the dispute, although the parties can agree in advance that the decision will not be binding. Arbitration is used with collective bargaining disputes, and both sides must realize that the arbitrator's decision, unlike the mediator's decision, becomes binding on both sides of the dispute.

Fact Finding

The *fact finding* alternative dispute resolution process is normally reserved for complex multistate and multiparty disputes. Again, a neutral party is employed to sort out the various facts of the dispute and to assist the parties in knowing all the facts of the dispute, from the perspective of all the parties to the dispute.

Summary Jury Trial

A *summary jury trial* is an abbreviated, privately held trial that may be used to give both sides of the dispute an indication of the strengths and weaknesses of their case and the potential outcome should they decide to seek trial resolution.

NURSES AND CONTRACTS

Understanding contracts may not significantly alter one's nursing care, but such an understanding can aid nurses in their decisions to accept positions and can increase job security and satisfaction by giving them some control within the work setting. Remember, however, that nurses must be satisfied with all the terms of the contract before accepting it. Nurses' bargaining power is in knowing exactly what they want in the work setting and in negotiating for it before the contract is accepted. There is no negotiating power once the contract is accepted. *Contract negotiation* is therefore an important skill for nurses.

Nurses can negotiate for individual employment contracts with health care facilities, as individual consultants for educational purposes, as consultants to improve effective management principles in a given facility, and as independent contractors. As the numbers of options increase for self-employed nurses, contracts will become more vital and prolific. Such self-employment contracts should specifically state the relationship of the parties, their duties and responsibilities, the payment schedule, the professional liability insurance payment, the length of contract, and dispute resolution provisions.

Nurses may also contract with other agencies during the course of operating a privately owned business. For example, a nurse or group of nurses may decide to open a home health care agency. Contracts are needed for employees hired as direct patient care givers, for clerical workers, for space rentals for the agency, and for dealing with other agencies who deal with the home health care agency as durable medical suppliers and suppliers of supplies and tangibles. Contracts also have to be made with the clients of the agency. The terms, both expressed and implied, must be understood and the home health care agency must ensure that all provisions are expressly contracted. Nurses entering such formal, multiparty contracts are encouraged to seek legal representation for all contract negotiations, particularly since state laws vary. A variety of nursing consultants specialize in this area of the law, and a variety of law firms offer this expertise.

For nurses negotiating or trying to understand individual employment contracts with health care agencies, the following guidelines are offered (see next page).

EXERCISE 16-2

You are negotiating a contract for work as an independent contractor to review legal cases for a large law firm specializing in medical malpractice law. What provisions should you insist be included in the contract? What other terms would you like to see negotiated into the contract? What are some advantages to being an independent contractor versus a part-time employee in this type of work?

CONTRACTS THAT ARISE AFTER EMPLOYMENT

Courts have held that contracts may arise after employment, even in states with employment-at-will doctrines and the absence of collective bargaining units. Statements in employee manuals or handbooks may serve to create a valid contract and prevent the discharge of an employee, just as oral statements made to entice a person to take the position may create contract language.

In *Sides v. Duke* (1985), a nurse moved from Michigan to North Carolina, accepting a position from which she was told she could be discharged only for cause, and incompetency was specified as the sole cause for discharge. While at the health care setting, she refused to administer a medication that she believed would injure a patient, and indeed the patient was injured after another nurse gave the medication. During that patient's malpractice suit against the hospital and physician, Ms. Sides was told not to tell the whole truth by the defendants and their counsel. When Ms. Sides testified to the true matter, she was discharged by the hospital.

Guidelines: Negotiating an Individual Employment Contract

Before accepting a contract with a potential employer:

1. Address employment practices and ensure that you are aware of the following:
   a. Exact work hours and schedules
   b. Time off, including individual days off, vacation time, and sick leave
   c. Float policies
   d. Mandatory or requested days off without pay
   e. Accruement of vacation and sick time
   f. Periodic evaluations, including their purpose and by whom they are made
   g. Style of nursing care, as primary or team nursing
   h. Philosophy of nursing
   i. Status of the institution, either as a collective bargaining unit or employment-at-will
   j. Classification of nurses as Staff Nurse I, II, or III and how to advance from one level to the next
   k. Orientation time and educational expectations
   l. Number of required hours of continuing education per year
   m. Leaves of absence such as bereavement, medical, jury duty, and personal leaves
   n. Seniority and how it is accrued, how it affects temporary and permanent work reductions, and how it is lost
   o. Grievance procedures
   p. Existence of clinical ladder programs, qualifications, and when the employee becomes eligible to apply for such programs
   q. Use of private car for transportation, as applicable
2. Understand the payment scale in the following areas:
   a. Base salary
   b. Differentials for evening and night shift work, charge nurse responsibilities, working specific units as intensive or intermediate care, weekend shift work, holiday pay, and salary differences for degrees, certification, and/or years of experience
   c. Raises, either as cost of living or merit

    d. Number of paid holidays per year and restrictions on when they may be taken

    e. Change in base scale for clinical ladder positions

    f. Reimbursement for usage of private car, as applicable

3. Ask about benefits and who pays the cost of such benefits as the following:

    a. Group hospitalization, vision, and dental plans

    b. Term life insurance policies

    c. Retirement plan

    d. Parking

    e. Savings programs and employer-sponsored credit union

    f. Conversion of accrued sick leave and vacation time to terminal pay

    g. Professional liability insurance

    h. Child care facilities

    i. Housing

    j. Formal education reimbursement programs

    k. Insurance for private car as needed to see patients in home settings

In her suit for wrongful discharge, she argued two theories of law: contract and tort. She successfully convinced the jury that the move from Michigan to North Carolina, plus the statement that she could be discharged only for incompetency created an employment contract. Her expectations, based on the employer's statements, changed an at-will employment to a contractual employment.

Some courts have also held that employee handbooks create a contractual relationship by language that offers continued employment. Coupling with the employee's continued work converts that offer to a formal contract (Aiken & Catalano, 1994).

SUMMARY

Contracts serve as a basis for employment relationships between businesses and the personnel they employ. Contracts also serve as a basis for independent practice by nurses such as contracts for self-employment, contracts for consultant roles, or contracts for nurse executive positions. An understanding and appreciation of this area of the law is needed to ensure that the contract effectively protects the professional nurse.

AFTER COMPLETING THIS CHAPTER, YOU SHOULD BE ABLE TO

- Define and describe the terms used in contract law.
- Describe the four elements of a valid contract.
- Define the statute of frauds and its relationship to contract law.
- Define the types of contracts, and give examples when each type would be used.
- Describe three remedies for breach of contract law.
- Describe the purpose of alternative dispute resolutions, and give four means by which resolutions may be performed.
- Describe how contracts may arise after employment.

APPLY YOUR LEGAL KNOWLEDGE

- What are the advantages of having all nursing contracts in writing as opposed to oral agreements?
- Why would one include alternative dispute resolutions in a contract? When would these provisions be used?
- How does having a formal contract with the employing hospital assist staff nurses in the delivery of competent, safe nursing care?
- What are three advantages for nurses in understanding contract law?

REFERENCES

Aiken, T. D. & Catalano, J. T. (1994). *Legal, ethical, and political issues in nursing.* Philadelphia, PA: F. A. Davis Company.

Sides v. Duke, 74 N. C. App.3d 331, 328 S.E. 2d 818 (North Carolina, 1985).

• seventeen

Federal Laws: The Americans with Disabilities Act of 1990 and The Civil Rights Act of 1991

PREVIEW

The Americans with Disabilities Act (ADA) of 1990 and the Civil Rights Act of 1991 were both signed into legislation during the term of President George Bush. Both acts have significant implications for health care delivery. The ADA affects health care providers as well as consumers, with various sections of the act addressing the hiring and retention of providers as well as access to health care. The Civil Rights Act of 1991 also affects both health care providers and consumers. This chapter explores both acts, defining the purposes, applications, pertinent case-law, and projected futures of both.

The Americans with Disabilities Act of 1990	essential job functions	quid pro quo sexual harassment
disability	Civil Rights Act of 1991	hostile work environment
reasonable accommodations	undue hardship	preferential treatment
	sexual harassment	

THE AMERICANS WITH DISABILITIES ACT OF 1990 (ADA)

Background of the Act

On July 26, 1990, George Bush signed *The Americans with Disabilities Act of 1990 (ADA)* into law, providing comprehensive protection to Americans with disabilities. The ADA is one of the most significant pieces of legislature since the Civil Rights Act of 1964 and was seen by its sponsors as "the Emancipation Act of disabled persons." The Act had been necessitated by the discrimination faced by HIV/AIDS individuals, since those persons identified loopholes not adequately addressed by previous laws, both state and federal.

Bills were originally introduced in the 100th Congress, with joint hearings on the bills occurring in September 1988. Although many senators and representatives cosponsored the legislation by the end of that Congressional term, the bills never came out of committee.

Stating that the bill was too vague as originally proposed, the 101st Congress conducted several hearings on the bill. The Senate, in September 1989, and the House of Representatives, in May 1990, passed the bill by overwhelming margins. A Conference Committee approved the bill on July 13, 1990, and the bill was enacted on July 26, 1990.

In enacting the ADA, Congress was faced with the challenge of combining two legal concepts: disability and equality. The aim was to assure equality for the disabled, without undue hardships being placed on those regulated by the Act.

Covered Entities

Title I primarily covers employment provisions and is perhaps the best known portion of the ADA. The Act defines a "covered entity" as an employer, employment agency, or labor organization of joint labor-management committee. While the act was originally restricted to employers of 25 or more employees, the act now applies to all employers who have 15 or more employees. The United States, corporations wholly owed by the United States, Indian tribes, and bona fide tax-exempt private membership clubs are not included within the definition of employer. State governments, governmental agencies, and political subdivisions, though not specifically included in the Act, were intended by Congress to be part of the ADA.

While the ADA does not exclude religious organizations, it does authorize them to give preference in employment to their own members and to require that applicants and employees conform to their religious tenets.

Definition of Disability

The ADA defines *disability* broadly. Individuals are covered if:

1. The disability is a physical or mental impairment that substantially limits one or more of the major life enjoyments of the person.
2. There is a record of such impairment.
3. The individuals are being regarded as having such an impairment.

A *physical or mental impairment* includes:

1. Any physiologic disorder or condition, cosmetic disfigurement, or anatomical loss affecting one or more of the following body systems: neurological, musculoskeletal, special sense organ, respiratory (including speech organs), cardiovascular, reproductive, digestive, genitourinary, hemic, lymphatic, skin, and endocrine.
2. Any mental or psychological disorder such as mental retardation, organic brain syndrome, emotional or mental illness, and specific learning disabilities. Conditions that would qualify under this definition include diabetes, cancer, heart diseases, AIDS, as well as those persons recovering from alcoholism and drug abuse.

The existence of a disability is determined without regard to the availability of alleviating measures such as medicines and prosthetic devices. Thus the fact that a physical or mental impairment may be successfully treated with a medicine or remedial device does not remove the impairment from the ADA coverage of disabilities.

The ADA does not regard advancing age as an impairment, but illnesses associated with advanced age such as hearing loss, arthritis, and impairment of gait would constitute impairments.

Major life events are defined as fundamental activities that the average person in the general population can perform with little or no difficulty such as caring for oneself, performing manual tasks, walking, seeing, hearing, speaking, breathing, learning, and working. *Substantially limits* is defined as (1) the inability to perform a major life activity that the average person in the general population can perform, or (2) a significant restriction as to the condition, manner, or duration under which a person can perform a particular major life activity as compared to the condition, manner, or duration under which the average person in the general population can perform that same major life activity.

A *record of impairment* is someone who has a history of, or has been classified as having, a mental or physical impairment that substantially limits one or more of the major life activities. This provision is intended to ensure that the covered entities do not discriminate against individuals because they have a history of a disability or because they have been misclassified as being disabled. This clause was included because Congress clearly intended to prohibit discrimination against individuals with disabilities based on society's myths and unfounded fears about disabilities.

A *qualified individual* is a person who can safely perform all aspects of the job with or without reasonable accommodations. The employer has the right to demand that individuals do not pose any threats to the safety of themselves or others.

Reasonable accommodations refer to the employers' responsibilities to provide the necessary structure, reassignment, and equipment modifications or devices, interpreters, or other reasonable needs that would allow the disabled person to perform the job satisfactorily. Employees and potential employees should be prepared to inform the employer of modifications or special needs that will accommodate them. Reasonable accommodations may be so simple as providing telephone devices so that the hearing-impaired person applying for the position of telephone switchboard operator can qualify for the position. Other reasonable accommodations include job restructuring, part-time or modified work, provision of qualified readers or interpreters, or reassignment to another position.

To meet the qualifications of this section, employers must also identify *essential job functions*. These functions are based on the employer's judgment, the job description, and amount of time performing the given function. The purpose of such a provision is to ensure that, if qualified disabled applicants apply for a job, they will not be discriminated against because of nonessential job functions that they are not able to perform. Note, though, if there are other, better or equally qualified nondisabled applications, the employer does not have to hire the disabled person. The issue arises when more qualified disabled applicants are passed over for less qualified, nondisabled applicants.

EXERCISE 17-1

Review all the components and skills used in nursing staff performance. If you were to author a list of the staff nurse's essential job functions, what essential job functions would you want to include? What are the staff nurse's nonessential functions? Explain your answers.

Exclusions from the Definition of Disability

There are many exclusions from the definition of disability under the ADA. The ADA excludes homosexuality and bisexuality from its coverage. It further excludes transvestism, transsexualism, pedophilia, exhibitionism, voyeurism, gender identity disorders not resulting from physical impairments, and other sexual behavior disorders. The ADA does not protect compulsive gamblers, kleptomaniacs, pyromaniacs, and those who currently use illegal drugs. Moreover, the employer may hold alcoholics to the same qualifications and job performance standards as other employees even if the unsatisfactory behavior or performance is directly related to the alcoholism.

PROVISIONS OF THE ADA

The ADA is closely related to the *Civil Rights Act of 1964* and incorporates the antidiscrimination principles established in Section 504 of the Rehabilitation Act of 1973. There are five titles in the ADA.

Title I

Title I of the ADA prohibits employment discrimination, adopting the remedies and procedures provided by Title VII of the Civil Rights Act of 1964. This title also incorporates the concepts of reasonable accommodation and undue hardship that was established in parts of the Rehabilitation Act.

The purpose of this section is to ensure that people with disabilities are not excluded from job opportunities or adversely affected in any other aspect of employment unless they are not qualified or otherwise unable to perform the job. This protects qualified and disabled individuals in regard to application, salary, promotions, discharge, transfer, and all other aspects of work.

The ADA's prohibition against employment discrimination extends to medical examinations and inquiries on applications. The employer is not allowed to ask about disabilities or to ask about the extent of obvious disabilities. The employer may make inquiries into the ability of the applicant to fulfill the job requirements. A medical examination may be conducted after a job offer has been extended to the disabled person and provided that all applicants for the position are subjected to the same examinations. Drug testing to determine the illegal usage of drugs may be performed since such screens are not considered medical examinations. Depending on the job, employers may make inquiries about disabilities if the inquiry is job-related and consistent with business necessity. Employers may also conduct voluntary medical examinations that are part of an employee health program made available to all employees at the work site.

Defenses that the employer has to the ADA include *undue hardship.* This provision is available if the accommodation to be made is extremely expensive or difficult to implement. The act provides that the employer must investigate the required accommodations and offer data proving this hardship.

Undue hardships are based on cost, numbers of employees, and type of business enterprise.

Other possible defenses include public safety defense and health and safety defense. Under these two defenses, the employer must show that reasonable accommodation cannot prevent potential compromised safety and health hazards to others in the workplace. For example, health care institutions have requirements that persons with contagious diseases may not work in the facility during the active phase of the illness. As stated earlier, religious employers may give preference to individuals of the same religious sect.

Title II

Title II of the ADA prohibits discrimination against disabled individuals by any state or local government entity without regard to the receipt of federal funds and includes comprehensive provisions designed to ensure access to and use of public transportation by disabled persons. Title II incorporates the remedies and procedures set forth by the Rehabilitation Act.

Title III

Title III prohibits discrimination by public accommodations against individuals on the basis of disability in the full and equal enjoyment of the entity's goods, services, facilities, privileges, advantages, or accommodations. This title mandates the removal of architectural and structural barriers and the provision of auxiliary aids and services in many cases. Public accommodations are required to remove barriers in existing facilities if such removal can be accomplished without substantial difficulty or expense. However, newly constructed facilities and major renovations of existing structures must be designed to be readily accessible to and usable by individuals with disabilities. Title III also includes provisions on discrimination in transportation services provided by private entities. The title incorporates remedies and procedures from the Civil Rights Act of 1964.

Title IV

Title IV is designed to ensure that individuals with speech and hearing impairments have meaningful access to and use of telephone services. The ADA requires common carriers that are engaged in intrastate and interstate communications to provide telecommunications relay services to individuals with hearing and speech impairments.

Title V

Title V contains miscellaneous provisions, including some construction clauses. Provisions under this section include the statement that the ADA does not invalidate or limit other federal or state laws, allows insurance carriers to continue classifying risks in the manner consistent with state laws, and prohibits retaliation against persons who file discrimination charges under the act or who assist others in filing such charges.

LAWSUITS UNDER THE ADA

Court cases have challenged various aspects of the ADA during the last five years. One of the early challenges to the ADA concerned mandatory HIV testing. In *Leckelt v. Board of Commissioners* (1990), the court upheld the dismissal of a nurse for refusal to take an HIV antibody test. The court reasoned that the nurse was not otherwise qualified because he refused to take a test that the court felt was consistent with appropriate infection control procedures. Even though the likelihood that Leckelt would transmit an HIV infection was low, the hospital policy was justifiable given the hospital's need to protect patients.

This view had been rejected by the Supreme Court in *School Board v. Arline* (1987), a pre-ADA case. In that case, the Supreme Court had rejected the claim that HIV presented a direct threat to the public, given the fact that HIV cannot, in most circumstances, be transmitted in the workplace. The *Arline* standard also prohibited discrimination against HIV-infected individuals, who with reasonable accommodations, could perform jobs in the workplace.

A 1994 court case held that asthma did not fit within the definition of handicapped since asthma did not constitute a "substantial limitation of a major life activity" within the meaning of the Rehabilitation Act of 1973 (*Heilweil v. Mount Sinai Hospital*). If brought under the ADA, asthma would qualify as a disability within the broad definition of qualified individuals. This case serves to point out difficulties with loopholes in previous acts meant to protect and assist the disabled.

A second 1994 case held that a former employee had no claim under the ADA when the employee failed to suggest reasonable accommodations (*Derbon v. United States Shoe Corporation*). The employee insisted that she needed no accommodation despite a medical report stating that she would. Her actions prevented the employer from considering any reasonable accommodations, and the court concluded that the plaintiff had failed to create a genuine issue of fact as to whether she could perform the essentials functions of her job with or without her employer's reasonable accommodations.

In a case brought against an independent contractor at a California hospital, the court held that Title III of the ADA did not apply to physicians who work in hospitals as independent contractors (*Aikins v. St. Helena Hospital*, 1994). The plaintiff, a deaf person, had brought this action alleging that the hospital and the attending physician had discriminated against her because of her disability when they failed to provide an interpreter for her.

The court centered its discussion on the regulation that Title III concerned entities owing, leasing, or operating a place of public accommodation. Thus, persons can be liable under this ADA provision only if they have some measure of control over the place providing the services. Since, in this case, the physician was an independent contractor, he had no control over the place providing the services and also had no liability.

The court noted the distinction between physicians providing care in hospitals, where they had no control, and providing care in their own offices, where they had control. The ADA defines a public accommodation as including the professional office of a health care provider. Additionally, the court held that the hospital could be held liable for the failure to provide an interpreter to the plaintiff, unless the hospital could show that the provision of such services was an undue hardship.

In *Bradley v. University of Texas M.D. Anderson Cancer Center* (1993), the court held that the reassignment by a hospital of an HIV-positive surgical assistant to another department within the facility did not violate the ADA. In this case, the court reasoned that, since his continued employment in the operating suite would pose a substantial threat of harm to patients, Bradley could not perform the essential functions of a surgical assistant.

An area that the courts are now attempting to define is the interaction between the ADA and the professional discipline of nursing. The impact of the ADA has forced alternatives in testing for impaired candidates and non–public disposition of nurses in treatment for substance abuse. The ADA appears to restrict discipline options in cases involving drug abuse, alcohol abuse, and other disabilities. Future case-law should decide such issues.

Enforcement of the ADA

Enforcement of the ADA is done primarily through the Equal Employment Opportunity Commission. Complaints are filed with this commission, and trials by jury may be a second option. The Department of Justice oversees Title III violations. Enforcement assures one of the primary purposes of the Act: that no one, either disabled or abled, will be given a greater advantage in employment opportunities, public services, transportation, and communications.

EXERCISE 17-2

A coworker of yours, also an RN, is HIV-positive and works in the emergency center at your hospital. Following the court's reasoning in the *Bradley* case, to which areas of the hospital could this nurse be transferred where the risk of infecting patients would be the least likely? Could he or she transfer to some areas of clinical nursing? What are the potential risks to the nurse?

Conclusion

The Act represents an expansive vision of the capabilities of disabled individuals and rightly regards them as productive members of society. Similarly, the Act holds that the societal costs of discrimination against and isolation of dis-

Guidelines: The ADA and Hiring Processes

1. To be a qualified individual with a disability under the ADA definition, applicants must be able to perform essential job functions. This allows employers to question individuals about their educational and experiential qualifications for the job, plus licensure and required certification if that is a prerequisite of all candidates for the position.

2. Applicants can be questioned about their ability to perform the job safely, with or without accommodation. No accommodations are necessary unless the disabled person requests them.

3. No accommodation is required if it would impose an undue hardship on the employer. Such undue hardships include costly or disruptive renovations to the existing facility, or costs disproportionate with the size of the employer, the numbers of other employees, and the nature of the business place.

4. Applicants may be questioned about their ability to perform essential job functions, and case scenarios can be devised to ascertain qualifications for clinical-based jobs. What cannot be asked are questions about disabilities, past medical problems, or previous workers' compensation claims.

5. Employment tests that would screen out disabled workers may not be used unless the test is shown to be job-related and consistent with business necessity. Tests that screen for illegal drug usage may be given, if required of all applicants for the position, not just disabled job applicants.

6. If preemployment physicals are part of the hiring process, they cannot be done until after the job is offered, conditioned on the applicant's passing the examination. The same medical examination requirements must be made of all persons applying for the position and all test data must be kept confidential. Only persons with a need to know may be told of the disabled persons' medical data following the examination.

7. All applicants should be queried about their qualifications for the position and have explained to them policies and procedures of the facility. The ADA does not mandate that disabled persons be hired. It mandates that all persons, both the disabled as well as the abled, be given the same advantages in job opportunities.

abled individuals far outweigh the economic costs of accommodation. The ADA's scope is vast, and over time the Act can be expected to effect major changes in the areas of employment, transportation, communications, access to public services and public accommodations, in all other areas where the disabled have been subject to discrimination, isolation, and segregation. The ADA offers an historic opportunity to fully integrate disabled individuals into the mainstream of American society.

EXERCISE 17-3

Review the hiring practices of your institution with the nurse manager who hires personnel on your unit. During the interview, what types of questions are asked? What information is imparted? Is there a preemployment physical and/or a mandatory drug screen? What essential job functions have been developed for the positions for which applicants are interviewed? Having read this section, what advice would you give the nurse manager?

CIVIL RIGHTS ACT OF 1991

Background of the Act

Congress, the federal courts, and numerous other courts have struggled with issues of sexual discrimination and harassment for this half of the 20th century. The culminating factor that brought the issue to a final showdown was the Clarence Thomas Supreme Court confirmation hearings in October of 1991, heightening awareness of concern about sexual harassment in the workplace. The Thomas hearings pushed sexual harassment to the top of the national agenda, and the act was signed into law on November 21, 1991.

Unlike the ADA, the Civil Rights Act of 1991 did not have smooth sailing in committee or in Congress. Following the Thomas hearings, Senator Danforth catalyzed the warring factions into temporary harmony, with most of the "rough edges" addressed. President Bush, in signing the Act, stated "most of the Act's major provisions have been subject to bipartisan consensus" (Sacher, 1992).

Definition of Sexual Harassment

The major portion of the act contains definitions of sexual harassment, identifying two categories of sexual harassment. Overall, *sexual harassment* is simply "unwelcome sexual conduct that is a term of employment" [29 *C.R.F.*, section 1604.11(a)]. The two categories of sexual harassment are discussed separately.

Quid Pro Quo Sexual Harassment

Quid pro quo sexual harassment occurs when submission to or rejection of the sexual conduct by an individual is used as a basis for employment decisions affecting the individual. To show quid pro quo sexual harassment, the individual must show that:

1. The employee was subjected to unwelcome harassment in the form of sexual advances or requests for sexual favors.
2. The harassment complained of was based on sex.

3. The employee's submission to the unwelcome advances was an express or implied condition for receiving job benefits or that the employee's refusal to submit to the supervisor's sexual demands resulted in tangible job detriment.
4. The individual is a member of a protected class (an employee in a lower position in the power chain of command).

Additionally, employers are strictly liable for the conduct of supervisory personnel in quid pro quo harassment suits.

Robinson v. Jacksonville Shipyards, Inc. (1991), a suit brought under quid pro quo harassment allegations, contains an excellent review of the types of prohibited conduct plus policies and procedures for preventing and investigating future allegations. A previous case, *Chaimberlain v. 101 Realty, Inc.* (1990) had enumerated the elements of a quid pro quo sexual harassment suit.

Hostile Work Environment

The majority of the cases brought under the Act concern the **hostile work environment** sexual harassment. In these instances, there are no tangible job benefits or detriment. Here the employee is subjected to sexual innuendos, remarks, and physical acts so offensive as to "alter the conditions of the employee's employment and create an abusive work environment (*Meritor Savings Bank v. Vinson*, 1986). Elements that must be shown in this type of case include the establishing (1) that the harassment unreasonably interfered with work performance, and (2) that the harassment would affect a reasonable person's work environment. The employer is not strictly liable in such a suit, but becomes liable when the individual alleging the harassment files complaints with the employer or when the harassment is so pervasive that knowledge can be inferred.

Because most issues in this area affect women, the court addressed the issue of a "reasonable woman standard." In *Robinson v. Jacksonville Shipyards, Inc.* (1991), the court concluded that "the cumulative, corrosive effect of their work environment over time affects the psychological well-being measured by the impact of the work environment on a reasonable woman's work performance or more broadly by the impact of the stress inflicted on her by the continuing presence of the harassing behavior. The fact that some female employees did not complain of the work environment or find some behaviors objectionable does not affect this conclusion concerning the objective offensiveness of the work environment as a whole" (at 1492). The *Robinson* case was the first to carve out the reasonable woman standard in dealing with sexual harassment cases since there is a gender issue in this area. *Ellison v. Brady* (1991) had concluded that a complete understanding of the victim's views requires an analysis of the different perspectives between men and women and what men may consider unobjectionable may offend many women.

In hostile work environment sexual harassment cases, the conduct need not be directed at the individual who files the complaint. It is enough that the behavior or condition was observed or known by the individual and that it affected the psychological well-being of the individual. For example, hostile work environment sexual harassment may be triggered by posting pornography in the office, displaying lewd cartoons labeled with a worker's name, making sexually demeaning comments or jokes, touching or attempting to touch the individual, and sexual propositions. The conduct/behavior complained of must be unwelcome and the victim's perspective is what is relevant.

Conduct akin to that of a quid pro quo sexual harassment case may also exist in this type of suit, but the offending employee has no direct supervision over the individual or there is no corresponding job benefit or detriment connected with the harassment. In *Ellison v. Brady* (1991), the employee was sent a letter in which a co-worker proclaimed his love for her and suggested a sexual liaison. The bizarre content of the letter so frightened the employee that she complained to the supervisor. The same type of letter could have formed the basis of a quid pro quo sexual harassment suit if the co-worker was a supervisor who then fired the employee when she failed to comply with his liaison.

Employees who sense some type of hostile environment sexual harassment should notify superiors or the employer directly, depending on the size of the facility/place of employment and organizational chart. The employer has a duty to investigate the report, maintaining confidentiality, then report back to the initiating complainant and document the investigation. While maintaining professionalism, the alleged victim, as well as the alleged harasser and other potential witnesses, should be interviewed. The employer must consider what action needs to be taken and communicate the results of the investigation to all parties involved.

Termination of the alleged harasser is not mandatory, and other remedial action may be taken, such as a transfer of the offender to other units or work sites and disciplinary warnings. Generally, courts have held that, for serious physical harassment, termination may be required, while less serious verbal harassment may justify lesser discipline. Most importantly, some action must be taken if a potential lawsuit is to be avoided.

Additionally, there is some evidence to support that courts may hold independent contractors, those with no direct employee-employer relationship, liable under this Act. Thus physicians and agency personnel, who have no direct employer-employee relationship to health care facilities, may make health care facilities liable for their actions or comments within these facilities.

Preferential Treatment or Sexual Favoritism

An employer may also be liable for unlawful sexual discrimination when an employee is denied a job opportunity or benefit due to the *preferential treatment* of another employee who submits to the employer's sexual advances. Additionally, there may be liability when employers promote employees who give sexual favors to supervisors, rather than other better qualified employees.

GUIDELINES: AVOIDING SEXUAL HARASSMENT CLAIMS

1. Try to prevent the harassment from occurring since this is the most cost-effective means to deal with the reality of workplace relationships.
2. Take affirmative action to prevent harassment, such as starting educational programs to alert persons about how to react to such advances and hostile environments, expressing strong disapproval, informing persons of their right to raise sexual harassment issues, and sensitizing all concerned.
3. Develop policies prohibiting either type of sexual harassment. The policy should include:

    Strong language prohibiting such actions and stating that such actions will not be tolerated.

    A procedure for reporting complaints.

    Notice that violators will be subject to stern disciplinary procedures, including discharge.

    Identification of an employee representative to whom complaints should be directed.

    A statement that all complaints and investigations will be treated in a confidential manner.
4. Communicate the policy, including placement in policy manuals, bulletin boards, interoffice memoranda, and employee handbooks.
5. Conduct training programs for supervisory personnel.

EXERCISE 17-4

For each of the following examples, are there grounds for a sexual harassment claim? If so, which type of claim could be brought (quid pro quo or hostile environment)?

1. John rejects a homosexual advance by David, a nurse manager, and is subsequently fired by the unit manager.
2. William, the hospital chief operating officer, asks Judy, the assistant director of nursing, for a date.
3. During a conference sponsored by the institution, Paul makes remarks and sexual physical contact with a female co-worker, Judy. Judy complains to her direct supervisor. Twelve hours later, the hospital director of nursing tells her that she needs to stay at the conference, but will no longer be required to work with Paul after the conference.

4. Marilyn and Jeff, both employed by the same institution, are having an affair. They are both upper-level managers, but work in different departments.
5. During a trip, Rita makes sexual innuendos and tells lewd jokes to a male co-worker named Richard. After Richard complains, the company transfers Richard and reprimands Rita.

SUMMARY

The ADA is a significant enactment because it impacts health care employers, health care personnel, potential employees, and consumers of the health care delivery system. Hiring practices should be changed to accommodate the new restrictions when interviewing potential employees, and necessary accommodations made for disabled persons, employees, or patients.

Although it is virtually impossible to eliminate sexual harassment from the workplace, an employer can implement policies and practices that will significantly limit its practice. An employer should have a written sexual harassment policy, promptly respond to allegations of sexual harassment, and take remedial actions as warranted.

AFTER COMPLETING THIS CHAPTER, YOU SHOULD BE ABLE TO

- Describe the conditions within the United States that caused both acts to be written and implemented.
- Describe the various sections of the two acts, the necessary definitions, and the intended purposes.
- Describe how the acts affect the health care delivery system in terms of consumers and providers.

APPLY YOUR LEGAL KNOWLEDGE

- How do staff nurses comply with these two acts in providing competent care to patients?
- Have these two laws had the desired affect that their drafters intended?

REFERENCES

Aikins v. St. Helena Hospital, 1994 WL 38971 (N.D. Cal., February 2, 1994).

Bradley v. University of Texas M.D. Anderson Cancer Center, 3 Fed. 3d 922 (5th Cir., 1993).

Chaimberlain v. 101 Realty, Inc., 915 F. 2d 777 (1st Cir., 1990).

Derbon v. United States Shoe Corporation, No. CIVA MJG-93-130, 1994 WL 631155 (D. M.D., September 7, 1994).

Ellison v. Brady, 924 F. 2d 872 (9th Cir., 1991).

Heilweil v. Mount Sinai Hospital, CA 2, No. 93-1548 *PA Jury Verdict*, *13*(4), 28 (1994).

Leckelt v. Board of Commissioners, 909 F. 2d 820 (5th Cir., 1990).

Meritor Savings Bank v. Vinson, 477 U.S. 57 (1986).

Robinson v. Jacksonville Shipyards, Inc., 760 F. Supp. 1486 (M.D. Fla., 1991).

Sacher, J. (1992). *Sexual harassment in the workplace.* Houston, TX: South Texas College of Law.

School Board v. Arline, 480 U.S. 273 (1987).

29 C.R.F., Section 1604. 11(A), 1991.

• eighteen

Nursing in Community Health Settings

PREVIEW

As nurses move from the traditional hospital setting, a variety of new and innovative opportunities are opening for professional nursing in many community health settings, including public health nursing, school health nursing, occupational nursing, and home health care nursing. All these opportunities offer new, exciting, and more autonomous roles for nursing, and all have some liability for nurses. This chapter presents legal liability in a variety of community settings, including cases in which nurses donate their services, either in disaster nursing or through volunteer services.

OVERVIEW OF COMMUNITY HEALTH NURSING

The primary purpose of community health nursing is to promote and maintain the health of aggregates (Miller, 1990). Everything that is done to promote and maintain this health has a basis in law and is subject to legal sanctions of one type or another. Perhaps the best starting point for understanding these legal concepts in community health nursing is to know and understand federal and state laws impacting the implementation of community health nursing.

FEDERAL STATUTES

Few pieces of legislation have impacted the health and welfare systems of the United States as have the Social Security Act of 1935 and the Public Health Service Act of 1994, with their respective amendments.

Social Security Act of 1935

The Social Security Act of 1935 was signed into legislation by President Franklin D. Roosevelt, as a result of the Great Depression of 1929. The Act was based on European health and welfare practices, and many of its roots can be traced back to early European poor laws.

The *Social Security Act of 1935* provided for the general welfare by establishing a system of federal old age benefits and by enabling states to make provisions for aged persons, blind persons, dependent and crippled children, maternal and child welfare, public health, and the administration of state unemployment compensation laws. Programs were both *contributory,* financed through taxation and individual contributions, and *assistance* or *noncontributory,* financed only through taxation. Historically, contributory programs have offered more comprehensive benefits than assistive programs.

The Act has been amended numerous times since its enactment, with Medicare and Medicaid being the most important health programs added in 1965. The Act affects the services that nursing provides to its clients. Through Medicare-reimbursable services, regulations specify which clients nurses see, what type of care is provided, how the care is provided, and how long the care is provided. Medicare benefits have changed greatly since their enactment. Alcohol detoxification facility benefits were added in 1980, hospice reimbursements were added in 1983, and a 1990 amendment has allowed Medicare Part B premiums to be paid for eligible beneficiaries.

Nurses must recognize their own personal values and attitudes in relation to the programs under the Act and realize that these attitudes and values may cause conflict for them. For example, if nurses believe that single mothers should not receive monetary support from the government, they may have difficulty working with mothers receiving Aid to Families of Dependent Children assistance or even letting clients know that they are eligible for the services.

Public Health Service Act of 1944

The *Public Health Service Act of 1944* consolidated all existing public health legislation under one law and became the major piece of health legislation for the country. This piece of legislation, through the original Act and its amendments, provides a variety of resources and services including the National Institutes for Health, nursing training acts, traineeships for graduate students in public health, health services for migratory workers, family planning services, health research facilities, and programs and services for the prevention and control of heart disease, cancer, stroke, kidney disease, sudden infant death syndrome, sickle-cell anemia, and diabetes. These services are administered by a number of federal and state agencies.

Implications for nurses of this broad and comprehensive Act are extensive. The Act provides funding for services to at-risk aggregates in the community, such as migratory workers, as well as persons with AIDS, tuberculosis, and other communicable diseases, and programs for persons with chronic problems, such as heart disease, stroke, kidney disease, and diabetes. This Act financially covers at least some aspect of nursing in all acute care, home health care, and institutional settings. It provides funding for nursing education and for all levels of disease prevention: primary, secondary, and tertiary.

The amendments to this Act have brought about numerous changes over the years since enactment. There are now block grants to states, allowing the individual states to decide which programs are most needed in their territories, and monies remain available for specific programs such as immunizations, family planning, and venereal disease programs. Table 18–1 depicts some of the more important aspects of these two acts.

TABLE 18–1. FEDERALLY LEGISLATED PUBLIC HEALTH LAWS

Title	Purpose of Act
Social Security Act and Amendments	
Social Security of 1935, Titles I-XI	Enabled each state to furnish financial assistance to the aged, needy individuals; additional titles allowed for payments to persons over 65, aid to dependent children, and maternal and child welfare.
Old Age and Survivors Amendments of 1939	Provided for payment of insurance benefits to qualifying survivors of workers.
Maternal and Child Health and Retardation Act of 1963	Amended the act to assist states and communities in preventing and combating retardation.
Social Security Amendments of of 1965, Title XIX (Medicaid)	Provided funding to states to establish medical assistance for the needy as defined under the act.
Social Security Amendments of 1965, Title XVIII (Medicare)	Established hospital and medical insurance benefits for persons over 65 who are residents of the U.S.
Social Security Amendments of 1977 (Health Clinic Services)	Authorizes reimbursement for clinic services in rural areas designed as a "health manpower shortage area."
Tax Equity and Fiscal Responsibility Act of 1982 (DRGs)	Set forth a system of prospective payment for Medicare Services, called Diagnostic Related Groups.
Child Support Enforcement Acts of 1984	Amended the act to allow mandatory income withholding and other improvements in child support enforcement programs.
Family Support Act of 1988	Reformed the system to emphasize work and child support; established child support programs, job opportunities, and basic skills and training programs.
Medicare Catastrophic Coverage Act of 1988	Amended act to protect Medicare recipients from catastrophic health care expenditures.
Public Health Services Act and Amendments	
Public Health Services Act of 1944	Created federally coordinated department to address the public health need of the nation; established the office of the Surgeon General, National Institutes of Health, Bureau of Medical Services, and Bureau of State Services.
Special Health Revenue Sharing Act of 1975	Amended the act to revise and extend the health sharing program, providing comprehensive public health services.
Omnibus Budget Reconciliation Act of 1981	Consolidated federal assistance to states for social services into a single grant to increase the states' flexibility in using grants to achieve the goals of preventing, reducing, or eliminating dependency; created block grants for social services.

Source: *Data from the* U.S. Code, Congressional and Administrative News *(1935, 1939, 1944, 1963, 1965, 1975, 1977, 1981)*. St. Paul, MN: West Publishing Company.

LEGAL RESPONSIBILITIES OF COMMUNITY HEALTH NURSES

Serving in a variety of settings, *community health nurses* care for persons in need of their services in the clinic (public health nurses), school (school health nurses), home (home health nurses), and workplace (occupational health nurses). Many of the legal responsibilities of these nurses differ slightly, depending on the setting. For ease of understanding, the various nurses working in the community will be discussed separately.

HOME HEALTH CARE NURSES

Home health care nursing has emerged as a key component of health care delivery in the 1990s. These nurses provide care that ranges from assistance with daily living to complex, highly technical nursing skills. And the care is provided in the client's home—a setting where the nurse has little control but many potential risks.

Federal Legislation

Federal legislation sets requirements for all home health care nurses. The 1987 provisions to the Omnibus Budget Reconciliation Act of 1986 substantially changed the federal law relating to participation of home health care agencies in the Medicare program. Clients must be screened for eligibility, and the signatures of the client must be witnessed after explaining client rights and legal contracts for service. Important provisions of the statute include an extensive listing of consumer rights. For example, the right to be fully informed in advance about the care and treatment to be provided by the agency, to be fully informed in advance of any changes in the care or treatment to be provided by the agency that may affect the individual's well-being, and to participate in planning care and treatment or changes in care or treatment. The Act also enumerates the right of individuals to confidentiality of clinical records, the right to have one's property treated with respect, and the establishment of a grievance hotline to be established by each state. A separate provision under this Act sets strict criteria of qualifications for home health care aides who have a predominant role in direct, hands-on contact with clients. Under this provision, the agency may not use any individual who is not a licensed health care professional, unless the individual has successfully completed a training and competency evaluation program that meets minimum federal standards and the individual is actually competent to provide the services assigned.

In 1987, amendments were also made to the Older Americans Act (Public Law 100-175), which directly affects home health care agencies. These amendments were aimed at developing demonstration projects to strengthen home care consumer protection mechanisms, such as the rights of the developmentally disabled person. Since these demonstration projects have been successful, regulations concerning home health care consumer protection and corresponding provider obligations are being developed.

Other federal legislation affecting home health care delivery of services is the Patient Self-Determination Act of 1991. Under this regulation, agencies that receive federal funds (including home health agencies) must inquire whether patients being admitted to their services have executed a living will and/or special directive such as a durable power of attorney for health care. If the patient has such a document, then the agency is obligated to abide by its provisions. If there is no such directive and the patient wishes to complete a directive, the agency must provide guidance on completing such directives.

State Legislation

State laws encompass a variety of issues that may arise within home health care settings. Home health care nurses are advised to explore individual state law in such areas as protection of the uninsured person, of the abused person, of the homeless person; the rights of renter or tenant; and the laws that protect individuals from eviction under certain circumstances. All care givers should be aware of the state abuse laws, knowing how and when to report suspected abuse. Family law issues, such as the right to decide for another, rights of guardians, and consent to perform procedures on minors or incompetent persons, also vary state to state.

One of the most important state legislative acts is the state nurse practice act. Home health nurses must practice within the scope of their nurse practice acts, including all relevant administrative rules and statutes, particularly with respect to standards of practice. Standards of practice or standards of care refer to both state and national standards concerning the minimum degree of care to be delivered to the client. Standards of care are established through the nurse practice act, relevant current literature, professional organizations, and agency policy and procedure manuals. Home health care nurses are responsible for ensuring that clients receive quality and competent nursing care.

EXERCISE 18-1

You are a community health care nurse and have been assigned to assess the potential health care needs of a family of five. The mother, age 36, is unemployed and cares for a 2-month-old child and an 8-year-old child. The 8 year old attends elementary school about four blocks away. A maternal grandfather, with insulin-dependent diabetes and congestive heart failure is unable to be employed outside the home. A 20-year-old daughter works at a commercial cafeteria and has been diagnosed with salmonella by stool culture. The mother receives Aid to Families with Dependent Children, and she would like to start a home day care center for additional income.

What state and federal law provides guidance for the health care worker in assessing this family group? Where would you find out about applicable laws? Speak with a public health nurse about applicable laws once you have decided which laws fit this scenario. Were you surprised at the number of laws applicable to this one family group?

Standing Orders

Because of the relative isolation of home health care, nurses should have written standing orders in case of emergencies or unexpected needs of clients. Standing orders complement verbal orders, and both types of orders should be clarified when used by the home health care nurse. Standing orders should be reviewed and updated on a regular basis and must be signed by the attending physician(s) before being implemented. Some agencies prefer protocols that are jointly written by nursing and medicine. Either standing orders or protocols must be specific about their implementation and approval by agency physicians.

If verbal orders are used, the home health care nurse should document the order and have the physician cosign the order as soon as practical. If a patient is injured when the nurse relied on a verbal order and no written documentation of the order is evident, the nurse may have difficulty in demonstrating that the physician's written order was accurately followed. The agency should develop a plan by which verbal orders are to be cosigned, such as a system to mail the order to the physician and have the physician mail the signed order back to the agency for inclusion in the client record.

Contract Law

Home health nurses must honor contracts made with clients. Contracts include both the written and oral agreements of understanding made between the agency and the receiver of health care services. Contracts made with clients include the advertised services included in agency brochures and advertisements, as well as formal contracts signed by clients and agency staff. Provisions that should be included in all contracts include:

1. Provider's and client's respective roles and responsibilities.
2. Length, type, frequency, and limitations of services.
3. Cost and payment schedules.
4. Provisions for informed client or surrogate consent for specific interventions on both an initial and a continuing basis.

Be careful of promises that one may not be able to meet, such as a provision in a brochure ensuring that clients will be evaluated within 12 hours of contacting the agency.

All the agency's legal duties to the client stem from the legal relationship formed between the two parties. Thus the referral as well as initial evaluation periods are crucial. Medicare and Joint Commission for Healthcare Organizations standards require that a home care agency accept clients based on a reasonable expectation that it can adequately meet the patient's medical, nursing, and social needs in the client's residence. New referrals must be carefully evaluated, from a referring physician aspect as well as a nursing aspect to ensure that:

1. The client is medically stable or a medically unstable condition, as with the dying client, can be managed.
2. There is a desire for home care.
3. The needs of the client can be safely and effectively met by the home care agency.
4. Satisfactory financial arrangements can be made.

Any deficiencies or inability to provide adequate care should be discussed with both the physician and potential client before entering a contract. Client education and informed consent issues, as well as client options and other available resources and services, should be discussed and agreed on before entering the contract.

At the initiation of the contract, clients should be instructed about the availability of 24-hour staffing, how to contact staff at other than routine office hours, and why 24-hour staff may be needed. Agencies are advised to have written guidelines on the appropriate use of 24-hour staffing and the financial responsibilities of the client if 24-hour staffing is used.

Clients may be transferred or their care terminated by the agency after a formal contract is entered. Before transferring the care of the client, a discussion about the advantages as well as disadvantages should be conducted between the client and agency. Issues such as adverse physical and mental reactions to the transfer must be considered, as well as better or more acceptable levels of care by the transferring agency.

Care must be taken to avoid *abandonment* of the client by unilaterally terminating the professional relationship without affording the client reasonable notice and health care services. Remember, though, that a contract is a two-way street and that both parties have roles and responsibilities. Agencies do not have perpetual, ongoing responsibilities to provide services in the absence of compensation. Nor do agencies need to continue to provide care if the safety of the agency staff is threatened. To avoid liability for client abandonment or dumping, the agency must develop and implement a satisfactory discharge program. Discharge planning should be started with the initial evaluation of the client and clients should remain involved in the plan throughout their care. Potential clients should be made aware of this discharge program before a formal contract is signed.

Confidentiality

As a general rule, home care workers and the agency must treat as confidential any information that becomes known as a direct result of the agency-client relationship. Persons and agencies violating this rule may be held liable in damages to the client.

There are some exceptions to this general rule. One exception is the sharing of information among the various health care providers who are responsible for the client's care, including professional staff members, home health care aides, occupational or physical therapy providers, social workers, and the like. It is advisable to obtain the client's written provision for sharing information at the time of the initial contract. If no such provision was made, then the client should sign a release form to authorize release. The release form should include exactly what information is to be released, to whom the information is to be given, and the time during which the release is valid. This latter provision may be time-related or event-related.

Other exceptions include the release of information to third-party payors. This is done by the client or client surrogate since release of this type of information is required before insurance companies and other third-party payors honor requests for payments. The client may also request information from the record, and the agency should have a written policy concerning the release of records to the client or client surrogate. Although the original record is the property of the agency, a copy may be given to clients for their records.

Refusal of Care

An issue of growing concern is clients' right of *refusal of care.* Even if clients have previously consented to treatment, they can later withdraw consent. Verbal withdrawal of consent is adequate. The agency staff should immediately communicate the withdrawal to other members of the health care team, and document the refusal or withdrawal in the agency record.

Refusal of care depends on informed consent. With informed consent, the client must be given sufficient information on which to base an informed choice. The information needed includes the purpose or expected outcome of the treatment or procedure, the risks and complications that accompany the treatment or procedure, who is to perform the treatment or procedure, and alternatives to the treatment or procedure. To refuse treatment, patients need this information as well as the potential and realistic expectations of the refusal or withdrawal of consent. Again, documentation of the refusal and the client education must be included in agency records.

Agency Policies

Home health nurses have a duty to inform themselves about written *agency policy* and/or procedures, because deviation from these policies may result in substandard care to clients. If the policies are outdated, communicate this to the agency so that changes can be made and policies made more current. Additionally, ensure that the policies do not require nurses to function outside of the scope of nursing practice. The employer's policies and procedures set the standard of care and will be used to show deviation from that standard if a lawsuit develops.

Malpractice and Negligence

One of the major roles of nurses is to assess and instruct patients and their families. Nurses must be able to identify significant changes in the client's condition and decide if further medical intervention or hospitalization is required. If changes occur, home health care nurses must convey clearly any concern and indication for further treatment. While the client has the right to refuse further interventions, nurses must ensure that the client or family members understand the nature and extent of change in the patient's condition. It may be necessary for home health care nurses to contact their supervisor, other family members, and the physician. Because they are working alone in the home setting, it is vital that they carefully assess and communicate concerns quickly and appropriately.

In a case that exemplifies negligent training of employees, a home health care aide left a patient unattended in the shower while she did other work in the patient's home. The patient, disabled and using a shower chair, was unable to control the temperature of the water and she was severely scalded. The aide applied ice to the burned areas and attempted to reach her supervisor, who was unavailable at the time. The aide waited before calling an ambulance, and the patient suffered severe third degree burns over a large portion of her body that required numerous operations and skin grafts (*Loton v. Massachusetts Paramedical Inc.*, 1989). This case also exemplifies the need to evaluate and call for assistance immediately when needed.

Much of the current case-law in this area concerns the duty to train and supervise in the home setting, particularly for home health care aides and nursing staff members. The *Loton* case showed the need to properly train personnel, particularly when the patient is disabled and placed in a position where harm is likely to occur. In a later case that shows this same need to train and supervise, a home health care aide lost control of a wheelchair on a hill and the 19-year-old quadriplegic was rendered unconscious (*R.W.H. v. W.C.N.S., Inc.*, 1992).

Both these cases also show the failure to adequately supervise, an issue that is of extreme importance yet difficult to manage, given the isolated nature of home health care nursing. Nursing personnel should institute a system of periodic visits in the home to identify the efficiency and level of care being delivered by the home health care aide and other nursing personnel. Patient satisfaction questionnaires may be another means to pinpoint potential trouble areas so that follow-up visits can be made.

The duty to instruct patients is paramount in the home setting, because patients and family members must rely on these instructions when nurses are not readily available in the setting. The education of the patient and family should include both preventative and self-care information, and the nurse must ensure that the patient or family member has understood the instructions. Asking for return demonstrations or ensuring that questions are answered appropriately are ways of validating patient understanding. Since references may not be available, nurses should refrain from answering ques-

GUIDELINES: HOME HEALTH CARE NURSING

1. Know areas of the law that pertain to home health care nursing, including federal and state laws, and adhere to the mandates of those laws. Request the agency to provide a continuing education program to ensure that all nurses in the agency are knowledgeable about laws affecting home health care nursing.

2. Practice within the scope of nursing practice. If in doubt, request that the agency clarify the issue before proceeding with the treatment or procedure in question.

3. Obtain permission (consent) before caring for clients in the home. This means being able to discuss with patients or their family the risks and benefits of the proposed procedure or intervention before initiation of the intervention.

4. Honor patients' right to refuse care, if that is their wish. If the patient has a living will or other advanced directive, honor the document. The patient in the home has the same rights as hospitalized patients to know about such advanced directives and to implement such directives. If the patient refuses care, make sure that the refusal is communicated to all members of the health care team.

5. Respect the patient's privacy rights, including confidentiality in the nurse–patient relationship. Release forms must be used if patient information is to be given to other health care agencies or health care providers.

6. Follow standing orders and protocols, particularly in times of emergencies or changes in the patient's status. Verbal orders may be secured as needed, and then signed by the physician according to agency protocol.

7. Client education is one of the responsibilities of the home health care nurse. Answer questions as much as possible, and tell patients that you will find out needed information and get back to them. Remember that you are most likely the patient's sole reference in health matters and that it is vital that you give correct information.

8. Follow agency policies and initiate change in policies as needed.

9. Document all pertinent information about the patient's condition, and information concerning teaching and referrals that you may have made. As with other health care settings, the one way to show and remember what was done is through effective and timely documentation.

10. Delegate wisely, supervise effectively, and train personnel in the delivery of competent patient care and how to respond to emergencies. Much of the case-law to date in this area of the law has concerned these three vital concepts. So ensure that all three issues are addressed.

tions or providing information until they are sure that the information is correct. Thus nurses in these settings must remain current in aspects of information that they will be responsible for teaching.

OCCUPATIONAL HEALTH NURSING

The expansion of *occupational health* nursing has greatly increased the potential for liability. This area of practice is greatly influenced by a variety of federal and state laws, particularly workers' compensation laws, mandatory reporting laws, and occupational safety and health laws. Because of the unique interplay between the worker's compensation laws and the doctrine of respondeat superior, nurses in this setting face a higher risk of personal liability than nurses in most other settings.

State workers' compensation laws mandate the compensation of employees who are injured while at work in accordance with specific compensation schedules. These same laws make this avenue the injured employee's sole remedy against the employer, and thus deny the employee the legal right to sue the employer for damages even if the employer's negligence was the prime cause of the injury.

In a minority of states, employees injured on the job may sue any person, other than their employer and including co-workers, whose negligence caused the resultant injury. In most states, the immunity extended to the employer is also extended to co-workers of the injured employee. Thus a nurse employed by a company in these states is protected from civil liability in much the same manner as the employer. Nurses may, though, work as independent contractors within companies and are thus not protected.

Occupational nurses have responsibilities in a variety of areas, including adequate and rapid assessment of clients, communications with other health care providers who are frequently not at the work site, delivery of nursing interventions using standing orders and protocols, and teaching preventative health and safety needs as well as the teaching involved with specific diseases and conditions, development of safety programs within the setting, and verification of employees' ability to work. Thus the job description of occupational health nurses is of vital importance.

It is also important for these nurses to have specific guidelines, standing orders, and protocols. Written standards guide nurses and prevent greater liability exposure for them. If they were allowed to work under a "do whatever you think is necessary" guideline, such a standard would open them to charges of practicing medicine without a license as well as increased malpractice liability. Remember that nurses retain personal accountability for their actions, as well as potentially making other persons liable.

A case that exemplifies some of the nursing responsibilities of this role is *Therrell v. Fonde* (1986). In that case, an employee suffered a crushing hand injury, which was examined by the occupational health nurse. She examined and wrapped the injured hand and gave him an injection of either Vistaril or Demerol. The patient was then directed to wait in the outer waiting room while transportation was being secured. During the patient's hour wait for transportation to arrive, the company-employed physician arrived, was told of the injury, and refused to see the patient.

Eventually the patient was seen at the health care facility that the company routinely used for their patients, and surgery was performed, resulting in a partial amputation of two fingers and the permanent disuse of the index and little finger of his left hand. The suit was brought for negligence, alleging that the company failed to transport promptly, that the company failed to adequately diagnose and treat his injury, and that such conduct was willful, outrageous, and wanton.

Occupational health nurses may also have some accountability for the action of nonhealth care providers who render first aid assistance in the work site. If occupational health care nurses have the responsibility to teach first aid or to ensure that needed supplies for first aid intervention are available, they may incur potential liability. Additionally, they will have potential liability if they note that first aid assistance is not being delivered correctly and fail to do anything about the lack of quality first aid assistance.

EXERCISE 18-2

Julio Ortis is an occupational health nurse employed in a state that has not granted immunity from co-workers of an employee injured on the job. Doctor Doe is the plant physician. A number of written protocols and standing orders guide Julio's practice in the absence of the Doctor Doe. A patient presented to the occupational health clinic, during Doctor Doe's absence, was misdiagnosed and negligently treated by Julio. As a result of the negligent nursing care, the patient suffered permanent and extensive injuries. Who has potential liability in this instance? Why? How would the liability change if Doctor Doe was present at the time of the patient's arrival, but was unable to see the patient because of a second worker's injuries? Would the liability change in the latter instance? Why or why not?

SCHOOL HEALTH NURSING

School health nurses face much of the same type of increased liability issues as occupational health nurses. In most jurisdictions, the school nurse is subjected to the same potential liabilities as other governmental workers, because of the relationship of the employing school district to the state. This exposes nurses to greater potential legal liability for injuries.

Because school nurses work in a nonmedical environment, they must exercise considerable independent judgment, and they must be able to recognize and treat or know when to seek immediate assistance. This includes the ability to assess the situation quickly, treat the child if that is appropriate, or make arrangements for the child to be taken for immediate medical attention.

Many children visit the school health nurse for traumatic injuries, and nurses must be competent to provide an emergency standard of care. If injuries occur after school hours, as they frequently do in schools with competitive sports teams, nurses will be functioning outside the scope of her employment. Again, the nurses are held to the standard of the reasonably prudent nurse in an emergency setting.

A recent court case that exemplifies this need to follow an emergency standard is *Schlussler v. Independent School District No. 200 et al.*, a 1989 Minnesota case. In that case, a child had come to the nurse's office, suffering from an asthmatic attack. The nurse assessed the situation, gave another child's inhaler to this child, and sent the child back to the classroom. After other children came to the office concerned about this child's breathing pattern, the nurse assessed the child and determined that neither supplemental oxygen nor emergency transportation via an ambulance were needed to transport this child to the physician's office. Within minutes after leaving the school, the child collapsed and died following a brief comatose period.

The court, on hearing evidence from nursing and asthma expert witnesses, concluded that school nurses have a higher duty of care than hospital nurses to make an assessment of the need for emergency medical services. While they are not expected to provide medical treatment, they are expected to determine the need for those services and for immediate, safe transportation to emergency medical care. The nurse's action also fell below the acceptable standard of care when she used another child's inhaler for this child.

Actions that could have been performed in the preceding case include competent assessment skills, performance to a standard of care and laws governing prescription medications, better monitoring of the student, adherence to school policy concerning the notification of parents (particularly in a case where the child has no prescription medications for asthmatic attacks), and consultation with other school health nurses and health care providers to develop written criteria for such emergency conditions.

VOLUNTEER SERVICES

Many health care providers routinely perform *volunteer services*, usually as a vital part of community services. A volunteer status may also arise when one agrees to care for a sick neighbor or a family member. Nurses may also be donating professional services and nursing skills when helping to conduct a hypertension screening program or presenting a lecture on juvenile diabetes for the local parent-teachers association.

Remember several points about volunteer status:

1. Legal status may not be well defined, because donated services do not fall within the auspices of the state nurse practice act. Most nurse practice acts apply only to compensated services. So the strict rules and regulations generated by the state board of nurse examiners do not apply to donated services.
2. Responsibilities and professional actions do not change. Nurses are still professionals and owe a minimum standard of care to patients or clients. The standard of care for professional nurses remains the same under most circumstances.
3. The donation of services does not exempt nurses from a possible lawsuit or from the standard of the reasonably prudent nurse. The state nurse practice act still guides one's professional responsibilities.
4. The state board of nursing may subject nurses to disciplinary action should the care delivered fall below minimum standards. This is true even if no ancillary civil action is filed.
5. The nurse–patient relationship is initiated when care is first given. Once established, the same duty of care owed a hospital or paying patient is owed this patient (*Lunsford v. Board of Nurse Examiners*, 1983).

To protect themselves legally, nurses should follow this basic advice:

1. Never administer any treatment or medication without first obtaining a doctor's order or, in the majority of jurisdictions, without a valid standing order. This is true even if the medication is an over-the-counter drug. Professional nurses are responsible for knowing indications, mechanisms of action, contraindications, dosages, adverse reactions, and drug interactions for all medications that they give to patients.
2. Reread carefully their professional liability insurance policy. Does it cover gratuitous services? Depending on the type of services volunteered (eg, to a large group as opposed to volunteering to care for a sick relative) and the number of lawsuits filed against nurses in the given geographic area, nurses may want to increase the dollar amount of the policy. They might also want to increase the coverage limits if they frequently volunteer professional services and come in contact during the donated work with large numbers of persons.
3. A system of record keeping should be initiated and accurate records maintained. Even though there is no formal chart, the records may prove to be invaluable should a lawsuit later be filed. The notes will help to refresh the defendant's memory and may make him or her a more reliable witness.
4. Know the state's Good Samaritan laws. Many states fail to cover nurses for voluntary work done outside of an emergency or away from an accident scene.
5. Above all, know the provisions of the nurse practice act. Understand standards of care, and perform to that minimal level or better at all times. If the purpose of the donated services is the better education of

GUIDELINES: VOLUNTEERING PROFESSIONAL SERVICES

Community/Neighborhood Services

Before donating professional services:

1. Reread your nurse practice act to see if the free services are covered by the nurse practice act.
2. Check your professional liability insurance policy to ensure that you are covered financially should such services result in a malpractice suit being filed against you.
3. Consider carefully the impact of your decision on public relations and the nursing community should you refuse.

If you decide to volunteer your professional services:

1. Stay within the confines of nursing scope of practice.
2. Refrain from crossing into a medical scope of practice; do not make medical diagnoses or distribute medical therapies and treatments.
3. Maintain the same standard of care you would maintain if you were a paid employee.
4. Keep accurate notes for your personal files.
5. Use this opportunity wisely to expand the positive image of nursing to the public at large.

the public, as with a mass hypertension screening program, carefully review with the sponsoring agency what the questionnaire should say and the types of questions normally asked. This review allows professional nurses to answer the questions and to conduct the mass learning program at an optimal standard-of-care level.

DISASTER NURSING

Some broad guidelines may be applied when a nurse either volunteers to give aid or is compensated for giving it during a disaster. The standard of care in *disaster nursing* usually becomes similar to the standard of care given in emergency situations. Once having decided to render aid, the level of skill and competency is that which a reasonably prudent nurse practitioner would do under the same or similar conditions. If the practitioner meets or excels these standards, there is no negligence.

GUIDELINES: DISASTER SITUATIONS

1. Be prepared. Know in advance your capabilities and what to do should a disaster occur. Know the limits of your professional liability policy and the provisions of your nurse practice act.
2. Maintain at least an emergency standard of care. Perform functions that you are qualified and skilled to do, even if they are outside your normal nursing actions, when instructed to do so by those in authority.
3. Take rests. If you are so exhausted that you cannot make valid judgments, no one benefits from your care or presence.
4. Make notes and record happenings as quickly as possible after rendering nursing care. These notes and records will refresh your memory, if necessary.

A second consideration concerns assuming duties that one ordinarily does not assume. In a true disaster, professional nurses may be asked to perform actions usually reserved for interns and residents or for nurses with advanced education and skills. Provided that the nurses have the knowledge and skills required to perform the actions competently, they are permitted to give such substituted care. Either an emergency exception to the nurse practice act or other statutory or common laws will allow the expanded scope of practice in emergency settings.

Health care providers, once committed to aiding those injured in a disaster, have a duty to give safe, competent care. No one can meet the standards of safe and competent care if they are physically or emotionally exhausted. Allow time for rest. The quality of nurses' work will greatly increase if they are able to reach sound decisions, and the probability of a negligent action will be diminished.

DONATING HEALTH-RELATED ADVICE

Every health care practitioner has been asked at some time for *health-related advice.* It may have been at a fashionable party, at the grocery store, or over the telephone. Although unlikely, a lawsuit could be filed if the advice given falls below the accepted nursing and community standard or actually endangers the person's life and future health. As with volunteer services, nurses must decide if they are willing to give free advice. There is no mandatory duty to do so, but, once it is started, nurses have a duty to give competent and safe advice. There is no duty under the state nurse practice act, since most nurse practice acts exclude gratuitous actions.

The advice given must reflect accepted nursing and community standards and be as current as possible. Be as open and honest as possible. If you are not sure of the best advice to give or if the person seeking advice asks about a field of nursing in which you have no expertise, it is advisable to avoid giving advice. It is perfectly acceptable to have a specialty area (eg, cancer nursing or pediatric nursing) and to be unfamiliar with other fields of nursing (eg, neurological nursing or rehabilitative nursing). There is no liability incurred if you honestly refrain from giving advice, but there may be liability if you guess and give incorrect information.

The advice given should be within the scope of nursing practice. Even though the advice is freely given, nurses may not make a medical diagnoses or interfere with the physician–patient relationship. Instead, nurses should make general statements such as, "From what you have described it could be a mild stroke or a prestroke condition. You should make an appointment and see your doctor as soon as possible," or "I'm not sure. It's been a long time since I had any experience with sick children." Such statements prevent problems with scope of practice issues. Likewise, a statement such as, "I don't know the doctor you mentioned. I always see Bob Smith" prevents charges that the nurse recommended changing physicians or that the nurse advised ignoring the primary physician's advice.

Another factor to consider concerns a possible nurse–patient relationship and the reliance of the other person in adhering to the health-related advice given. For example, a next door neighbor calls and asks a nurse about her son's cut elbow. The son had attempted to catch a ride on the hood of a moving car and fell into the street. The nurse examines the obvious wound and applies a sterile dressing, telling the mother that an antibiotic cream should help prevent an infection and that a doctor's visit at this time is unwarranted. The nurse also questions the son about the fall, asking exactly how he hit the pavement, and he reassures the nurse that he took the full brunt of the fall on his arm and elbow. The next day the mother calls to say that the injured arm looks better, but she is concerned with her son's erratic gait. He is bumping into doors and furniture. Now the nurse's professional advice is to have the son immediately see his physician. The mother's reliance on the nurse for advice demands that the advice is kept current and specific as the situation changes.

This reliance type of relationship seldom follows a casual party or a one-time encounter. Remember two points: (1) if health care questions are asked in an informal manner, the answers given must meet the standard of any reasonably prudent nurse, and (2) there is no duty to recontact the person to see how or if the advice was implemented. It is always acceptable to suggest that the person seeking advice consult with a physician. For example, "If it were me, I would see my doctor immediately" is an appropriate response. The law does not require nurses to make such a suggestion if, in their professional judgment, such a suggestion is not necessary or if a reasonably prudent nurse would likewise not make the suggestion. Similarly, the law does not place liability if the person seeking advice fails to follow the advice. The person asking advice can choose to ignore the advice given.

GUIDELINES: HEALTH-RELATED ADVICE

1. Before the situation ever arises, reread both the state nurse practice act and your professional liability insurance policy to see if you are covered financially and if the nurse practice act covers free advice.

2. If you decide to give advice:
   a. Give only current, up-to-date advice.
   b. Stay within the nursing scope of practice and refrain from medical diagnoses and treatments.
   c. Refrain from suggesting that the physician currently being seen is giving wrong advice.
   d. Refrain from false reassurance.
   e. Keep a personal written account of your advice.

3. If you are unsure of what to say or how the advice will be taken, suggest that the person seeking advice see a physician, or state that you are unqualified to answer. You will not be sued for advice not given, but you can be sued for incorrect or potentially harmful advice.

A final word of caution: Always refrain from reassuring the person who has asked about a particular disease or symptom that there is nothing to worry about. Reassurance is appropriate only if the condition is indeed minor. As a general rule, ask yourself the following question: If you were at your regular employment and a patient asked the identical question, how would you answer it? That very same answer should be given to the person asking for free health care advice.

EXERCISE 18-3

Your neighbor knocks on your door late one night, stating that his wife has fallen, has hit her head, and is asking that you come see her. When you arrive, you find her conscious, inebriated, and bleeding from a 4-cm gash over the left eyebrow. She hit her head on a sharp object, and she was dazed and unconscious for about a five-minute period. You help her bandage the cut, and advise her to seek medical help. The next day you discover that the neighbor did not seek medical help and that she is lightheaded and unsure on her feet. She still refuses to see a doctor or to go to the local emergency center.

What are your potential legal liabilities if further harm comes to the neighbor? Are you liable? If so, what is the neighbor's cause of action against you? Does the husband also have any reason to name you in a lawsuit?

SUMMARY

Nursing in community health settings is both fluid and dynamic. As laws continue to evolve in community health care, nurses are cautioned to remain current on state and federal laws, as well as on pertinent court decisions within their geographic areas. Treating the client with respect and competent nursing care allows nurses to remain free from potential liability and encourages them to communicate with the client and family. People—not events or bad outcomes—bring lawsuits, and the client who feels that nurses are caring, trusting individuals is less likely to bring suit even if a bad outcome occurs.

AFTER COMPLETING THIS CHAPTER, YOU SHOULD BE ABLE TO

- Describe the provisions of the Social Security Act of 1935 and the Public Health Service Act of 1944, with their respective amendments, and give examples of how each act has changed community health nursing.
- Describe the legal responsibilities of community health nurses, including
    Home health care nurses.
    Occupational health nurses.
    School health nurses.
- Describe nurses' legal liabilities when volunteering nursing services, including:
    Disaster nursing services.
    Donating health-related advice.

APPLY YOUR LEGAL KNOWLEDGE

- How have the Social Security Act of 1935 and the Public Health Service Act of 1944, with their respective amendments, changed the health care delivery system in the past ten years?
- What advice should be given to nurses seeking employment in occupational health or school health about their potential legal liability?
- What are three reasons why nurses should donate their services and three reasons why they should not?

REFERENCES

Loton v. Massachusetts Paramedical, Inc. (Mass. Sup. Ct., 1987). *National Jury Verdict Review and Analysis.* (1989).

Lunsford v. Board of Nurse Examiners, 648 S.W. 2d 391 (Tex. Civ. App.-Austin, 1983).

Miller, T. W. (1990). Political involvement and community health advocacy. In B. S. Spradley (ed.). *Community health nursing: Concepts and practice.* Boston: Little, Brown and Company.

Public Law, 100-175. (1987).

R.W.H. v. W.C.N.S., Inc. (1992). No. 88-CV-18315, *Medical Malpractice Verdicts, Settlements and Experts*, (6), 34.

Schlussler v. Independent School District No. 200 et al. Case No. MM89-14V, *Minnesota Case Reports.* (Minnesota, 1989).

Therrell v. Fonde, 495 So. 2d 1046 (Alabama, 1986).

• nineteen

Nursing in Academic Settings

PREVIEW

Students, including nursing students, frequently ask questions about their rights to an education, their rights to matriculate and graduate, and their rights in disputes concerning clinical settings or clinical grades. Likewise, faculty have rights, including those in the academic setting, academic freedom, and employment rights. While there is some overlap between the rights of students and faculty, legal issues can be separated. This chapter addresses issues affecting both students and faculty, giving guidelines for effective communication between them. Employment issues of faculty, including promotion and tenure, are not addressed since they are outside the scope of this book.

NURSING STUDENTS

The rights of *nursing students* are not as comprehensive as those of faculty. Many of the faculty rights are derived from the employer–employee relationship, a relationship that students do not enjoy. Some of the faculty rights are also derived from their professional and licensure status. Students' rights come through statutes and constitutional law, including the right of due process.

Admission Requirements

Applicants have few rights in applying to schools of higher education. Schools are not allowed to discriminate against potential applicants. Areas that are usually concerned with discrimination are race, gender, age, and national origin, and states may add other areas under the general category of discrimination. Since the passage of the Americans with Disabilities Act, schools cannot discriminate against the disabled and must make reasonable accommodations that allow disabled students to attend classes. These reasonable accommodations include making buildings and rooms within buildings wheelchair accessible, providing readers for blind students, providing specialized communication devices for hearing-impaired students, and allowing alternate means of testing for the visually impaired or for students who have learning handicaps.

Admission requirements should be based on the school's or program's mission statement, and all admission requirements must be reasonable. Schools of nursing usually establish health requirements, immunization requirements, and prerequisite course requirements. These prerequisite requirements allow students to more quickly move through the beginning nursing courses, and they may include courses such as chemistry, anatomy and physiology, sociology, and psychology. Health and immunization requirements are established since the students will be functioning in patient settings during the course of their study. In the past, schools denied admission to the visually impaired, hearing impaired, and other disabled students. Now schools are required to make reasonable accommodations for these students, although they may still deny admission if no accommodations are reasonable. For example, the wheelchair-dependent person is generally unable to meet clinical requirements.

Disciplinary and Grievance Procedures

Schools should have written *disciplinary and grievance procedures.* One component of these procedures is a *policy on grievances,* outlining the steps the student may elect to take in grade disputes, probation, or suspension from the program. Generally, the courts see the academic institution as having the expertise in handling and deciding grade disputes, and their issues are whether the student was afforded due process rights, if a public institution, and whether the school adhered to its own policies and procedures.

Courts often hold that the *school catalog* creates a contract with the student. The catalog must state the grading policy for the institution and what grades must be achieved to be considered passing. Students must have a copy of the catalog or handbook, and the institution must abide by its stated policy.

One of the leading cases in this area is *The University of Texas Health Science Center at Houston, School of Nursing v. Babb* (1982). In that case, the student entered the program under a catalog stating that each course must be passed with a D or better. The student was advised before the end of the term that she was failing a course and that she should resign from the program and then request readmission. She followed that advice and was subsequently readmitted the following year. During the time before her readmission, the program changed the catalog to read that courses must be passed with a C or better. The student earned two Ds during her first semester after admission. She brought this action, alleging that the school was unfair in changing its policy and that she should be allowed to continue under the catalog requirements in effect when she first entered the program. The court agreed, holding that there was a contract between the student and the school and that the contractual agreement dated from the time she first entered the program. The court further held that schools have the right to change and amend catalogs, that this cannot cancel contracts previously existing, and that the student need only fulfill the requirements of the initial requirement.

One of the more antagonizing decisions for faculty concerns students' lack of competence or minimal competence in the clinical setting. Because evaluations of clinical students are subjective, faculty may be reluctant to place students on probation or to fail them in the clinical practicum. Case-law upholds the faculty member's expertise in accurately evaluating student abilities.

An Ohio case, *Morin v. Cleveland Metro* (1986), exemplifies the courts' reluctance to interfere with faculty members' professional judgments, particularly in matters that relate to clinical evaluations. In that case, a student during her final medical-surgical course was observed by the clinical faculty as providing six separate instances of what the faculty believed to be unsafe nursing practices. The student was given instructions and evaluations with each occurrence, and later dismissed from the program based on the unsafe nursing practices, a poor pattern of performances evidenced by previous probation and failure to meet the school's curriculum requirements. The student subsequently completed her nursing education at another program.

In the court's final analysis, the justices were reluctant to interfere with the professional's judgment as it pertains to subjective clinical grading. As long as the decision is made with clear deliberation and students are given an opportunity to be heard and to understand the allegations against them, judicial interference in academic decision making is minimal. The court also noted that, with each instance of unsafe practice, the student was counseled and an honest attempt was made to assist her in learning. There was no indifference on the part of the faculty, nor was there evidence that the faculty member had anything but the patient's ultimate safety and the student's learning as motivating factors.

Arbitrary Treatment

The courts look very differently if students have been subjected to *arbitrary treatment*, which includes the lack of clear criteria in the school catalog concerning grading policies, passing grades, or grievance procedures. Students are to receive course syllabi at the beginning of courses, specifying how the final grade will be determined, the content of the course, and what is expected of students. If students can demonstrate that the course syllabus is not followed, particularly in grading procedures, they may file a discrimination charge against the institution.

To avoid such a happening, faculty are required to prepare course syllabi with care and to follow them as written and distributed. Documentation through the keeping of anecdotal notes should be encouraged, since it assists the faculty member in giving students concrete examples of when and how they either met or failed to meet the course criteria.

Safe Environment

The school has a responsibility to ensure a *safe environment* to students, and students may reasonably expect that they will have a certain degree of safety on school property. Schools have a responsibility to alert students of unsafe or potentially dangerous situations and to assist in alleviating these situations. For example, if the school administration knows of unsafe or potential dangers and fails to alert students to the dangers, the school may be held liable. In a 1987 case, there had been attacks on students in the campus dormitory and the school was held liable when a subsequent student was attacked because of failure to alert students to the possibility of such attacks (*District of Columbia v. Doe*).

Confidentiality of Records

Schools are required to maintain *confidentiality of records* with respect to materials received during the admission process and during the course of the student's studies. This includes references that may have been submitted, student's grades earned before and during the course of the program, and clinical evaluations. Students can sue for defamation if faculty inadvertently or inappropriately reveal to third parties confidential information that is false and that is damaging to their reputation or career.

Because of the possibility of sensitive information, *medical records of students* should be placed apart from their academic files and access to medical records restricted. Such confidentiality of medical records further assures that information will not be revealed except to a few individuals.

STANDARD OF CARE

The *standard of care* owed by nursing students to patients for whom they care is identical to the standard of care owed the patient by the RN. This applies even though the nursing faculty have assigned the patient to the student, not a member of the clinical facility. The rationale underlying this standard of care is that the patient has the right to expect that professional services supplied by the hospital or health care facility will be provided by persons with the prerequisite degree of professional skill and competence.

LIABILITY FOR NEGLIGENCE BY STUDENTS

Nursing students have the ultimate responsibility for their own actions and may be liable for their own negligence. *Student liability* holds true even if students are not adults under state law. The often quoted adage that students practice on their instructor's license is not a true or valid statement because only the individual rewarded the license practices on the license. Individual students always retain accountability, and nurse practice acts allow nursing students to perform professional actions without being awarded a license to practice professional nursing. If it were any other way, nursing students could not be allowed to learn their profession until after graduation and licensure.

The licensure exception places great accountability on the nursing student, since the same competent care that the reasonably prudent nurse would give must be the standard of care of the professional nursing student also. The student as well as the faculty must know hospital policies and procedures, and remain current in medical and nursing knowledge. The licensure exception further requires that unprepared nursing students or students who need additional supervision inform the faculty instructor of their special needs or inadequate preparation for clinical practice.

While nursing students remain accountable for their knowledge and skills, faculty or staff may become accountable for individual student incompetence or unpreparedness. For example, in *Blanding v. Richland Memorial Hospital* (1988), an 18-year-old patient suffered a cardiac arrest and died following a simple skin graft surgery. The nursing student who was caring for him at the time of the arrest had failed to place his head in a position so that he could breathe and also failed to notice that he was not breathing. There was student liability in the case, as well as liability to the instructor and nursing staff at the institution.

In a similar case, *Anonymous v. Anonymous Obstetrician* (1994), an infant suffered gangrene of the testicles and scrotal sac following a circumcision. The physician had given a verbal order to the nurse not to discharge the infant until after he voided. Rather than writing the order, the nurse relayed the order to the nursing student caring for the infant. The nursing student then consulted her instructor as to whether the child could be discharged, and finding nothing in the orders to countermand the infant's discharge, the child was discharged. Though liability was not found against the nursing student, the case illustrates that nursing students must act accountably in clinical settings.

Students are also charged with following hospital policy and procedure. Faculty must ensure that students understand and are aware of hospital policy. If students then exceed their student role and a patient suffers harm because of their actions, they are more likely to incur sole responsibility since no liability will be imputed to the faculty or the hospital staff member.

Hospital liability may be further decreased by an existing contract between the clinical institution and the educational institution. Usually the hospital agrees to accept a predetermined number of clinical nursing students in its various departments, and the educational institution agrees to prescreen the nursing students prior to their clinical assignments. Only nursing students whose academic and clinical records meet the standard of care of the reasonably prudent nursing student will be allowed to practice under close faculty supervision.

Thus a duty arises for the faculty and educational institution to allow only competent students the right to practice in the clinical setting. A duty also arises for the clinical institution to maintain safe, competent clinical sites. Both have an equal duty to monitor the other, and both parties may incur liability for allowing substandard conditions or substandard care to persist.

Students also have potential liability for course materials that they have mastered and passed successfully. These skills and competencies should be evaluated and documented by faculty as students complete the skills and competencies. Documentation of competencies can be done by meeting skills objectives, test scores, and evaluation performances, both in the clinical facility and in the skills laboratory. This documentation can then be used to attest to the fact that the faculty delegated appropriately should a subsequent patient injury occur.

Much of the early case-law concerning negligence and accountability of nursing students centered on whether students are employees of the hospital or of the educational institution. Today, in a collegiate atmosphere in which nursing students receive no compensation from the clinical institution but rather pay for the right to attend classes, it would seem that they have more of a relationship with the institution of higher education. This is especially true because the school has a duty to adequately supervise and teach its students, and incurs potential liability for failure to prevent unsafe nursing practices by its students.

GUIDELINES: NURSING STUDENTS' CLINICAL PERFORMANCE

1. Understand the institution's policies and procedures prior to undertaking any clinical assignment. Prepare adequately for clinical settings, ensuring that you are knowledgeable about the patient's condition, interventions, medications, and treatment.

2. If you are unprepared for the clinical setting, inform the clinical instructor. Never undertake to demonstrate skills, perform procedures, or give medications for which you are unprepared. Remember, the patient's ultimate safety is the first priority.

3. When unsure of a procedure or skill, ask for help before beginning the skill or procedure, even if this delays the intervention. If the instructor is not readily available, allow the staff nurse to complete the intervention. Again, the patient's ultimate safety is the primary goal.

4. Never allow yourself to be bullied into performing skills or procedures with which you are unfamiliar or that are not listed by the institution as those that nursing students may perform. Staff members may be hurried and ask you to assist them. That's appropriate as long as you are knowledgeable about the skill and the skill is approved by the institution as one that students can perform. You may want to volunteer to assist in another way, rather than refusing entirely. For example, you might volunteer to give the patient's bath so that the staff member is free to perform other interventions.

EXERCISE 19-1

You are a junior nursing student on a busy surgical unit. On your third clinical day, you are well prepared to take care of the patient assigned to you, but your clinical experience is limited. The nurse manager stops you, hands you a posey belt and soft wrist restraints, telling you to, "Go restrain that wacko in 502!" You have never cared for a patient who was restrained, nor have you ever seen a posey belt in use. What is your response? Do you restrain the patient? How do you later report the incident to your clinical instructor?

NURSING FACULTY

Several issues concern *nursing faculty,* their employer institutions, and the hospitals or health care settings in which they supervise students. Probably the most important factor is that individual faculty members are licensed to practice professional nursing within the given jurisdiction, and as such they owe the same duty of care to the patients or clients that they encounter as would any professional nurse.

Since the primary responsibilities of nursing faculty are to teach and supervise students, faculty owe themselves and those they encounter the duty of remaining current in medical matters such as diagnoses, etiologies, therapies, current treatments, and innovative nursing interventions and of continually reevaluating and reassessing students in the clinical area. Not all faculty will be interesting lecturers or outstanding role models, but all faculty should teach current concepts and be competent practitioners. Many nursing schools are now encouraging nursing faculty to have a *concurrent clinical practice*, since technologies and interventions are continuously being upgraded and updated. A clinical concurrent practice allows instructors to remain current in their clinical field.

The Faculty–Student Relationship

The faculty's role is critical in the education of nursing students. Individual faculty members determine the nursing students' capabilities and skills, and ultimately they determine if the patients' needs can be entrusted to a particular nursing student. Thus faculty must know the given hospital's policies and procedures, teach necessary skills to the students, and evaluate student performance on a continuing basis. Faculty must also be willing to counsel students and/or fail those who cannot meet clinical expectations or who fail to follow safe nursing practices. The patient's safety is the ultimate goal of both faculty and students.

To foster student–faculty relationships and to keep students current in their performance grades, faculty should meet the following evaluation guidelines.

1. Specify course requirements and expectations at the onset of the course. This is best accomplished by clear and complete course syllabi that are inclusive of attendance requirements, methods of evaluation, penalties for late work, and availability of faculty by phone, office hours, and times for individual and group student conferences. Refrain from changing syllabus requirements during the semester since that encourages unsuccessful students or those who make lower grades in the course to challenge the final grade.

2. Allow students the opportunity to review all evaluation data and reports that will become part of their permanent files. Forms signed by both the faculty member and the student ensure student review as well as the accountability of the faculty member. Students may wish to add their own accounts of occurrences and happenings, and they should be encouraged to do so. This further opens communications and shows the desire on the part of the faculty to work with students.

3. Retain all graded papers, tests, case studies, and care plans. It is advisable to retain such data rather than return the papers to the student during the course, although students should be able to see the graded paper. Retained data further support the faculty's assignment of grades, and the

papers should be retained for a period equal to that in which the student may appeal the grade. Allow students adequate time to review the paper data so that they can gain insight into the faculty's grading scale, methods, and areas of mastery versus areas where they need more study.

4. Conduct regular student–faculty conferences for feedback to the students. There should be at least a midcourse and a final course evaluation conference, especially for clinical courses. These conferences allow faculty the opportunity to discover areas where they could concentrate their efforts in assisting students to learn, and give students the opportunity to ask questions and offer explanations in a private setting.

5. Establish and publish as part of the student policies a review of the grading policy and steps in the school's grievance policy. Such policies allow students a formal recourse and prevent a charge of arbitrary treatment from occurring.

6. Maintain anecdotal notes for reference. These allow for specific examples and help to refresh the faculty member's memory should a grade be appealed or a grievance filed. These may also be used to give students examples showing how they were effective in the clinical setting or their need for improvement. Anecdotal notes, because of their content, should be kept in secure areas, preferably locked.

Academic versus Disciplinary Dismissal

Given the subjective nature of student performance evaluations, many faculty hesitate to put students on probation or to fail them. When dealing with students demonstrating no or low competence, faculty may wish to consider the distinction between academic and disciplinary issues.

1. To dismiss students for *disciplinary reasons,* such as for infractions of the school's rules and regulations, they should be accorded due process. Specifically, oral or written notices of the charges have to be made. If students deny the charges, the faculty must explain the evidence and give students an opportunity to present their side. Even in private schools where the Fourth Amendment due process rights do not attach, it is advisable to afford such rights to the student.

2. If students are to be dismissed for *academic reasons,* such as failure to pass a required course, they must only be given the opportunity to present their objections before the academic body responsible for dismissal. The faculty themselves are the best judges of students' academic performance. Courts have been reluctant to override this idea of faculty's professional judgment (*Morin v. Cleveland Metro,* 1986).

Records that should be required when reviewing disputes between students and faculty include the following, as applicable:

1. The school catalog.
2. Attendance records.

3. Grading appeals procedures and policies and/or grievance policies and procedures.
4. Student papers, examinations, and written clinical care plans.
5. Student handbooks.
6. Clinical or student evaluations.
7. Course syllabi.
8. Committee minutes.

It is of extreme importance for faculty to categorize whether a student dismissal is for academic or disciplinary reasons. If academic dismissal is forthcoming, the faculty may wish to counsel the student, to aid the student in pursuing other academic programs or careers, or to withdraw the student from the course with a passing grade. For disciplinary dismissal, students should still be counseled, placed on probation or informed of grade expectations for the course, and given an opportunity to present their side formally. Students may appeal through the dean of the school as well as through the president of the institution or equivalent. At all stages, written minutes and records of the various proceedings should be kept and signed by all concerned parties.

Evaluating noncognitive aspects of student performance is indeed difficult. Clinical competence, interpersonal relationships, and professionalism are vital components of the professional nurse. The grading of these is subjective, and students should be afforded ample safeguards. Such safeguards may be in the form of adequate conferences and unambiguous course requirements. Perhaps the most important factor for faculty to remember is that open communication lines must be maintained. Counsel students as needed when an incident occurs, give frequent evaluation conferences, and be open and constructive with them. A close family member of the student may also want to attend the conference, and faculty should make the ultimate determination to either allow or refuse such a request. Students and their parents or spouse seldom sue a faculty who is perceived as fair, impartial, and accessible. Just as adequate communications may prevent patient lawsuits, the same type of communications may keep a student from filing suit or may be instrumental in helping faculty prevail if a suit is tried.

Lastly, faculty should carry professional liability insurance coverage in an adequate dollar amount. Since legal action could come from either a dissatisfied student or an injured party within the clinical setting, faculty are well advised to maintain sufficient coverage, even if covered by the institution.

EXERCISE 19-2

For the fifth time in the last month, the nursing instructor has decided to change the number of written care plans you are expected to do, their due dates, and information needed to complete each one. How might this issue best be addressed? Can the issue be addressed so that both the students' learning and the faculty member benefit?

GUIDELINES: FACULTY–STUDENT ACCOUNTABILITY

1. Delineate course requirements at the onset of the course. Both faculty and students should be clear on the following:
   a. Credit hours.
   b. Lecture and clinical schedules.
   c. Methods and tools of evaluations.
   d. Assignment deadlines and penalties for late submission.
   e. Course description and specific requirements.
   f. Standards for students as identified in the school catalog or in a student policy manual.
   g. Conference times.
2. Conduct frequent, individual student–faculty conferences. Include in each conference:
   a. Written evaluation forms.
   b. Opportunity for both sides to clarify particular expectations and instances or happenings.
   c. Written identification of any deficiencies.
   d. Opportunity for students to respond orally or in writing to evaluator's comments or suggestions.
   e. A signed conference sheet that will become part of the student's permanent file.
3. Maintain current policies and procedures of the institution, and ensure that students have a mechanism to recommend new policies to faculty.
4. Maintain a permanent file of all student written work, including tests, papers, case studies, and written care plans. The students should be allowed to take responsibility for reviewing these materials at a time convenient to both instructor and student.
5. Establish a formal grievance policy. Both students and faculty share responsibility for knowing and implementing the policy.
6. Allow sufficient time for open communications. Faculty and students alike benefit from honest and open discussions.

SUMMARY

Issues relating to student–faculty interactions can pose difficult questions for everyone concerned. The ultimate goals of such interactions are to ensure that adequately prepared students will be able to care for patients competently and to ensure future nursing professionals.

AFTER COMPLETING THIS CHAPTER, YOU SHOULD BE ABLE TO

- Describe student rights, including:
  Admission requirements.
  Disciplinary and grievance procedures.
  Arbitrary treatment.
  Safe environment.
  Confidentiality of records.
- Describe the standard of care owed patients by nursing students.
- Describe areas of negligence for which nursing students may be held accountable.
- Describe faculty responsibilities in relationship to nursing students.
- Differentiate between academic and disciplinary issues in assisting students.

APPLY YOUR LEGAL KNOWLEDGE

- How should faculty react to admissions of clinical unpreparedness?
- What responsibilities do students have for their continual learning?
- When should students volunteer to assist staff nurses in the performance of clinical interventions? Why?

REFERENCES

Anonymous v. Anonymous Obstetrician. (1994). *Medical Malpractice Verdicts, Settlements and Experts,* 10(4), 35.

Blanding v. Richland Memorial Hospital, No. JR 155725. (1988). *Medical Malpractice Verdicts, Settlements and Experts,* 4(5), 22.

District of Columbia v. Doe, 524 A.2d 30 (District of Columbia, 1987).

Morin v. Cleveland Metro, 516 N.E.2d 1257 (Ohio, 1986).

The University of Texas Health Science Center at Houston, School of Nursing v. Babb, 646 S.W.2d 502 (Texas, 1982).

IV

ETHICS AND THE LAW

· twenty

Ethics

PREVIEW

Every day, nurses make ethical decisions in their professional practice. Some of the decisions are clear-cut and easily made, such as when all health care deliverers agree that life-saving measures will not be initiated for a terminal patient. Often, however, nurses find themselves trapped in the midst of ethical dilemmas among physician, patients, family members, and even their own peer group, such as when a patient refuses treatment. This chapter explores the distinction between law and ethics, discusses various ethical theories and principles, and gives the nurse an ethical framework on which to base ethical decisions.

DEFINITIONS OF ETHICS AND VALUES

Ethics is the science relating to moral actions and moral values. Ethics encompasses "principles of right or good conduct" or "a body of such principles" (Boyer et al., 1991, p. 253). A broader conceptual definition is that ethics is concerned with motives and attitudes and the relationship of these attitudes to the good of the individual. "Ethics has to do with actions we wish people would take, not actions they must take" (Hall, 1990, p. 37). Many people envision ethics as dealing solely with principles of morality—that which is good or desirable as opposed to that which is bad or undesirable. The problem faced by such a right or wrong definition is who decides what is good and what is evil: individuals, professionals, or cultures?

A broader conceptual definition of ethics is concerned with motives and attitudes and their relationship to the good of the individual. Thus values become interwoven with ethics. *Values* are personal beliefs about the truths and worth of thoughts, objects, or behavior. With values come value clarification, a process aimed at understanding the nature of one's own value system and its vast impact on the individual nurse's delivery of health care services.

DISTINCTION BETWEEN ETHICS AND THE LAW

The *legal system* is founded on rules and regulations that guide society in a formal and binding manner. Although man-made and capable of being changed by the judiciary or legislative enactments, the legal system is a general foundation that gives continuing guidance to health care providers, regardless of their personal views and value system. For example, the law recognizes the competent patient's right to refuse therapy. The patient retains this right whether health care deliverers agree or disagree with the choice.

This right, though, is not absolute. If there are overriding state interests, treatment may be mandated against a patient's or parent's wishes. Jehovah's Witness cases, mandatory immunization statutes, and fluoridation of water enactments are three examples of overriding state interests.

Ethical values are subject to philosophical, moral, and individual interpretations. Both the health care provider and the health care recipient have a system of rights and values. Can one justify allowing competent adult patients to refuse therapy if the cost is their lives? Does ethics allow the refusal of health care therapies and treatments based on one's religious convictions that all medications and therapies are against God's law?

Most health care providers have difficulty in areas that transect both the law and ethics, such as the issues of death and dying, genetics, abuse of others, and futility of health care. Table 20–1 attempts to distinguish these two opposing concepts.

Ethics and legal issues often become entwined so that it becomes difficult to separate the two. Both legal and ethical issues assist nurses in decision making and in the delivery of competent, quality curing care. Thus, nurses must be cognizant of both areas in clinical settings.

ETHICAL THEORIES

A variety of different ethical theories have evolved to justify moral principles. These so-called *normative theories* are universally applicable, involve questions and dilemmas requiring a choice of action, and entail a conflict of rights and obligations on the part of the nurse–decision maker. Most normative approaches to ethics fall into two broad categories, although a third category is currently evolving.

TABLE 20–1. DISTINCTION BETWEEN LAW AND ETHICS

	Law	Ethics
Source	External to oneself; rules and regulations of society	Internal to oneself; values and beliefs, and individual interpretations
Concerns	Conduct and actions; what a person did or failed to do	Motives, attitudes and culture; reasons for why one acted as he or she did
Interests	Society as a whole as opposed to the individual	Good of the individual within the society
Enforcement	Courts, statutes, and boards of nursing	Ethics committees and professional organizations

Source: Adapted from Hemelt, M.D. and Mackert, M.E. (1982). *Dynamics of Law in Nursing and Health Care* (2nd ed.). Reston, Va: Reston Publishing Company.

GUIDELINES: MAINTAINING LEGAL RIGHTS WITHIN ETHICAL DILEMMAS

1. Recognize the difference between legal rights and ethical views. While both concepts are important, legal rights must be afforded patients. For example, consent may be obtained for an abortion within the first trimester from both prospective parents, but only the prospective mother must sign the consent form.

2. Nurses must realize that their ethical views and values may differ greatly from the patient's value system. Such an understanding allows nurses to remain objective when caring for patients and when serving as consultants for decision making by the patient.

3. Nurses must remain current about recent judicial decisions in their jurisdiction and incorporate these standards and rights into their nursing care.

4. If the courts have not reviewed a case involving a particular ethical issue, then a legal standard may not exist. In such an instance, nurses are guided by the ethics of the profession and by personal moral values.

5. It is recommended that nurses remove themselves from patients' nursing care if values come into major conflict, such as when a terminally ill patient is kept alive by life support measures solely because the family cannot bear to let the patient die. If the nurse feels the patient should be allowed to die without further resuscitation efforts, the best solution may be to remove oneself from this patient's care.

6. Ethical dilemmas have no perfect answers, just better answers. Legal questions have right and wrong answers. When in conflict, follow the established legal principles.

Deontological (from the Greek *deon* for "duty") *theories* derive norms and rules from the duties human beings owe one another by virtue of commitments that are made and roles that are assumed. Generally, deontologists hold that a sense of duty consists of rational respect for the fulfilling of one's obligations to other human beings. The greatest strength of this theory is its emphasis on the dignity of human beings.

Deontological ethics look not to the consequences of an action, but to the intention of the action. One's good intentions ultimately determine the praiseworthiness of the action.

A branch of deontological ethics is commonly referred to as *situation ethics*, wherein decision making takes into account the unique characteristics of each individual, the caring relationship between the person and the care giver, and the most humanistic course of action given the circumstances. Situational ethics is frequently relied on when the nurse has cared for a particular patient for a long time.

Deontological theories can be subdivided into act and rule deontology. *Act deontology* is based on the personal moral values of the person making the ethical decision, while *rule deontology* is based on the belief that certain standards for ethical decisions transcend the individual's moral values. An example of such a universal rule could be "all human life has value" or "one should always tell the truth."

Teleological (from the Greek *telos* for "end") *theories* derive norms or rules for conduct from the consequences of actions. Right consists of actions that have good consequences, and wrong consists of actions that have bad consequences. Teleologists disagree, though, about how to determine the goodness or wrongness of an action.

This theory is often referred to as *utilitarianism;* what makes an action right or wrong is its utility and useful actions bring about the greatest good for the greatest number of people. An alternate way of viewing this theory is that the usefulness of an action is determined by the amount of happiness it brings.

Utilitarian ethics can then be subdivided into rule and act utilitarianism. *Rule utilitarianism* seeks the greatest happiness for all; it appeals to public agreement as a basis for objective judgment about the nature of happiness. *Act utilitarianism* attempts to determine, in a given situation, which course of action will bring about the greatest happiness, or the least harm and suffering, to a single individual. As such, utilitarianism makes happiness subjective (Guido, 1989).

An emerging theory is *principalism,* which incorporates various existing ethical principles and attempts to resolve conflicts by applying one or more of them. Ethical principles actually control professional decision making much more than do ethical theories. Principles encompass basic premises from which rules are developed. Principles are the moral norms that nurses both demand and strive to implement daily in clinical practice. Each of the principles can be used solely, although it is much more common to see the principles used in combination.

APPLYING ETHICAL THEORIES IN CLINICAL DECISION MAKING

While ethical theories do not provide easy, straightforward answers, they form an essential base of knowledge from which to proceed. Without ethical theories, the decision revolves solely on personal emotions and values. Because most nurses do not ascribe to either deontology or teleology exclusively, but to a combination of the two theories, principalism is growing in popularity.

EXERCISE 20-1

In a clinical setting, a patient refuses surgical intervention in favor of medical management. The health care delivery team and the patient's family favor surgical intervention. Could this ethical dilemma be resolved using the principles of deontology or teleology? Why or why not? How would you resolve this situation?

ETHICAL PRINCIPLES

Nurses apply eight ethical principles in everyday clinical practice, some to a greater degree than others. Each principle is discussed separately.

Autonomy addresses personal freedom and self-determination, the right to choose what will happen to one's own person. The legal doctrine of informed consent is a direct reflection of this principle. Autonomy involves health care deliverers' respect for patients' rights to make decisions affecting care and treatment, even if the health care deliverers do not agree with the decisions made. Since autonomy is not an absolute right, restrictions may be placed on a person's right to endanger others, as in the instance of communicable diseases.

The *beneficence* principle states that the actions one takes should promote good. In caring for patients, good can be defined in a variety of ways, including allowing a patient to die without advanced life support. Good can also prompt nurses to encourage the patient to undergo extensive, painful treatment procedures if these procedures will increase both the quality and quantity of the patient's life. Nurses frequently consider this principle when viewing the long-term outcomes of invasive and noninvasive procedures. The difficulty with this principle is in defining "good."

The corollary of beneficence, *nonmaleficence* states that one should do no harm. Many nurses find it difficult to follow this principle when performing treatments and procedures that bring pain to patients. Even the act of giving an intramuscular injection to relieve postoperative pain brings some immediate pain to most patients. Nurses frequently choose the principle of beneficence to follow rather than nonmaleficence. Ethicists frequently reserve this principle for issues of major impact as, "Can one preserve the life of anencephalic infants merely as a source for organ transplantation?"

Veracity concerns truth telling and incorporates the concept that individuals should always tell the truth. This principle also compels that the whole truth is told. This principle is followed when one completely answers patients' questions, giving as much information as possible and telling the patient when information is not available or known.

Fidelity is keeping one's promises or commitments. Staff members know not to promise patients what they cannot deliver or what they do not control, such as when the patient asks that nothing be done, should he or she stop breathing, before consulting the patient's physician for such an order. Keeping one's promises may become an issue in that patients are assured that they will be kept comfortable in the postoperative period, but complications may occur that prevent their being medicated, such as when the patient is hemodynamically unstable following surgery.

Paternalism (also known as *parentialism*) allows one to make decisions for another and is often seen as an undesirable principle. By definition, paternalism allows no collaboration on the decision, but totally removes the decision making from the patient or patient's family members. Called the *standard of best interest,* this principle may be used to assist patients in making a decision about their health care when they are unable to have full or complete knowledge on which to base the decision (Aiken & Catalano, 1994). Derived from the best interest test, this principle allows health care personnel to assist in decision making when patients lack the expertise or data to make decisions. When the entire decision is taken from the patient, the principle is to be avoided.

Justice states that people should be treated fairly and equally. This principle frequently arises in times of short supplies or when there is competition for resources or benefits, such as when two patients require intensive care beds and only one bed is available.

Respect for others, seen by many as the highest principle, incorporates all other principles. Respect for others acknowledges the right of individuals to make decisions and to live or die by those decisions. Respect for others transcends cultural differences, gender issues, religious differences, and racial concerns. Nurses positively reinforce this principle daily in actions with peers, interdisciplinary health team members, patients, and family members.

EXERCISE 20-2

Give an example of how each of the eight principles just discussed is used daily by nurses. How does the incorporation of all the principles strengthen the health care delivery system and further assure quality, competent nursing care?

ETHICAL DECISION-MAKING FRAMEWORK

Ethical decision making involves reflection on the following questions:

1. Who should make the choice?
2. What are the possible options or courses of action?
3. What are the available options or alternatives?
4. What are the consequences, both good and bad, of all possible options?
5. Which rules, obligations, and values should direct the choices?
6. What are the desired goals and outcomes?

When making ethical decisions, nurses need to combine all the elements using an orderly, systematic, and objective method. Ethical decision-making models assist toward this end.

The various models for ethical decision making have five to fourteen ordered steps that begin with fully comprehending the ethical dilemma and conclude with the evaluation of the implemented decision. Perhaps the easiest model to use at the bedside is the MORAL model, developed by Thiroux (1977) and refined for nursing by Halloran (1982). Many nurses prefer this model because the letters of the acronym remind nurses of the subsequent steps of the model.

The model is as follows:

M *Massage the dilemma.* Identify and define the issues in the dilemma. Consider the opinions of the major players—patients, family members, nurses, physicians, clergy, and other interdisciplinary health care members—as well as their value systems.

O *Outline the options.* Examine all options fully, including the less realistic and conflicting ones. This stage is designed to fully comprehend the options and alternatives available, not to make a final decision.

R *Resolve the dilemma.* Review the issues and options, applying basic ethical principles to each option. Decide the best option based on the views of all those concerned in the dilemma.

A *Act by applying the chosen option.* This step is usually the most difficult because it requires actual implementation, while the previous steps had allowed only for dialog and discussion.

L *Look back and evaluate the entire process, including the implementation.* No process is complete without a thorough evaluation. Ensure that those involved are able to follow through on the final option. If not, a second decision may be required and the process must start again at the initial step.

EXERCISE 20-3

Jody Smith, a retired nurse with three adult children and numerous adult grandchildren, lives in a small rural area on a limited income. Two months ago, she fell and broke her left hip. After surgery for an artificial hip replacement, she was transferred to a rehabilitation center where she had a left-sided cerebrovascular accident (CVA). Upon her readmittance to the acute care facility, she received aggressive therapy for the CVA.

Completely paralyzed on her left side, Mrs. Smith has decided that she no longer desires aggressive therapy and frequently asks the staff why she cannot die in peace. "The rehabilitation is so painful and I'll never walk again. What's the use?"

Both the doctors and her family are much more optimistic. The orthopedic surgeon is convinced that she will walk again, and the neurologist believes that she will make a full recovery and be able to return home and care for herself. Both doctors have excluded Mrs. Smith from their conversations, assuring her children that she will be "as good as new," and ignoring her requests to discontinue anticoagulant and rehabilitative therapy.

Mrs. Smith refuses to cooperate with the physical and occupational therapists, will not take her medications, and refuses to perform simple tasks, relying instead on staff members to meet her activities of daily living. Using the MORAL model, how would you resolve this dilemma?

Ethical decision making is always a process. To facilitate this process, use all available resources, including the ethics committee if your institution has one, and communicate with and support everyone involved in the process. Some decisions are easier to reach and support than others. It is important to allow sufficient time for a supportable option to be reached.

HOSPITAL ETHICS COMMITTEES

With the increasing numbers of legal and ethical dilemmas in patient situations today, health care providers are considering guidance with decision making. Perhaps one of the best solutions for both long-term and short-term issues is the creation and use of an institution ethics committee. *Ethical committees* can (1) provide structure and guidelines for potential problems, (2) serve as open forums for discussion, and (3) function as true patient advocates by placing the patient at the core of the committee discussions.

To form such a group, the proposed committee should first begin as a bioethical study group so that ethical principles and theories as well as current issues can be explored by its members. The composition of the committee should include nurses, physicians, clergy, clinical social workers, nutritional experts, pharmacists, administrative personnel, and legal experts. Once the committee has become active, individual patients or patients' family members may also be invited to the committee deliberations.

Ethics committees generally follow one of three distinct structures, although some institution ethics committees blend the three structures, and others differ in their approach depending on the individual case:

1. The *autonomy model* facilitates decision making for the competent patient.
2. The *patient benefit model* uses substituted judgment and facilitates decision making for the incompetent patient.
3. The *social justice model* considers broad social issues and is accountable to the institution.

In most settings, ethics committees are already a reality because of the complex issues in health care. In many medical centers, *ethical rounds*, which are

GUIDELINES: HOSPITAL ETHICS COMMITTEES

1. The hospital ethics committee should consist of a core group of health care professionals who are knowledgeable about legal and ethical issues within the institution.

2. The patient is the focus of ethical dilemmas. Decisions are based on the patient's values, desires, needs, and capabilities.

3. The hospital ethics committee serves as an objective body to provide assistance to those in need during difficult decision-making times. Hospital ethics committees are supportive of patients and patients' families, staff, and physicians.

4. The hospital ethics committee projects a positive public image through its committees and decisions. Such committee meetings aid in closing the gap between unrealistic societal expectations and the reality of everyday health care delivery.

5. The hospital ethics committee serves in a preventive capacity against potential litigation by being knowledgeable of current court decisions and by incorporating the same into its deliberations. This is especially true in the broad area of risk management.

6. The hospital ethics committee must guard against breaching patient privacy by ensuring that confidential matters are discussed only when vital and only with staff members and medical personnel who are directly concerned with the patient's care.

conducted on a weekly or monthly schedule, allow staff members, who may be involved in later ethical dilemmas, to begin viewing all the issues and to become more comfortable with ethical issues.

EXERCISE 20-4

If your health care institution has an active ethics committee, attend one of their sessions. Who is on the committee? Were family members or patients allowed to attend? Which structural model was used in the deliberations? Was their final recommendation consistent with your expectations? Would you have changed the outcome based on your use of the MORAL model?

SUMMARY

In ethics, unlike legal situations, there are frequently no easy answers, and sometimes there are no definable answers. Nurses must explore new issues and develop novel solutions. The better versed nurses are in ethical principles and everyday ethical issues, the more confidence they will have in working with difficult situations. As a starting point in developing their own ethical values and positions, nurses should be encouraged to attend ethics committee hearings and ethical grand rounds.

AFTER COMPLETING THIS CHAPTER, YOU SHOULD BE ABLE TO

- Distinguish law from ethics.
- Compare and contrast the three different ethical theories of deontology, teleology, and principalism.
- Define and apply to nursing practice the eight ethical principles of autonomy, beneficence, nonmaleficence, veracity, fidelity, justice, paternalism, and respect for others.
- Analyze the MORAL model in ethical decision making.
- Discuss the importance and role of hospital ethics committees and ethics grand rounds.

APPLY YOUR LEGAL KNOWLEDGE

- How can the professional nurse employ the concepts of ethics and law in clinical practice settings?
- Do professional nurses use ethical theories or ethical principles in clinical practice settings?
- Can the MORAL model be used truly at the bedside?
- What types of ethical dilemmas do professional nurses face on a daily basis?

REFERENCES

Aiken, T. D. & Catalano, J. T. (1994). *Legal, ethical, and political issues in nursing.* Philadelphia, PA: F. A. Davis Company.

Boyer, M., Ellis, K., Harris, D. R., & Soukhanov, A. H. (eds.). (1991). *The American heritage dictionary.* (2nd ed.). Boston: Houghton Mifflin Company.

Guido, G. W. (1988). *Legal issues in nursing: A source book for practice.* Norwalk, CT: Appleton & Lange.

Guido, G. W. (1989). Ethical and legal principles affecting decision-making in critical care nursing. In Dolan, J. *Critical care nursing: Clinical management through the nursing process.* Philadelphia, PA: F. A. Davis Company.

Hall, J. K. (1990). Understanding the fine line between law and ethics. *Nursing 90, 20*(10). 37.

Halloran, M. C. (1982). Rational ethical judgments utilizing a decision-making tool. *Heart and Lung, 11*(6), 566–570.

Thiroux, J. (1977). *Ethics: Theory and practice.* Philadelphia, PA: Macmillan.

Glossary

Abandonment: Unilateral termination of a professional contract without affording the client reasonable notice and services.

Abuse: Incorporates physical, mental, and sexual assaults as well as physical, emotional, and medical neglect; most often seen as child abuse or elder abuse.

Access laws: Group of statutory disclosure laws that permit a person to obtain medical records and information about an individual patient without first obtaining the patient's permission; examples include Medicare and Medicaid reimbursement and workers' compensation laws.

Act deontology: Based on the personal moral values of the person making the ethical decision.

Act utilitarianism: Attempts to determine, in a given situation, which course of action will bring about the greatest happiness, or the least harm and suffering, to a given individual.

Adequate staffing: Accreditation standards mandate that sufficient numbers of qualified staff must be provided by health care institutions.

Administrative agency: An arm of the government that administers or carries out legislative enactments; may be federal, state, or local.

Administrative laws: Rules and regulations originated and enforced through administrative agencies, whether federal, state, or local; administrative laws are created to enforce statutory laws.

Admission requirements: Statements of requirements that students must fulfill before being allowed admission to a school or institution.

Admitting privileges: Rights granted by individual health care institutions that allow physicians and other independent practitioners the ability to admit patients to the facility.

Advanced Directives: The various methods used by competent adults to indicate their choices in health care treatment decisions. These include but are not limited to express verbal communications, living wills, durable powers of attorney, and trust agreements.

Advanced practice roles: Areas of practice beyond the scope of B.S.N. and A.D.N. nurses; includes nurse practitioners, nurse midwives, nurse anesthetists, and clinical nurse specialists.

Agency personnel: Nurses who are hired by health care institutions to work a specific shift and are not full- or part-time workers of the institution, by employees of agencies that provide temporary help.

Agency policy: Written communications that set the standard of care for a given health care agency.

Affidavit: Voluntary written statement made or taken under oath before an officer of the court or a notary public; usually a sworn statement of facts.

Affirmative action: Federal mandate that enhances employment opportunities of protected groups of people, such as veterans, women, and minorities.

Age Discrimination in Employment Act: Mandates that it is illegal for employers, unions, and employment agencies to discriminate against men and women over the age of 40 in hiring practices.

Age of majority: Statutory or legal age of adulthood, generally 18 years of age.

Agency: The relationship in which one person acts for or represents another; an employer may act as the agent of an employer.

Agent: The person authorized by another to act for him or her.

Allegation: A statement, charge, or assertion that a person expects to be able to prove.

Alteration of records: Entries added to a patient record necessary to ensure a truthful and accurate report; two types of alterations may occur: minor (spelling, notations of laboratory data) and substantive (omitted progress notes, incorrect orders, incorrect laboratory data).

Alternative liability: Used in conjunction with products liability; applies when two or more manufacturers commit separate, wrongful or unreasonable actions, only one of which harms the plaintiff, but the plaintiff cannot show the actual cause-in-fact defendant.

Amended pleadings: Pleadings that alter or improve on previous pleadings; additions or subtractions from already existing pleadings in a lawsuit.

Americans with Disabilities Act of 1990 (ADA): Federal legislation that combines the doctrines of disability and equality in a variety of issues, including employment and public transportation issues.

Antitrust issues: Arise whenever there is an exclusion of a class of practitioners from membership on a medical or hospital staff, or where there are questions about the fair market value of a service, or where there are attempts by a society to restrict its members' use of a second class of practitioners.

Appeal: A legal proceeding in which a higher court is asked to reverse or correct the decision of a lower court.

Arbitration: Process by which an impartial person, chosen by the parties to a dispute, attempts to resolve the dispute.

Arbitrary treatment: Manner of student treatment that differs student to student or that is not included in official school documents.

Articulation with medical practice acts: Scope of practice that may be performed by either nurses or physicians, such as patient diagnoses and treatment by independent advanced practice nurses.

Assault: Any action that places another in apprehension of being touched in a manner that is offensive, insulting, or physically injurious without consent or authority; an intentional tort.

Attorney General's Opinion: Official statements of an executive officer issued in accordance with his or her authority; merely advisory and not mandatory orders to public officials; requested in instances where there is no clear-cut law on an issue in a given jurisdiction.

Autonomy: Personal freedom to make choices or decisions.

Autonomy model: In hospital ethics committees, this model facilitates decisions for the competent individual.

Battery: Contact with another or with their immediate "personage" (e.g., clothes, cane, car keys, purse) without consent or authority; the touching of another without permission; an intentional tort.

Bench trial: Official hearing in which no jury is sworn in; the judge serves as the trier both of facts and of law.

Beneficence: The ethical duty to do good.

Best interest test: An objective test that looks at personal preferences made while the now incompetent patient was rational and capable of stating what he or she would want in the event of a catastrophic happening; frequently relied on in the incompetent person's right-to-die issues.

Borrowed servant doctrine: A special application of the doctrine of respondeat superior, it applies when one employer lends the services or skills of an employee to another employer and serves to shift the vicarious liability from the primary to the borrowing employer; most frequently seen in the operating room when the hospital-employed nurse is acting under the exclusive control of the surgeon. Sometimes called the "captain of the ship" doctrine.

Breach: Failure of performance by a party of some agreed-on act or legal duty owed to another person.

Breach of duty: Deviation from standard of care owed.

Burden of proof: Duty of a party to legally substantiate an allegation by a preponderance (majority) of the evidence; usually the duty of the party bringing the lawsuit, although the burden of proof may shift to the defendant in limited circumstances.

Captain of the ship doctrine: Doctrine by which the physician, as "captain," is held liable for the actions of all members of the health care team; traditionally applied to a surgeon in an operating room; in most states has been discarded.

Causation: The injury for which the plaintiff complains must be directly linked with the breach of duty owed the plaintiff; may be subdivided into cause-in-fact (direct causation) or proximate case (indirect causation).

Cause of action: Claim in law and fact sufficient to demand judicial attention; facts that give rise to the right of action or the legal right to sue.

Caveat: Literally, "let him beware"; a caution or warning.

Certification: Programs sponsored by private, nongovernmental, professional organizations or agencies that recognize the attainment of advanced, specialized knowledge and skills beyond what is necessary for safe practice.

Charting by exception: Newer system of patient documentation that requires only entries of significant or abnormal findings and previously entered standardized or expected results are not entered into the record; dependent on extensive preprinted guidelines and standardized care plans and protocols.

Civil law: Used to distinguish that part of the law concerned with noncriminal matters; the branch of law that pertains to the rights and duties of persons in contracts, torts, patents, and the like.

Civil Rights Act of 1964: Legislation that affected equal employment opportunities for protected classes of people.

Civil Rights Act of 1991: Extended the protection given by the act of 1964 to include sexual harassment in the workplace.

Claims-made policies: Insurance policies that provide coverage for injuries arising from incidents that occurred during the active policy period.

Collective bargaining: Mechanism for settling labor disputes by negotiation between the employer and representatives of the employees.

Collective liability: Used in conjunction with products liability, holds several manufacturers in a wrongful activity that by its nature requires the participation of more than one wrongdoer liable to the injured party.

Common law: The system of jurisprudence that originated in England and was later applied to all of the United States except Louisiana; generally derived from principles rather than rules and regulations; consists of broad and comprehensive principles based on justice, reason, and common sense.

Community health nursing: Nurses who care for individuals in a variety of settings, including home health care settings, school health settings, occupational health settings, and public health settings.

Comparative negligence: Proportional sharing between plaintiff and defendant or between defendants of compensation for injuries incurred based on the relative negligence of the parties involved.

Competency at law: Seen with informed consent issues, means that the court has not declared the person to be incompetent and the person is generally able to understand the consequences of his or her actions.

Complaint (or petition): An application in writing addressed to a court or judge, stating the facts and circumstances relied on as a cause for judicial action and containing a formal request for relief.

Computerized charting: Newer methods of patient documentation that allows for more accurate recording of facts and for more prompt entries into the patient record; opposite of manual charting methods.

Concurrent jurisdiction: More than one court has the authority to hear a particular lawsuit; also known as overlapping or equal jurisdiction.

Confidentiality of medical records: Right of patients that no part of the medical record will be disclosed without the proper authority to do so or that the record will not be disclosed to persons without authority to the knowledge contained in the record.

Consent: A voluntary action by which one agrees to allow someone else to do something; may be oral, written, or implied based on the circumstances.

Constitutional law: Law that establishes the organization of a government, grants certain powers to a government, and places limits on the actions of a government; may be either federal or state.

Continuing education: Either mandatory or voluntary, specified hours of education that further ensure the continuing competency of the nurse.

Contract: Transaction involving two or more parties wherein each becomes obligated to the other; a binding agreement made between two or more parties to do or refrain from doing certain actions.

Contract negotiation: Ability of both parties to a contract to press for conditions or terms favorable to that party; may only be done when first writing the contract or in re-signing the contract.

Contract termination: Conclusion of the contract either at the mutual request of both parties to the contract, at the end-date of the contract, or because of breach of contract by one of the parties.

Contributory negligence: Conduct on the part of plaintiffs that falls below the standard to which they should conform for their own protection and that is a legally contributing cause cooperating with the negligence of the defendant in bringing about the plaintiffs' harm.

Conversion of property: Interference with the right of possession of a person's own property; an intentional tort.

Corporate liability or negligence: Concept wherein the hospital as an entity is directly liable in tort action; the established standard of conduct to which the hospital as a corporation or business should conform; a relatively new concept in tort law.

Counterclaim: An individual cause of action made by a defendant against the plaintiff, the purpose of which is to oppose or deduct from the plaintiff's claim.

Court order: A direction by the court on some matter incidental to the main proceeding.

Coverage conditions: Section of an insurance policy that outlines the insured nurse's duties to the carrier in the event that a lawsuit is filed, provisions for cancellation of the policy, subrogation of rights, and prohibition of assignment of the policy; such as the duty to give written notice to the carrier.

Covered injuries: Section in an insurance policy that outlines the types of injuries and provisions that the insurance carrier will honor; such as physical injuries and that the lawsuit must be for monetary damages.

Credentials: Proof of qualifications, stating that an individual or organization has met certain standards; licensure and certification are two means of credentialing.

Criminal law: Law pertaining to conduct that is offensive or contrary to the public good and conduct that is harmful to society as a whole, such as murder, theft, rape; prosecuted by and in the name of the state or local government. Also includes conduct that is expressly forbidden or prohibited by statute or common law; opposite of civil or private actions.

Cross-examination: The examination of a witness by an attorney for the opposing side.

Damages: Money awarded by the court to the plaintiff.

Decisional law: Rules and modes of conduct established by courts of law; also known as judicial law.

Declarations: First section of an insurance policy which includes the policyholder's name, address, covered professional occupation, and the covered time period.

Deductibles: Amounts that the insurance carrier subtracts for the total amount available to pay for plaintiffs' damages; for example, the amount paid for the legal defense of the defendant may be deducted from the total limits of liability.

Defamation: Publication of anything injurious to the good name or reputation of another or that tends to bring about another's disreputation; includes libel (written) and slander (oral); a quasi-intentional tort.

Default judgment: A judgment entered against a defendant for failure to respond to plaintiff's action or to appear at trial of the plaintiff's actions; judgment given without the defendant being heard in his or her own defense.

Defendant: The person against whom a civil action or criminal action is instituted.

Defense: A denial, answer, or plea opposing the truth or the validity of the plaintiff's cause of action; instances wherein one may commit a tort without incurring liability.

Defense costs: Reasonable and necessary costs incurred in the investigation, defense, and negotiation of any covered claim by insurance carriers.

Defense of others: Act by which one protects persons in the same area against harm; reasonable force may be used.

Delegation: The assignment by one person of specified tasks to another, often to a person who is lower in rank and theoretically less qualified.

Deontological theories: In ethics, these theories derive norms and rules from the duties human beings owe one another by virtue of commitments that are made and roles that are assumed.

Deposition: An oral interrogation of someone before trial regarding issues involved in a matter, given under oath and transcribed by a court reporter who is usually a notary public.

Direct access to patient populations: Often curtailed by medical practitioners, is the ability of independent nurse practitioners to practice in all areas of the health care delivery system.

Directed verdict: Returned by the jury when directed to do so by the judge or magistrate because the evidence or law is so clearly in favor of a given party and to continue the trial would be pointless.

Disability: Physical or mental impairment that substantially limits one or more of the major life enjoyments of a person.

Disaster nursing: Nursing done during natural or man-created disasters such as hurricanes, floods, fires, or bombings of buildings.

Disciplinary actions: Taken by boards of nursing, used to enforce licensure requirements against nurses who have violated provisions of nurse practice acts.

Disciplinary and/or grievance procedures: Written policies that outline the steps students may take in grade disputes, probation, and suspension from a program or school.

Disclosure statutes: Mandate the reporting of certain types of health-related information to protect the public at large; serve as defenses against defamation and invasion of privacy.

Discovery: Pretrial procedure by which one party gains vital information concerning the case held by the adverse party; disclosure by the adverse party of facts, documents, deeds, and the like that are exclusively within his or her possession or knowledge and that are necessary to the other person's defense.

Discovery rule: A rule by which patients have two years from the time that they become aware of an injury to file a personal injury lawsuit.

Diversion programs: Programs endorsed by state boards of nursing for the rehabilitation of nurses psychologically unable to function or who are addicted to drugs or alcohol.

Do-not-resuscitate directives: Executed by patients on admission to health care institutions, these directives allow patients to determine, while still competent, to what extent that will allow resuscitative measures.

Dual servant doctrine: Principle that serves to allow liability for an employee to flow to both the primary employer as well as to a second employer who borrowed the employee's skills or services.

Due process of law: Applies only to state actions and not to private actions; guarantees procedural fairness in instances in which the government could easily deprive one of liberty or property; due process does not have a fixed meaning, but adjusts with changing jurisprudence values.

Durable Power of Attorney for Health Care: Statutory directive that allows competent patients to appoint a surrogate or proxy to make health care decisions for them in the event that they are incompetent to do so.

Duty of care: Involves the manner in which one conducts oneself; obligation owed to conduct oneself in such a manner as to avoid negligent injury to others.

Duty to orient, educate, and evaluate: Usually seen as the responsibility of education departments within a health care setting, this duty assures that nurses give competent and quality nursing care to patients.

Effective documentation: Information from case law concerning what must be documented and how to document the information so that it is accessible and useful in preventing malpractice suits.

Emancipated minors: Persons under the legal age of adulthood who are no longer under the control and regulation of their parents and who may give valid consent for medical procedures; examples include a married teenager, underage parents, and teenagers in the armed forces.

Emergency: A sudden, unexpected occurrence or event causing a threat to life or limb. It is liberally interpreted to extend to serious illnesses, impairment of faculties, and permanent disfigurement, as well as potential death. It creates a form of implied consent where a person is unable to consent to treatment.

Employer-sponsored coverage: Insurance coverage provided by health care institutions for the benefit of its employees; narrowest of coverage for nurses.

Employment-at-will: Allows employers to hire, retain, and discharge employees for any reason and allows employees to either take or refuse employment opportunities.

Employment contract: Valid contract between two parties creating an employer-employee relationship.

En banc: By the full court; usually noted in case cites if the full court has heard the case.

Endorsement: Process for granting licensure from one state to an already licensed nurse in another state if the two state licensure requirements and qualifications are similar; differs from reciprocity in that no previous agreement exists between the two involved states.

Equal Employment Opportunity Commission: Known as the EEOC, federal agency that is concerned with utilizing employment practices that do not discriminate against or impair employment opportunities of protected groups.

Equal Pay Act of 1963: Made it illegal to pay lower wages to employees of one gender when jobs required equal skill, equal responsibility, and were performed under similar working conditions.

Equal protection of the law: Constitutional guarantee ensuring that all persons in the state must be equally affected by statutes and interpretations of those statutes; restricted to state actions and has no reference to private, nonstate agencies.

Error-in-judgment rule: Allows courts of law to evaluate the standards of care given a patient even if there was an honest error; evaluation of the care given and whether the care met the prevailing standards is evaluated, not whether the judgment was correct.

Essential job functions: Areas of a job that are seen as vital for employment; depends on the employer's judgment, the job description, and the amount of time performing the given function.

Ethical committees: In health care settings, such groups of persons provide structure and guidelines for potential problems, serve as an open forum for discussion, and function as true patient advocates.

Ethics: Science relating to moral actions and moral values; rules of conduct recognized in respect to a particular class of human actions.

Evidence: All the means by which an alleged matter of fact, the truth of which is submitted to investigation at judicial trial, is established or disproved; includes testimony of witnesses, introduction of records, documents, exhibits, objects, and the like.

Exclusions: Items not covered in an insurance policy.

Exculpatory contracts or clauses: Initiated and signed to limit the amount of damages one receives in a given lawsuit or to prevent future lawsuits based on the practitioner's actions; they violate public policy in most jurisdictions.

Expert witness: A witness having special knowledge of the subject about which he or she is to testify; knowledge of an expert witness must generally be such that it is not normally possessed by the average person; contrasts with lay witness.

Expressed consent: Oral or written consent.

Expressed (oral) contract: Written or orally agreed upon conditions constituting a valid contract at law.

External standards of care: Level or degree of quality considered adequate by a profession; set by state boards of nursing, professional and specialty nursing organizations, and federal organizations and guidelines. Synonymous with national standards.

Fact-finder: Person or group of persons that has the responsibility of determining the facts relevant to decide a controversy; usually synonymous with trier of fact.

Failure to act as a patient advocate: Deviation in the standard of care owed the patient when professional nurses fail to develop and implement nursing diagnoses, fail to exercise judgment in monitoring care given patients by physicians, and fail to report care that jeopardizes the health care of patients.

Failure to adequately access, monitor, and communicate: Can occur in all aspects of nursing, involve the falling below a standard of care either by failing to note changes in patients' conditions or in failure to let the primary health care provider know of the changes.

Failure to warn: A newer area of potential liability for nurse managers, this concept involves the responsibility to warn subsequent or potential employers of nurses' incompetence or impairment.

False imprisonment: The unjustified detention or confinement of a person without legal warrant; an intentional tort.

Family and Medical Leave Act: Federal law that allows up to 12 weeks of unpaid leave from work sites for qualified family and medical needs.

Federal Tort Claims Act: A statute that allows the federal government to be sued for the negligence of its employees.

Felony: Crime of a serious nature usually punishable by death, life imprisonment, or confinement greater than one year; examples include murder, rape, and grand theft.

Fidelity: In ethics, keeping one's promises or commitments.

Float personnel: Health care employees who are required to rotate to other than their usual unit of practice in times of staffing shortage in other areas of the institution.

Foreseeability: Doctrine by which an individual is liable for all natural and proximate consequences of any negligent acts to another individual to whom a duty is owed.

Formal contract: One that is required by law to be in writing; usually written on special paper and stamped with an official seal.

Fraud: Intentional misleading of another person so as to cause legal injury to the person. May include false representation, false or misleading allegations, concealment, deception, or other means that serve to get advantage over another human being.

Fundamental rights: Rights given by the First Amendment, such as freedom of speech and freedom of religious preference.

Good Samaritan laws: Individual state legislative enactments passed to encourage health care providers and citizens trained in first aid to deliver needed medical care at accident sites and roadside emergencies without unnecessary fear of incurring criminal or civil liability.

Grandfather clause: Process that grants certain persons working within a profession for a given period of time or prior to a deadline date the privilege of applying for licensure without having to meet all the specific requirements for licensure.

Guardian-ad-litem: An impartial guardian appointed by the court to ensure that the incompetent person's rights are respected and enforced; a guardian for the purpose of litigation.

Harm: See injury.

Health related advice: Statement regarding health issues made by a health care professional to another person.

Hiring practices: Statements, interviews, and measures taken by nurse managers to acquire new staff in health care settings.

Holographic will: A handwritten will, not valid in most states.

Home health care: Nursing care provided in the client's home.

Hospice: A philosophy that allows the terminally ill to receive required nursing and medical care without fear that they will be placed on life-support systems at the hour of death but will be allowed to die naturally when the time comes.

Hostile work environment: Type of sexual harassment claim in which the employee is subject to sexual innuendos, remarks, and physical acts so offensive as to alter the conditions of the employee's employment and create an abusive work environment.

Indemnification: The obligation resting on one person to make good any loss or damages that another has incurred; refers to the total shifting of the economic loss to the party chiefly or primarily responsible for that loss.

Immunity: A right of exemption from a duty or a penalty; a favor or benefit granted to one and contrary to the general rule.

Implied consent: Permission is inferred by the patient's actions (nodding of the head, extension of an arm) or may legally be presumed, as in the instance of emergency consent.

Implied contract: Terms or conditions of the contract that each party anticipates, but are never actually discussed or expressed.

Incident (variation, situation, or unusual occurrence) forms: Mandated by the Joint Commission on the Accreditation of Healthcare Organizations, these forms are part of the overall risk management of the institution; the main functions of these forms are review and evaluation of patient care.

Incorporation by reference: Referring to outside reports or writings in medical records allows that outside record to become part of the permanent medical record of the patient.

Indemnity: Claims brought by employers for monetary damages from the nurse or nurses whose actions or failure to act caused the original patient injury.

Independent contractor: One who makes an agreement with another to perform a service or piece of work and retains in himself or herself control of the means, method, and manner of producing the result to be accomplished; sometimes called an independent practitioner.

Informed consent: Consent only after full notice is given; person must be apprised of the nature, risks, benefits, alternative therapies, and potential complications of a medical procedure before true and valid informed consent is obtained.

Informed refusal: Extension of the rule of informed consent to ensure that patients are made aware of the risks and potential consequences of not consenting to a proposed therapy or diagnostic screening test.

Injunction: The judicial remedy awarded for the purpose of requiring a party to refrain from doing a particular act or activity; a preventive measure that guards against future injuries rather than affording a remedy for past injuries.

Injury (or harm): Wrong or damage done to another, either to the person, rights, representation, or property; as the fifth element of negligence, must be physical damage to the person.

In loco parentis: Literally, "in the place of the parents."

Institutional licensure: Process by which health care institutions are granted the authority to regulate staff members' practice as well as to direct requirements for administration, equipment specifications, fire safety, and the like; process that allows nonprofessionals to control the practice of a professional; contrasts with professional licensure.

Intentional infliction of emotional distress: May be called extreme and outrageous conduct; an intentional tort wherein the conduct goes beyond that which is tolerated by society, and the conduct is calculated to cause the mental distress.

Intentional tort: Wrongful conduct that is intentional in nature and designed to cause harm or damage to another; examples include assault, battery, false imprisonment, libel, and invasion of privacy.

Internal standards of care: Level or degree of quality considered adequate by a profession; set by the nurse's job description, education, and expertise, and the institution's policy and procedure manual.

Interrogatories: A pretrial discovery procedure in which written questions are asked by one side in a controversy of the adverse side in the controversy; an effective and inexpensive means of establishing important facts that are known only to the plaintiff or the defendant at the outset of the lawsuit; the written replies are sworn to under oath and the questions may be asked only of named parties to the controversy.

Invasion of privacy: Violation of the right to protection against unreasonable and unwarranted interference of one's solitude; the violation of one's right to be left alone; a quasi-intentional tort.

Joint Commission for the Accreditation of Healthcare Organizations: Sets nursing standards of care on a yearly basis in its *Accreditation Manual for Hospitals;* also known as JCAHO.

Joint statements: Means of increasing the nursing role, joint statements are issued between the disciplines of nursing and medicine and serve as a basis for expanding nursing practice.

Judgment: Determination of a court of competent jurisdiction to matters submitted to the court; a final determination of the rights of the parties to an action.

Judicial law: Rules and modes of conduct established by courts of law or the judiciary; also known as decisional law.

Jurisdiction: The authority to both hear and decide a lawsuit; may be either subject matter jurisdiction (cause of action and amount of money damages) or jurisdiction over the parties to the suit (residency of the plaintiffs and defendants). Frequently refers to particular legal systems, such as "the law varies in different jurisdictions" and in a sense of territoriality, such as "within the jurisdiction of a given state."

Jurisprudence: Science of the law; study of the structure of the legal system; sometimes used synonymously with "the law."

Justice: In ethics, states that people should be treated fairly and equally.

Labor union: Association of workers that exists for the purpose of bargaining on behalf of the workers, either in whole or in part, with management about the terms of the employment.

Landmark decision: A departure by a court from precedent or stare decisis; such a decision signifies that the precedent has been changed.

Law: From the Anglo-Saxon term *lagu,* meaning that which is fixed or laid down; the total of rules and regulations by which society is governed; the rules and regulations established and enforced by authority or custom within a given community, state, or nation.

Law reporters: Published volumes containing the decisions and opinions of state and federal courts; commonly, such decisions are first published in advance sheets and thereafter in bound reports or reporter volumes; they may be either official reporters (published by state or federal governmental agencies) or unofficial reporters (published by private publishers).

Lay witness: A person who testifies to what he or she has seen, heard, or otherwise observed; contrasts with an expert witness.

Legal consultant: An expert whose name and reports are not disclosed to the opposing side in a lawsuit.

Legal guardian or representative: A person legally responsible for giving or refusing consent for the incompetent patient; appointed through the court system for incompetent patients.

Liability: Refers to one's responsibility for his or her own conduct; an obligation or duty to be performed; differs from strict liability in that the latter involves liability without a showing of fault.

Liability insurance: A contract issued by a casualty insurance company to an individual under which the company, in return for a premium, agrees to defend all claims and pay all sums the policyholder is legally liable to pay third persons because of his or her negligent conduct.

Liable: To be responsible for; to be obligated in law.

Libel: Written defamation.

Licensure: A right granted that gives licensees permission to do something that they could not legally do absent such permission; as a personal right, it is generally nontransferable and is not assignable.

Licensure by examination: Licensing in which the requesting nurse must meet all the requirements for licensure of a given state plus successfully complete a licensing examination.

Licensure by waiver: If the petitioning nurse meets and exceeds some of the requirements for licensure, the portion previously demonstrated may be waived while the nurse successfully demonstrates other requirements for licensure.

Limits of liability: Section in an insurance policy that specifies the dollar amount that a company will pay during a given policy period; usually is expressed as two separate figures indicating limits per single claim and per aggregate amounts.

Living will: A directive from competent individuals to medical personnel and family members regarding the treatment they wish to receive when they can no longer make the decision for themselves; has no legal enforcement as such.

Locality rule: Existence of a prevailing community standard; establishes a standard within a fixed geographic area; in nursing today has been replaced by a national standard.

Malice: The intentional doing of a wrongful act without just cause or excuse, with an intent to injure another, or under circumstances that the law will imply an evil intent.

Malpractice: Professional misconduct, the improper discharge of duties, or failure to meet the standard of care expected of a reasonably prudent member of that profession in his or her dealings with clients or patients, any of which causes harm to the latter.

Mandatory licensure: All persons who are compensated as members of a licensed profession must obtain a valid license prior to practicing the profession; both the title and the actions of the profession are protected by law.

Mature minor: A person under the legal age of adulthood who is able to fully comprehend the nature and consequences of medical therapy or lack of therapy and is allowed to sign or refuse to sign a consent form.

Mediation: Allows disputing parties to a contract to resolve their differences while maintaining a professional relationship; done through a mediator who is a neutral third party.

Medical community standard: Requires that the physician or independent practitioner disclose facts that a reasonable medical practitioner in a similar community and of the same school of medical thought would disclose in assuring informed consent; also know as the reasonable medical practitioner standard.

Medical or physician directive: Directive authorized by states that lists a variety of treatments and allows patients to decide what they would want in the event that they become incompetent; has legal worth comparable to that of the living will; not approved in all states.

Medical disclosure laws: Laws that mandate that certain risks and consequences be printed on the face of informed consent forms in language that the patient can reasonably be expected to understand; statutory attempt to bypass the three more standard tests of disclosure; these laws are not applicable in all states.

Medical records: Mandated by governmental and nongovernmental agencies, these documents contain a verbatim account of the care of a patient while in health care settings.

Medication errors: Deviations from the standards of care owed patients in the area of correct medication delivery; includes omitted doses, incorrect doses, incorrect time of administration, incorrect patient, improper injection techniques, or incorrect route of administration.

Minor: A person who has not yet reached the age of majority; 17 or younger in most states.

Misdemeanor: Crime of a lesser nature, involving fines of less than $1,000 and/or confinement of a year or less; examples include minor traffic violations, theft, and violations of some city ordinances.

Monetary damages: Injuries for which compensation can be assessed in dollar figures.

Moral turpitude: Baseness or dishonesty of a high degree; conviction of such a crime usually leads to licensure suspension; examples include larceny, bribery, and perjury.

Motion: Application to the court requesting an order or ruling in favor of the applicant, as in a motion to dismiss.

Motion for directed verdict: Formal request for the conclusion of a lawsuit based on the failure of the plaintiff to meet the burden of proof or of the defendant to present the necessary defense to the plaintiff's cause of action.

Motion to dismiss: Application to the court, by either the plaintiff or the defendant, requesting the court to set aside the case because there is no valid cause of action or form of relief.

Napoleonic code or law: Derived from the civil law of the French, Romans, and Spaniards; the basis of Louisiana law; may also be known as the Justinian code (Codex Justinianens).

National Labor Relations Act: Passed in 1935 and amended throughout the years since 1935, this federal act defines and protects the field of collective bargaining.

National Practitioner Data Bank (NPDB): Created by the Health Care Quality Improvement Act of 1986, records three types of information about professional practice; instituted to further protect consumers through the mandatory reporting of unsafe practitioners.

National standards: Based on reasonableness, are the average degree of skill, care, and diligence exercised by members of the same profession regardless of the locale of the health care delivered.

Natural death act: Legally recognized living will; a directive of a competent person that allows the person to die without use of extraordinary life-support systems; protects the health practitioner from civil or criminal liability for following the directive.

Necessity: Allows one person to interfere with a second person's property rights if the intent of the interference is to avoid threatened injury.

Negligence: Failure to exercise the degree of care that a person of ordinary prudence, based on the reasonable man standard, would exercise under the same or similar circumstances; also known as ordinary negligence.

Negligent hiring and retention: Provides for employer liability if the injured party can show that the employee was incompetent or unsafe for the position and that the employer knew or should have known that the employee was incompetent or unsafe; often invoked where the doctrine of respondeat superior is inapplicable to provide for hospital liability.

Next of kin: Those persons who by the law of descent would be adjudged the closest blood relative of a decedent or person.

Non compos mentis: Literally, "not of sound mind"; a person suffering from a mental disorder such that he or she is not competent to handle his or her own affairs.

Nonsuit: Judgment rendered against a plaintiff who proceeds to trial or who is unable to prove his or her case; also used to designate a defendant dropped from the lawsuit by the plaintiff.

Nonmaleficence: The duty to do no harm.

Normative ethics: Are universally applicable, involve questions and dilemmas requiring a choice of actions, and entail conflicts of rights and obligations on the part of the nurse decision maker.

Nurse practice acts: Statutory enactments that define the practice of nursing and give guidance with scope of practice issues; passed on a state-to-state basis.

Nurse registration acts: Permissive precursors to nurse practice acts.

Nursing faculty: Nurses holding advanced degrees hired by schools of nursing to teach in programs in nursing.

Nursing students: Student officially admitted to a course of study in the nursing discipline; may be at the entry or advanced levels of nursing.

Occurrence-based policies: Insurance policies that cover claims for injuries arising out of incidents that occurred during the policy period, the time that the policy was in effect.

Occupational health nursing: Nursing at business or work settings, such as factories.

Occupational Safety and Health Act: Known as OSHA, this act assures the healthful and safe working conditions in the workplace.

Omnia prasumuntur contra spoliatorem: Literally, "all things are presumed against a despoiler," the doctrine applies when medical records or portions of medical records are lost or unretrievable as a presumption of guilt against the physician or institution (maker of the record) and in favor of the injured party.

Opening statements: Initial statements by both parties in a litigation that indicate what each side intends to show by the evidence to be presented.

Ordinance: Law passed by a municipal legislative body (city council).

Original jurisdiction: Authority of a higher court to hear cases dependent on constitutional law, as the federal courts always have jurisdiction over bankruptcy cases (Art. III, Sec. 2 of the U.S. Constitution).

Ostensible authority: An application of agency law, it allows a principle to be liable for acts and omissions by independent contractors working at the principle's place of business and who are misinterpreted by a third party as being an employee of the principle; also known as agency by estoppel.

Overlapping jurisdiction: More than one court has the authority to hear a particular lawsuit; also known as concurrent or equal jurisdiction.

Parens patriae: Literally, "the state as parents"; protects both children and adults under the police power of the state; automatic guardianship powers to protect persons under a legal disability to act for themselves.

Paternalism: In ethics, allows one to make decisions for another; also known as parentialism.

Patient access to medical records: State laws that determine when the patient or authorized surrogate is allowed to view and obtain copies of the medical record.

Patient benefit model: In ethics committees, this model uses substituted judgment and facilitates decision making for the incompetent patient.

Patient self-determination: Enacted into law in November 1991, mandates that patients are informed about advanced directives when admitted to health care settings and given the opportunity to enact such directives.

Patient safety: Duty owed patients by nurses that assure protecting patients against falls, from injuring themselves, from medication errors, and from faulty equipment or unsafe conditions.

Permissive licensure: Regulates only the use of the title; nursing actions may be performed as long as one does not use the protected title of registered nurse (RN).

Personal liability: Serves to make persons accountable and responsible for their actions.

Petition: Or complaint; an application in writing addressed to a court or judge, stating facts and circumstances relied on as a cause for judicial action and containing a formal request for relief.

Plaintiff: Party bringing a civil lawsuit seeking damages or other relief; at trial level, the injured parties or their representative.

Pleadings: Statements of the facts that constitute the plaintiff's cause of action and the defendant's grounds of defense.

Policies and procedures: Part of risk management, the written documents that set standards of care for a given health care institution.

Policyholder: Person insured in an insurance policy; also known as the insured.

Policy period: Time frame in which an insurance policy is valid.

Precedent: A rule of law decided by the court in a prior lawsuit that serves as legal authority in subsequent similar cases. Also known as stare decisis.

Preferential treatment: Different treatment of one employee over another employee because the employee submits to the employer's sexual advances.

Preponderance of the evidence: Sufficient credible evidence to convince a court or jury that the essential allegations made are more probably true than not.

Prelitigation panel: A screening panel that hears allegations before proceeding to court litigation.

Prescriptive authority: Right of practitioners to prescribe medication treatment for patients; concerns the full range of medications used today.

Pretrial hearing (or conference): An informal session during which the judge and attorneys agree on the issues to be decided and settle procedural matters.

Principalism: An emerging theory in ethics, incorporates the various ethical principles in attempting to resolve conflicts in clinical settings.

Privacy right: See invasion of privacy.

Privilege: A defense to defamation; a disclosure that might ordinarily be defamatory, but that is allowable to protect or further public and private interests recognized by law; examples include the reporting of certain diagnoses and diseases to public health officials and to the Centers for Disease Control.

Privileged communications: Communications that occur in an air of legal or other recognized professional confidentiality; for example, spousal communications, and patient–physician communications.

Procedural: Legal method; the legal process for each step of a lawsuit; mechanics of the legal process, as opposed to the substance and content of the law.

Procedural law: Law that governs the procedure or rules to create, implement, or enforce substantive law.

Products liability: An area of tort law dictating that manufacturers are strictly liable when an article they place in the marketplace, knowing that it is to be used without inspection for defects, proves to have a defect that causes injury to a human being.

Professional liability insurance policy: Insures professionals while functioning in the capacity of their scope of practice; formal contract between the insurer and the insured party.

Protocols: Statements written and used by nurses in expanded roles that outline and authorize particular practice activities.

Public Health Services Act of 1994: Consolidated all existing public health legislation under one law.

Public law: The branch of law concerned with the state in its political capacity.

Punitive damages: Awarded over the actual amount of proven damages to punish the negligent party.

Qualified privilege: Permits persons to release information that would ordinarily be defamatory if there is a legal duty to release such information; an example is the reporting of a violation of the nurse practice act to the state board of nursing.

Quasi-intentional tort: Volitional action that has direct causation, but where intent to commit an intentional wrong is lacking; commonly seen quasi-intentional torts in health care settings are defamation and invasion of privacy.

Question of fact: Disputed contention that is traditionally left for the jury to decide; for example, in a battery case, a question of fact would be whether A touched B.

Question of law: Disputed legal contentions that are traditionally left for the judge to decide; the occurrence or nonoccurrence of an event is a question of fact, and their legal significance is a question of law.

Quid pro quo sexual harassment: Submission or rejection to sexual conduct is the basis for employment decisions affecting an individual.

Rational basis test: States that persons in the same class must be treated alike.

Reasonable accommodations: Employer's responsibility to provide necessary structure, reassignment, and equipment modifications of devices to allow the disabled person to perform a job satisfactorily.

Reasonable or prudent patient standard: Test of informed consent based on the needs of what a prudent person in the patient's position would deem material about the disclosure of risks and benefits of a proposed treatment; may be divided into objective patient standard and subjective patient standard.

Reciprocity: Process by which individual states grant recognition of licensure as issued by other states' boards of nursing; licensing requirements are equivalent and a previous agreement to grant the recognition of licensure previously existed; contrasts with endorsement in that in endorsement no previous agreement exists between the involved states.

Refusal of care: Ability of the client to withdraw consent for procedures or nursing care.

Reimbursement: Ability to be paid for services by other than those directly provided the care; maybe insurance companies and other governmental agencies as Medicare and Medicaid.

Release: Signed statement relinquishing a right or claim against another person, usually for valuable consideration; accompanies a settlement to prevent a future lawsuit on the same issues or occurrence.

Reporting statutes: Laws that mandate health care providers or their employees to give certain information to proper state or federal agencies; examples include vital statistics, deaths, persons with diagnosed venereal diseases, etc.

Reservation of rights: Section in an insurance policy that allows the company to deny coverage for named exclusions.

Res ipsa loquitor: Literally, "let the thing speak for itself"; a rule of evidence whereby negligence of the alleged wrongdoer may be inferred from the mere fact that the occurrence happened, provided: (1) the character of the occurrence and the circumstances attending it lead reasonably to the belief that in the absence of negligence, it would not have occurred; and (2) the thing that caused the injury is shown to have been under the exclusive management of the alleged wrongdoer.

Res judicata: Literally, "a thing or matter settled by judgment"; applies only when a legal dispute has been decided by a competent court of jurisdiction and no further appeals are possible.

Respect for others: In ethics, the highest principle as it incorporates all the other principles; transcends cultural differences, gender issues, religious differences, and racial concerns.

Respondeat superior: Literally, "let the master respond" or "let the superior reply"; the employer is given accountability and responsibility for an employee's negligent actions incurred during the course and scope of his or her employment.

Restraints: Use of chemical or physical measures that prevent patient freedom.

Retention of records: Obligation of health care facilities to maintain and protect patient medical records for a given time frame that is set by the individual state or state statute of limitations.

Right of refusal: Inherent in informed consent is the right of the patient to refuse consent, even after the original consent is given.

Right-to-die law: A law that upholds a patient's right to choose death by refusing extraordinary treatment. Also referred to as a natural death law or living will law.

Right of discovery: The right of both parties in a lawsuit to uncover relevant written materials and other information prior to the court hearing.

Rule deontology: In ethics, is based on the belief that certain standards for ethical decisions transcend the individual's moral values, such as all human life has value.

Rule utilitarianism: In ethics, seeks the greatest happiness for the greatest number.

Safe environment: Responsibility of an institution to provide an environment that will not be injurious to another's health or well-being; also the duty to alert others about potentially dangerous situations.

School health nursing: Nursing at primary and secondary institutions of education.

Scope of practice: Refers to legally permissive boundaries of practice for a health professional; the allowable scope is defined by statute, rule, or a combination of rule and statute; to go outside one's allowable scope of practice usually means that one is practicing another profession without the necessary licensure, such as a nurse practicing medicine without a license.

Self-defense: Act of protecting oneself against harm to one's person; justifiable to protect oneself from persons and areas of harm.

Service: Delivery of a petition or complaint, pleading, notice, or other paper in a lawsuit to subject the person to its legal effect.

Settlement: Conclusive fixing or resolving of a matter; a compromise achieved by the adverse parties in a civil suit prior to final judgment; by settling out of court one does not admit liability or establish nonliability.

Sexual harassment: Unwelcome sexual conduct that is a term of employment.

Situation ethics: A branch of deontological ethics, this theory takes into account the unique characteristics of each person and seeks the most humanistic course of action given the circumstances.

Slander: Oral defamation.

Social Security Act of 1935: Provided for general welfare by establishing a system of federal benefits for qualified persons.

Social justice model: In ethics committees, this model considers broad social issues that affect the entire health care institution.

Specific performance: A court-ordered action to be taken in a civil suit, in lieu of and in addition to monetary awards.

Standards of care: Level or degree of quality considered adequate by a profession; skills and learning commonly possessed by members of a profession; minimal requirements that define an acceptable level of care.

Standards of disclosure: Tests that have evolved to assure that patients are informed about the risks and consequences of their decisions for the purposes of informed consent; may be a medical community standard or a reasonable patient standard.

Standards for record keeping: Set by JCAHO, these standards ensure the adequacy of the entire record.

Standing orders: Medical orders written by a doctor that instruct nurses what treatment should be rendered under given circumstances when the doctor is not present.

Stare decisis: Literally, "let the decision stand"; a doctrine wherein a previously decided case is recognized as the authority for deciding future cases; a rule that causes courts to be slow to interfere with principles announced in former decisions and often to uphold them, even though they would decide otherwise were the question a new one. Also known as precedent.

State appellate court: Court that hears appeals and that bases its decisions on evidence as presented in the record of the trial hearings.

Statutory laws: Rules and regulations created by legislative bodies such as Congress, state houses, and city councils; also referred to as statutes.

Statute of frauds: Legal principle in contract law that certain contracts must be written to be valid and enforceable, such as marriage contracts and contracts for the sale of goods over a certain dollar figure.

Statute of limitations: Any law that fixes the time within which parties must take judicial action to enforce rights or else be thereafter barred from enforcing them; behind these laws is the belief that there is a point beyond which a prospective defendant should no longer need to worry about possible future lawsuits.

Statutes: Rules and regulations created by legislative bodies, such as Congress, state houses, and city councils; also known as statutory laws.

Strike: Walk-out by employees following the expiration of a work contract; means by which employees stop work when arbitration fails.

Student liability: Potential liability incurred in a student role.

Subpoena: Court order requiring one to appear in court to give testimony.

Substantive law: Defines the substance of the law; may be divided into civil, administrative, and criminal law.

Substituted judgment: A subjective determination of how persons, were they capable of making their opinions and wishes known, would have chosen to either accept or refuse medical therapy; frequently relied on in the incompetent person's right-to-die issues.

Suicide prevention: Obligation of nurses to protect patients from self-destruction.

Summary jury trial: Abbreviated, privately held trial used by both sides to a contract dispute to ascertain the strengths and weaknesses of their case and the potential outcome should they decide to seek trial resolution.

Sunset laws: Process that calls for an automatic review of a given act or law at a fixed time; prevents the outdating of an act or law because of the automatic review process.

Supplemental payments: Section in an insurance policy that provides for additional payments to the insured for named instances, such as costs of appeal bonds and reasonable lost earnings.

Supplemental pleadings: Pleadings that add to those already before the court; allows the original pleading to stand while supplying additional facts.

Technology and equipment: Issues that have created special problems of liability for nurses; nurses must know the capabilities, limitations, hazards, and safety features of a variety of machines and devices.

Therapeutic privilege: Concept that allows health care providers to withhold information and other disclosures that they feel would be detrimental to the patient's overall health status; informed consent is considered to have been obtained even though pertinent information is withheld.

Temporary licensure: Time frame during which a qualified practitioner may practice while preparing to either take the examination needed for licensure or during which the test is being evaluated and full licensure awarded the practitioner.

Testimony: The statement of a witness given under oath; may be written or oral.

Tort: Private or civil wrong or injury independent of contract, resulting from a breach of a legal duty; may be intentional, quasi-intentional, or nonintentional (negligent).

Tort law: A branch of civil law concerning legal wrongs committed by one person against another or against another's property.

Tortfeasor: One who commits a tort.

Trial court: The court of original jurisdiction.

Trier of fact: Synonymous with fact-finder; person or group of persons that has the responsibility of determining the facts relevant to decide a controversy.

Truth: Valid defense against defamatory statements.

Two schools of thought doctrine: Supports the nurse who chooses among alternative interventions in delivering quality health care; issue is whether the nurse met the standards of care in delivering the intervention chosen, not that other nurses would have chosen the same intervention.

Uniform act: A model act concerning a particular area of the law created by a nonlegal body in the hope that it will be enacted in all states to achieve uniformity, for example, the American Nurses Association's Model Practice Act.

Unlicensed assistive personnel (UAP): Individuals employed in health care settings to augment patient care; persons without licensure under state nurse practice acts.

U.S. district courts: The original trial court in the federal court system; normally hears cases involving federal questions.

U.S. Supreme Court: Highest level in the federal court system; its decisions are binding on all state and federal courts.

Utilitarianism: Ethical theory that allows decisions to be made based on their utility.

Values: Personal beliefs about the truths and worth of thoughts, objects, or behavior; motives and attitudes and the relationship of these motives and attitudes to the good of the individual.

Veracity: In ethics, truth telling.

Verdict (or decision): The formal declaration of a jury's findings of fact, signed and presented to the court.

Vicarious liability: The imputation of accountability upon one person for the actions of another; substituted liability; may also be called imputed liability.

Voir dire: The selection of the jury.

Volunteer services: Nursing care given without monetary compensation; outside the scope of nurse practice acts.

Waiver: Intentional giving up of a right, such as a waiver to privileged communications information.

Writ of certiorari: Written petition to the U.S. Supreme Court to hear a specific case.

Writ of habeas corpus: Literally, "you have the body"; procedure for obtaining a judicial determination of the legality of an individual's custody or confinement.

Wrongful discharge: An exception to the employment-at-will doctrine, wrongful discharge may be brought against an employer who fires an employee for less than good cause, if there is a good cause provision in the employment contract.

· appendix a

ANA Code of Ethics

1. The nurse provides services with respect for human dignity and the uniqueness of the client unrestricted by considerations of social or economic status, personal attributes, or nature of health problems.
2. The nurse safeguards the client's right to privacy by judiciously protecting information of a confidential nature.
3. The nurse acts to safeguard the client and the public when health care and safety are affected by the incompetent, unethical, or illegal practice of any person.
4. The nurse assumes responsibility and accountability for individual nursing judgments and actions.
5. The nurse maintains competence in nursing.
6. The nurse exercises informed judgment and uses individual competence and qualifications as criteria in seeking consultation, accepting responsibilities, and delegating nursing activities to others.
7. The nurse participates in activities that contribute to the ongoing development of the profession's body of knowledge.
8. The nurse participates in the profession's efforts to implement and improve standards of nursing.
9. The nurse participates in the profession's efforts to establish and maintain conditions of employment conducive to high quality nursing care.
10. The nurse participates in the profession's efforts to establish and maintain conditions of employment conducive to high quality nursing care.
11. The nurse collaborates with members of the health professions and other citizens in promoting community and national efforts to meet the health needs of the public.

Source: Reprinted by permission from *Code for Nurses.* Kansas City, MO, 1976.

· appendix b

International Code for Nurses

The fundamental responsibility of the nurse is fourfold: to promote health, to prevent illness, to restore health, and to alleviate suffering.

The need for nursing is universal. Inherent in nursing is respect for life, dignity, and rights of man. It is unrestricted by considerations of nationality, race, creed, color, age, sex, politics or social status.

Nurses render health services to the individual, the family and the community and coordinate their services with those of related groups.

NURSES AND PEOPLE

The nurse's primary responsibility is to those people who require nursing care.

The nurse, in providing care, promotes an environment in which the values, customs and spiritual beliefs of the individual are respected.

The nurse holds in confidence personal information and uses judgment in sharing this information.

NURSES AND PRACTICE

The nurse carries personal responsibility for nursing practice and for maintaining competence by continual learning. The nurse maintains the highest standards of nursing care possible within the reality of a specific situation.

The nurse uses judgment in relation to individual competence when accepting and delegating responsibilities.

The nurse when acting in a professional capacity should at all times maintain standards of personal conduct which reflect credit upon the profession.

NURSES AND SOCIETY

The nurse shares with other citizens the responsibility for initiating and supporting action to meet the health and social needs of the public.

NURSES AND CO-WORKERS

The nurse sustains a cooperative relationship with co-workers in nursing and other fields. The nurse takes appropriate action to safeguard the individual when his care is endangered by a co-worker or any other person.

NURSES AND THE PROFESSION

The nurse plays the major role in determining and implementing desirable standards of nursing practice and nursing education.

The nurse is active in developing a core of professional knowledge.

The nurse, acting through the professional organization, participates in establishing and maintaining equitable social and economic working conditions in nursing.

Source: From International Council of Nurses. (1973). International Council of Nurses Code for Nurses. Geneva, Switzerland: Author. Used by permission.

· appendix c

Sample Professional Liability Insurance Policy

In consideration of payment of the premium, in reliance upon the statements in the declarations and subject to all of the terms of this policy, agrees with the named insured as follows:

COVERAGE AGREEMENTS

The company will pay on behalf of the insured all sums that the insured shall become legally obligated to pay as damages because of:

COVERAGE—INDIVIDUAL PROFESSIONAL LIABILITY

Injury arising out of the rendering of or failure to render, during the policy period, professional services by the individual insured, or by any person for whose acts or omissions such insured is legally responsible, except as a member of a partnership, performed in the practice of the individual insured's profession described in the declarations including service by the individual insured as a member of a formal accreditation or similar professional board or committee of a hospital or professional society.

EXCLUSION

This insurance does not apply to:

1. Liability of the insured as a proprietor, superintendent, or executive officer of any hospital, sanitarium, clinic with bed and board facilities, laboratory or business enterprise other than as stated in the above declarations;
2. Liability of the insured as a nurse-anesthetist or as a nurse midwife.

LIMITS OF LIABILITY

Individual Professional Liability

The limit of liability stated in the declarations as applicable to each claim is the limit of the company's liability for all damages because of each claim or suit covered hereby. All claims arising from the same rendering of or failure to render the same professional services shall be considered a single claim for the purposes of this insurance. The limit of liability stated in the declarations as aggregate is, subject to the above provision respecting each claim, the total limit of the company's liability under this coverage for all damages. Such limits of liability shall apply separately to each insured.

SUPPLEMENTARY PAYMENTS

The company will pay, in addition to the applicable limit of liability:

1. All expenses incurred by the company, all costs taxed against the insured in any suit defended by the company, and all interest on the entire amount of the judgment therein which accrues after entry of the judgment and before the company has paid or tendered or deposited in court that part of the judgment that does not exceed the limit of the company's liability thereon.
2. Such premiums on appeal bonds required in any such suit, premiums on bonds to release attachments in any such suit for an amount not in excess of the applicable limit of liability of this policy, and the cost of bail bonds required of the insured because of accident or traffic law violations arising out of the use of any vehicle to which this policy applies, not to exceed $250 per bail bond, but the company shall have no obligation to apply for or furnish such bonds.
3. Reasonable expenses incurred by the insured at the company's request in assisting the company in the investigation or defense of any claim or suit, including actual loss of earnings not to exceed $25 per day.

DEFINITIONS

"Insured" means any person or organization qualifying as the policyholder in the person's insured provision of this policy. The insurance afforded applies separately to each insured against whom claim is made or suit is brought, except with respect to the limits of the company's liability.

"Damages" means all damages, including damages for death, which are payable because of injury to which the insurance applies. "Named insured" means the person or organization named in the declarations of this policy.

CONDITIONS

Insured's duties in the event of occurrence, claim or suit:

1. Upon the insured becoming aware of any alleged injury to which this insurance applies, written notice containing particulars sufficient to identify the insured and also reasonably obtainable information with respect to the time, place, and circumstances thereof, and the names and addresses of the injured and of available witnesses, shall be given by or for the insured to the company or any of its authorized agents as soon as practicable.
2. If claim is made or suit is brought against the insured, the insured shall immediately forward to the company every demand, notice, summons, or other process received by him or his representative.
3. The insured shall cooperate with the company and, upon the company's request, assist in making settlements, in the conduct of suits and in enforcing any right of contribution or indemnity against any person or organization who may be liable to the insured because of injury or damage with respect to which insurance is afforded under this policy; and the insured shall attend hearings and trials and assist in securing and giving evidence and obtaining the attendance of witnesses. The insured shall not, except at his own cost, voluntarily make any payment, assume any obligation, or incur any expense.

SUBROGATION

In the event of any payment under this policy, the company shall be subrogated to all of the insured's rights of recovery therefore against any person or organization, and the insured shall execute and deliver instruments and papers and do whatever else is necessary to secure such rights. The insured shall do nothing after loss to prejudice such rights.

ASSIGNMENT

The interest hereunder of any insured is not assignable.

CHANGES

Notice to any agent or knowledge possessed by any agent or by any other person shall not effect a waiver or change in any part of this policy or stop the company from asserting any right under the terms of this policy; nor shall the terms of this policy be waived or changed, except by endorsement issued to form a part of this policy, signed by a duly authorized representative of this company.

• appendix d

Model Practice of Nursing Acts

1955 MODEL ACT

The practice of professional nursing means the performance for compensation of any act in the observation, care, and counsel of the ill, injured, or infirm, or in the maintenance of health or prevention of illness of others, or in the supervision and teaching of other personnel, or the administration of medications and treatments as prescribed by a licensed physician or dentist; requiring substantial specialized judgment and skill and based on knowledge and application of the principles of biological, physical, and social science. The foregoing shall not be deemed to include acts of diagnosis or prescription of therapeutic or corrective measures (American Nurses Association, 1955).

1976 MODEL PRACTICE ACT

The practice of nursing means the performance for compensation of professional services requiring substantial specialized knowledge of the biological, physical, behavioral, psychological, and sociological sciences and of nursing theory as the basis for assessment, diagnosis, planning, intervention, and evaluation in the promotion and maintenance of health; the casefinding and management of illness, injury or infirmity; the restoration of optimal function; or the achievement of a dignified death. Nursing practice includes but is not limited to administration, teaching, counseling, supervision, delegation, and evaluation of practice and execution of the medical regimen, including the administration of medications and treatments prescribed by any person authorized by state law to prescribe. Each registered nurse is directly accountable and responsible to the consumer for the quality of nursing care rendered (American Nurses Association, 1980).

1990 MODEL PRACTICE ACT

The "practice of nursing" means the performance of services for compensation in the provision of diagnosis and treatment of human responses to health or illness.

"Professional nursing practice" encompasses the full scope of nursing practice and includes all its specialties and consists of application of nursing theory to the development, implementation, and evaluation of plans of nursing care for individuals, families, and communities. Professional nursing practice requires substantial knowledge of nursing theory and related scientific, behavioral, and humanistic disciplines. Professional nursing practice includes, but is not limited to:

(1) assessment, diagnosis, planning, intervention, and evaluation of human responses to health or illness;

(2) the provision of direct nursing care to individuals to restore optimum function or to achieve a dignified death;

(3) the procurement, coordination, and management of essential client resources;

(4) the provision of health counseling and education;

(5) the establishment of standards of practice for nursing care in all settings, including the development of nursing policies, procedures, and protocols for a specific setting;

(6) the direction of nursing practice, including delegation to those practicing technical nursing;

(7) the supervision of those who assist in the practice of nursing;

(8) collaboration with other independently licensed health care professionals in case finding and the clinical management and execution of intervention as identified to be appropriate in a plan of care; and

(9) the administration of medication and treatments as prescribed by those professionals qualified to prescribe under the provision of (cite state statute[s]);

"Technical nursing practice" includes the skilled application of nursing principles in the delivery of direct care to individuals and families within organized nursing services. Technical nursing practice requires the study of nursing within the context of the applied sciences. Technical nursing practice includes, but is not limited to:

(1) participation in the development, evaluation, and modification of a plan of care;

(2) the provision of direct care to individuals to restore optimum function or to achieve a dignified death;

(3) patient teaching;

(4) the supervision of those who assist in the practice of nursing;

(5) the administration of medication and treatments as prescribed by those professionals qualified to prescribe under the provisions of (cite state statute[s]).

REFERENCES

American Nurses'Association approves a definition of nursing practice. (1955). *American Journal of Nursing, 55*(12), 1474.

American Nurses'Association. The Nursing Practice Act: Suggested State Legislature (1980). Kansas City, KS: Author.

American Nurses'Association. (1990). *Suggested state legislation: Nursing practice act, nursing disciplinary diversion act, prescriptive authority act.* American Nurses Association.

Index